Emergency and Trauma Radiology

A Teaching File

Emergency and Trauma Radiology

A Teaching File

Editor

Daniel B. Nissman, MD, MPH, MSEE
Assistant Professor of Radiology
Division Chief, Musculoskeletal Imaging Division
Department of Radiology
University of North Carolina at Chapel Hill
Chapel Hill, North Carolina

Associate Editors

Katherine R. Birchard, MD
Associate Professor of Radiology
Cardiothoracic Imaging Division
Director, Medical Student Education
Department of Radiology
University of North Carolina at Chapel Hill
Chapel Hill, North Carolina

Benjamin Y. Huang, MD, MPH
Associate Professor of Radiology
Director, Neuroradiology Fellowship
Neuroradiology Division
Department of Radiology
University of North Carolina at Chapel Hill
Chapel Hill, North Carolina

Ellie R. Lee, MD
Assistant Professor of Radiology
Abdominal Imaging Division
Department of Radiology
University of North Carolina at Chapel Hill
Chapel Hill, North Carolina

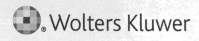. Wolters Kluwer

Philadelphia · Baltimore · New York · London
Buenos Aires · Hong Kong · Sydney · Tokyo

Acquisitions Editor: Ryan Shaw
Product Development Editor: Lauren Pecarich
Production Project Manager: David Orzechowski
Design Coordinator: Terry Mallon
Manufacturing Coordinator: Beth Welsh
Marketing Manager: Dan Dressler
Prepress Vendor: S4Carlisle Publishing Services

9 8 7 6 5 4 3 2 1

Printed in China

978-1-4698-9948-0
1-4698-9948-5
Library of Congress Cataloging-in-Publication Data
available upon request

LWW.com

RRS1601

Scott S. Abedi, MD
Resident, Diagnostic Radiology
Department of Radiology
University of North Carolina at Chapel Hill
Chapel Hill, North Carolina

Ana Lorena Abello, MD
Neuroradiologist
Hospital Universitario del Valle
Cali, Colombia

Michael K. Altenburg, MD, PhD
Resident, Diagnostic Radiology
Department of Radiology
University of North Carolina School of Medicine
Chapel Hill, North Carolina

Bryan E. Ashley, MD
Resident, Diagnostic Radiology
Department of Radiology
University of North Carolina School of Medicine
Chapel Hill, North Carolina

Christopher J. Atkinson, MD
Resident, Diagnostic Radiology
Department of Radiology
San Antonio Military Medical Center
San Antonio, Texas

Andrew F. Barnes, MD
Resident, Diagnostic Radiology
Department of Radiology
University of North Carolina at Chapel Hill
Chapel Hill, North Carolina

Mustafa R. Bashir, MD
Director of MRI
Associate Professor of Radiology
Center for Advanced Magnetic Resonance Development
Duke University Medical Center
Durham, North Carolina

Katherine R. Birchard, MD
Associate Professor of Radiology
Cardiothoracic Imaging Division
Director, Medical Student Education
Department of Radiology
University of North Carolina at Chapel Hill
Chapel Hill, North Carolina

Kelsey R. Budd, MD
Resident, Diagnostic Radiology
Department of Radiology
University of North Carolina School of Medicine
Chapel Hill, North Carolina

Kaleigh L. Burke, MD
Resident, Diagnostic Radiology
Department of Radiology
University of North Carolina School of Medicine
Chapel Hill, North Carolina

Lauren M.B. Burke, MD
Assistant Professor of Radiology
Abdominal Imaging Division
Department of Radiology
University of North Carolina School of Medicine
Chapel Hill, North Carolina

Lazaro D. Causil, MD
Research Fellow
Department of Radiology
University of North Carolina
Chapel Hill, North Carolina

Andy K. Chon, MD
Fellow, Abdominal Imaging and Intervention
Department of Radiology
Brigham and Women's Hospital
Boston, Massachusetts

Wui Chong, MD
Associate Professor of Radiology
Abdominal Imaging Division
Interim Chief, Abdominal Imaging
Fellowship Director, Abdominal Imaging
Associate Professor of OB-GYN
Chief of Diagnostic Ultrasound
Department of Radiology
University of North Carolina School of Medicine
Chapel Hill, North Carolina

Richard L. Clark, MD, FACR
Professor Emeritus
Department of Radiology
University of North Carolina School of Medicine
Chapel Hill, North Carolina

Stephanie F. Coquia, MD
Assistant Professor of Radiology and Radiological Science
Department of Radiology
The Johns Hopkins Hospital
Baltimore, Maryland

James C. Darsie, MD
Resident, Diagnostic Radiology
Department of Radiology
University of North Carolina at Chapel Hill
Chapel Hill, North Carolina

John Duncan, MD
Resident, Diagnostic Radiology
Department of Radiology
St. Barnabas Medical Center
Livingston, New Jersey

Ryan E. Embertson, MD
Resident, Diagnostic Radiology
Department of Radiology
University of North Carolina at Chapel Hill
Chapel Hill, North Carolina

Elena Fenu, BS
Medical Student
University of North Carolina
Chapel Hill, North Carolina

Joseph C. Fuller III, MD
Resident, Diagnostic Radiology
Department of Radiology
University of Washington
Seattle, Washington

Sam A. Glaubiger, BS
Medical Student
University of North Carolina at Chapel Hill
Chapel Hill, North Carolina

Rajan T. Gupta, MD
Assistant Professor of Radiology
Director, Abdominal Imaging Fellowship Program
Duke University Medical Center
Durham, North Carolina

Tamar Gurunlian, BSc
Medical Student
Ross University School of Medicine
Portsmouth, Dominica

Brian D. Handly, MD
Assistant Professor of Radiology
Abdominal Imaging Division
Department of Radiology
University of North Carolina at Chapel Hill
Chapel Hill, North Carolina

Kelly L. Hastings, MD
Resident, Diagnostic Radiology
Department of Radiology
University of North Carolina at Chapel Hill
Chapel Hill, North Carolina

Bryan M. Hoag, MD
Resident, Diagnostic Radiology
Department of Radiology
University of North Carolina at Chapel Hill
Chapel Hill, North Carolina

Benjamin Y. Huang, MD, MPH
Associate Professor of Radiology
Director, Neuroradiology Fellowship
Neuroradiology Division
Department of Radiology
University of North Carolina at Chapel Hill
Chapel Hill, North Carolina

Sheryl G. Jordan, MD
Associate Professor of Radiology
Director GME
Department of Radiology
University of North Carolina School of Medicine
Chapel Hill, North Carolina

Christopher J. Karakasis, MD
Fellow, Neuroradiology Division
Department of Radiology
University of North Carolina at Chapel Hill
Chapel Hill, North Carolina

Eun Lee Langman, MD
Assistant Professor of Radiology
Division of Breast Imaging
Department of Radiology
University of North Carolina School of Medicine
Chapel Hill, North Carolina

Ellie R. Lee, MD
Assistant Professor of Radiology
Abdominal Imaging Division
Department of Radiology
University of North Carolina at Chapel Hill
Chapel Hill, North Carolina

Sheila S. Lee, MD
Assistant Professor of Radiology
Division of Breast Imaging
Department of Radiology
University of North Carolina School of Medicine
Chapel Hill, North Carolina

E. Matthew Lopez II, DO
Fellow, Neuroradiology
Department of Neuroradiology
University of North Carolina
Chapel Hill, North Carolina

Troy H. Maetani, MD
Assistant Professor of Radiology
Division of Musculoskeletal Imaging
Department of Radiology
University of North Carolina School of Medicine
Chapel Hill, North Carolina

Brian P. Milam, MD
CPT, U.S. Army, Medical Corps
Orthopaedic Surgery Resident
Department of Surgery
Madigan Army Medical Center
Tacoma, Washington

Ho Chia Ming, MBBS (Singapore), FRCR (London)
Consultant, Diagnostic Radiology
Department of Diagnostic Radiology
Singapore General Hospital
Adjunct Associate Professor
Duke-National University of Singapore
Singapore

Aaron Moore, BS
Medical Student
University of North Carolina School of Medicine
Chapel Hill, North Carolina

Eduardo V. Moroni, MD
Fellow, Abdominal Imaging Division
Department of Radiology
University of North Carolina School of Medicine
Chapel Hill, North Carolina

Malik Mossa-Basha, MD
Resident, Diagnostic Radiology
Department of Radiology
University of North Carolina School of Medicine
Chapel Hill, North Carolina

Niyati Mukherjee, MD
Assistant Professor of Radiology
Abdominal Imaging Division
Department of Radiology
University of North Carolina at Chapel Hill
Chapel Hill, North Carolina

Brett R. Murdock, MD
Fellow, Cardiothoracic Imaging Division
Department of Radiology
University of North Carolina at Chapel Hill
Chapel Hill, North Carolina

Abdul O. Nasiru, MD
Resident, Diagnostic Radiology
Department of Radiology
Emory University
Atlanta, Georgia

Daniel Nissman, MD, MPH, MSEE
Assistant Professor of Radiology
Division Chief, Musculoskeletal Imaging Division
Department of Radiology
University of North Carolina at Chapel Hill
Chapel Hill, North Carolina

Peter J. Noone, BS
Medical Student
University of North Carolina at Chapel Hill
Chapel Hill, North Carolina

Renato H. Nunes, MD
Neuroradiologist
Neuroradiology Division
Santa Casa de Sao Paulo
Sao Paulo, Brazil
Neuroradiologist
Neuroradiology Division
Grupo Fleury
Sao Paulo, Brazil

Kwaku A. Obeng, MD
Fellow, Neuroradiology Division
Department of Radiology
University of North Carolina at Chapel Hill
Chapel Hill, North Carolina

Jorge D. Oldan, MD
Assistant Professor of Radiology
Division of Nuclear Medicine
Department of Radiology
University of North Carolina School of Medicine
Chapel Hill, North Carolina

Parth C. Patel, MD
Resident, Diagnostic Radiology
Department of Radiology
University of North Carolina at Chapel Hill
Chapel Hill, North Carolina

Kavya E. Reddy, MD
Resident, Diagnostic Radiology
Department of Radiology
University of North Carolina at Chapel Hill
Chapel Hill, North Carolina

Kenny E. Rentas, MD
Fellow, Neuroradiology Division
Department of Radiology
University of North Carolina at Chapel Hill
Chapel Hill, North Carolina

Lana M. Rivers, MD
Resident, Diagnostic Radiology
Department of Radiology
University of North Carolina at Chapel Hill
Chapel Hill, North Carolina

Adam T. Ryan, MD
Fellow, Musculoskeletal Imaging Division
Department of Radiology
University of North Carolina at Chapel Hill
Chapel Hill, North Carolina

Shaun R. Rybak, MD
Resident, Diagnostic Radiology
Department of Radiology
University of North Carolina at Chapel Hill
Chapel Hill, North Carolina

Cassandra M. Sams, MD
Assistant Professor of Radiology
Pediatric Imaging Division
Department of Radiology
University of North Carolina at Chapel Hill
Chapel Hill, North Carolina

Denny Scaria, BS
Medical Student
University of North Carolina School of Medicine
Chapel Hill, North Carolina

Cody J. Schwartz, MD, MPH
Resident, Diagnostic Radiology
Department of Radiology
University of North Carolina at Chapel Hill
Chapel Hill, North Carolina

Francisco Sepulveda, MD
Research Fellow
Department of Radiology
University of North Carolina
Chapel Hill, North Carolina

Tiffany M. Sills, MD, PhD
Resident, Diagnostic Radiology
Department of Radiology
University of North Carolina School of Medicine
Chapel Hill, North Carolina

Jiheon Song, MSc
Medical Student
University College Cork School of Medicine
Cork, Ireland

Ami V. Vakharia, MD
Resident, Diagnostic Radiology
Department of Radiology
University of North Carolina at Chapel Hill
Chapel Hill, North Carolina

Daniel M. Varón, MD
Neuroradiologist
Hospital Universitario del Valle
Cali, Colombia

Audrey R. Verde, PhD
Medical Student
University of North Carolina School of Medicine
Chapel Hill, North Carolina

Shaun R. Wagner, DO
Fellow, Neuroradiology Division
Department of Radiology
University of North Carolina at Chapel Hill
Chapel Hill, North Carolina

Joshua A. Wallace, MD, MPH
Resident, Diagnostic Radiology
Department of Radiology
University of North Carolina Hospitals
Chapel Hill, North Carolina

Sarah B. Wilson, BS
Medical Student
University of North Carolina School of Medicine
Chapel Hill, North Carolina

Alexander D. Wyckoff, MD
Resident, Diagnostic Radiology
Department of Radiology
University of North Carolina at Chapel Hill
Chapel Hill, North Carolina

Teaching files are one of the hallmarks of education in radiology. When there was a need for a comprehensive series to provide the resident and practicing radiologist with the kind of personal consultation with the experts normally found only in the setting of a teaching hospital, Wolters Kluwer was proud to have created a series that answers this need.

Actual cases have been culled from extensive teaching files in major medical centers. The discussions presented mimic those performed on a daily basis between residents and faculty members in all radiology departments.

This series is designed so that each case can be studied as an unknown. A consistent format is used to present each case. A brief clinical history is given, followed by several images. Then, relevant findings, differential diagnosis, and final diagnosis are given, followed by a discussion of the case. The authors thereby guide the reader through the interpretation of each case.

Cases have been randomized to better prepare the reader for the challenges of the clinical setting. In addition, to answer the growing demand for electronic content, we have included more cases online, which has left us, in turn, able to offer a more cost-effective product.

We hope that this series will continue to be a trusted teaching tool for radiologists at any stage of training or practice and that it will also be a benefit to clinicians whose patients undergo these imaging studies.

The Publisher

The field of radiology is traditionally subdivided into body systems, which allows for both ease of study and specialization. Imaging of the acutely ill patient, the subject of emergency and trauma radiology, cuts across all of these traditional organ-based subdivisions. Historically, very few case review texts have been written exclusively on the imaging of the acutely ill patient. Instead, radiologists, including residents, who cover the emergency department must draw on their experience in each of the traditional body systems to interpret the wide variety of acute imaging pathology. This text is intended fill this gap. Our survey of the field of emergency and trauma radiology will be most useful for residents preparing for and taking call. Naturally, this work will also interest those preparing for board examinations and practicing radiologists desiring additional exposure to emergency radiology.

This text is a collaborative work. Expert subspecialty radiologists have selected and edited the cases within one of four general areas: Dr. Lee – abdominal, Dr. Huang – central nervous system, Dr. Nissman – musculoskeletal, and Dr. Birchard – thoracic. Both adult and pediatric cases are represented. The complete collection of 300 cases is contained in the online version of this work. A subset of 100 of these cases is presented in the print version and represents a sampling of true emergencies, urgencies, and concepts that the editors felt needed to be emphasized for the radiology resident. Cases are presented in random order to mimic the appearance of cases in a real emergency radiology practice.

Each case is presented in a sequence that models the actual interpretive process: one to four images, an image description, a differential diagnosis, the diagnosis, and a discussion. These are followed by brief sections summarizing what the referring physician needs to know, reporting responsibilities, and one or more questions for further thought. The questions for further thought may expound on the differential diagnosis, the mechanism of injury, anatomical considerations, or technical factors related to imaging.

In the acute care setting, there are certain expectations regarding reporting. True emergencies require immediate direct communication with the referring clinician whereas all other cases require a timely report. The definition of timely is often dependent on patient setting, modality, and contractual obligations. The "Reporting Responsibilities" section of each case assumes that the patient is in a high volume emergency department where cases not meeting the definition of a true emergency will still be acted on in a timely fashion. Alternatively, in an outpatient setting, some non-emergent diagnoses may merit a phone call to ensure expedited subspecialty care or that the implications of an unusual diagnosis are appreciated.

Many acute pathological entities have been classified, graded, and typed with the hope of predicting prognosis and/or guiding management. This is particularly true of orthopedic trauma. Unfortunately, very few classification systems are able to achieve these goals in all situations. When appropriate, the most commonly used classification system is described with the recognition that it is often not perfect and that there may be other classifications that are used by practicing physicians. Unless there is one universally accepted classification system for an entity, it is better to know the elements that serve as the bases for these systems and describe those in the report; this allows the referring physician to make an assignment based on their own preferences.

In summary, it is our hope that after you have studied all the cases in this book (print and online) that you will be well prepared to handle the variety of pathology seen in the acute care setting with confidence.

Daniel B. Nissman, MD, MPH, MSEE

Katherine R. Birchard, MD

Benjamin Y. Huang, MD, MPH

Ellie R. Lee, MD

This book would not be possible without the hard work of all of our contributors, including medical students, residents, fellows, and faculty. In particular, we would like to acknowledge the participation of the faculty contributors who have done so in the face of very high clinical workloads in addition to other teaching, research, and administrative responsibilities.

Daniel B. Nissman

Katherine R. Birchard

Benjamin Y. Huang

Ellie R. Lee

CLINICAL HISTORY *25-year-old female with history of Crohn's disease presenting with nausea, dehydration, and headache.*

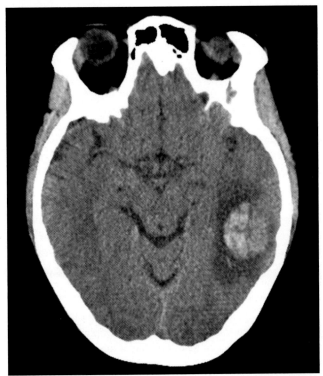

FIGURE 1A

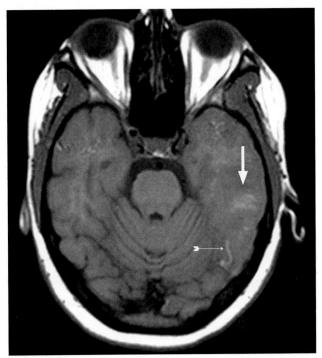

FIGURE 1B

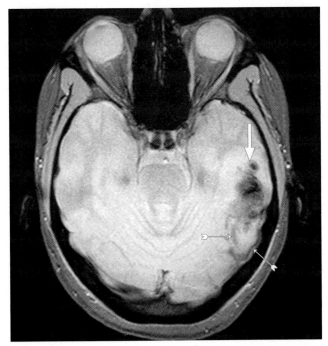

FIGURE 1C

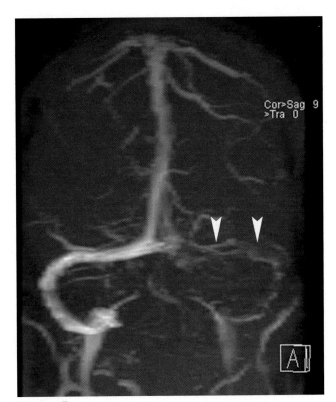

FIGURE 1D

FINDINGS Figure 1A: Axial unenhanced computed tomography (CT image) demonstrates a posterior left temporal lobe hemorrhage. Figure 1B: Axial T1 precontrast magnetic resonance imaging (MRI) demonstrates the hematoma (*larger arrow*) to be of heterogeneous iso- to slightly hyperintense signal relative to the adjacent brain parenchyma. In addition, there is a T1 hyperintense curvilinear cordlike structure posterior to the area of edema in the left temporal lobe (*small hatched arrow*). Figure 1C: Axial GRE image demonstrates an area of signal dropout with blooming (*larger arrow*) in the area of the hematoma. There are also thin curvilinear, cordlike structures posterior to the hematoma (*small hatched arrows*). Figure 1D: Anteroposterior maximum intensity projection (MIP) reconstruction from a magnetic resonance venography (MRV) of the head demonstrates loss of flow-related signal in the left transverse sinus (*arrowheads*) and sigmoid sinus.

DIFFERENTIAL DIAGNOSIS The findings on the images provided are diagnostic of a hemorrhagic venous infarction caused by cerebral venous thrombosis. Based on the CT alone, a hemorrhagic metastasis, hemorrhagic primary brain malignancy, or ruptured arteriovenous malformation (AVM) could be considered; however, the ancillary findings allow the correct diagnosis to be made. Amyloid angiopathy can also cause peripheral parenchymal hemorrhages, but this disease occurs in a much older patient population.

DIAGNOSIS Cerebral venous sinus thrombosis with hemorrhagic venous infarction.

DISCUSSION Cerebral venous thrombosis (including the dural venous sinuses and cortical veins) can be caused by a long list of entities that may induce a hypercoagulable state in patients. These include genetic causes (including factor V Leiden mutation, which is thought to be the most common cause of sporadic CVT), pregnancy, dehydration, oral contraceptives, infection/inflammation, and malignancy.

The pathophysiology behind the hemorrhagic infarct usually occurs as follows: dural sinus thrombosis → clot progresses into cortical veins → increased venous pressure → blood–brain barrier breakdown with vasogenic edema and hemorrhage → venous infarct with cytotoxic edema.

Although it can occur at any age, almost 90% of cerebral venous thrombosis in adults occurs between the ages of 16 and 60 years, with most occurring between 21 and 50 years. Roughly 75% occur in women. The thrombosis is usually seen in more than one sinus, with thrombus identified in the transverse sinus 86% of the time, in the superior sagittal sinus 62% of the time, and in the other sinuses much less often.

Signs and symptoms are nonspecific and include headache, seizure, altered mental status, intracranial hypertension, and focal neurologic deficit.

Imaging findings include a dense and expanded dural sinus on noncontrast CT, a "cord" sign of a dense cortical vein on CT or MRI, filling defects within the dural sinuses on postcontrast MRI or computed tomography venography (CTV) images, loss of signal within the sinuses on time-of-flight or phase contrast MRV, and peripheral or cortical edema or hemorrhage that may not correspond to a typical arterial vascular territory. Bilateral infarction may occur with a parasagittal distribution because of thrombosis of the veins draining into the superior sagittal sinus, or in a bithalamic distribution if the deep venous system is involved. On unenhanced MRI, one may see loss of the normal flow void on T2 spin echo sequences, or the T1 hyperintense thrombus in the affected sinus or cortical vein (evident in this case as curvilinear high signal corresponding to thrombus within cortical veins in Fig. 1B). The thrombus blooms on T2*, GRE, and SWI sequences (Fig. 1C).

There are many imaging pitfalls that can mimic or obscure the potential cerebral venous thrombosis. For example, slow flow can cause T1/T2 hyperintensity, mimicking a subacute thrombus. Flow voids on contrast-enhanced MRI can look like thrombus (compare with your MRV phase contrast images). Time-of-flight imaging can show signal loss owing to in-plane flow or show simulated flow by T1 shine-through of methemoglobin within the thrombus, causing a false-negative on time-of-flight images. On phase contrast MRV images, a hypoplastic transverse sinus can look like a thrombosed sinus. It helps in these instances to look for a small jugular foramen which is seen with hypoplastic transverse sinuses. Slow flow can also look like a thrombosed sinus on phase contrast MRV. Chronic thrombus may enhance. The lesson is to review all your images and modalities in conjunction when considering cerebral venous thrombosis.

Treatment of cerebral venous thrombosis is the same as that of almost any other venous clot in the body: anticoagulation. Care must be taken with patients who have hemorrhagic infarct when using anticoagulation; however, the critical point is that, unlike hemorrhagic conversion of ischemic arterial infarctions, hemorrhage caused by venous occlusion is not a contraindication to anticoagulation. These patients are usually monitored in the ICU setting by means of frequent neuro checks to evaluate for worsening hemorrhage. Endovascular thrombectomy can also be performed in patients who fail to respond to anticoagulation.

Complications of cerebral venous thrombosis include dural arteriovenous fistula (DAVF), intracranial hypertension, and long-term disabilities from the initial stroke. Progression to development of a DAVF may require embolization for cure. In some instances, surgery, observation, and radiation can also be considered.

Questions for Further Thought

1. What additional imaging clues should you look for as potential causes of cerebral venous thrombosis, especially in young patients? How about in older patients?
2. What do the neonatal dural sinuses look like?

Reporting Responsibilities

The findings of cerebral venous thrombosis should be immediately communicated to the ordering physician so that the patient can receive appropriate and timely care.

What the Treating Physician Needs to Know

- Is cerebral venous thrombosis present? If so, which sinuses are involved? Does the thrombus involve the deep venous system, the superficial venous system, or both?
- Is there evidence of edema or hemorrhage?
- Is there evidence of significant mass effect or impending brain herniation?
- Is there any evidence of infection or malignancy that could be contributing to a hypercoagulable state?

Answers

1. Infections such as otitis/mastoiditis, sinus infection, and meningitis are common causes of CVT, particularly in younger patients. In older patients, as with any venous thrombus, you should look especially hard for a cancer as the cause of the hypercoagulability.

2. Neonatal dural sinuses are hyperdense and can mimic CVT secondary to normal polycythemia in the dural sinuses and increased fluid content of the brain.

CLINICAL HISTORY *55-year-old female with fatigue.*

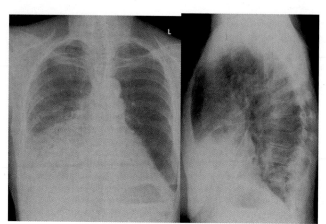

FIGURE 2A

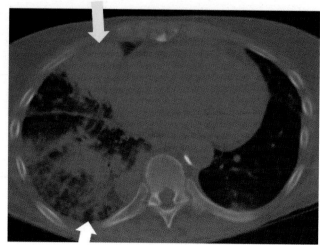

FIGURE 2B

FINDINGS Figure 2A: Posteroanterior and lateral chest films show heterogeneous opacities in the right middle and right lower lobes, silhouetting the right heart border and right hemidiaphragm. Normal right hilar structures are obscured. Lateral film shows opacities in the middle lobe are denser than in the right lower lobe. Thickening of right minor and major fissures also evident. Figure 2B: Axial CT image of the lungs shows dense focal opacity in right middle lobe (*yellow arrow*) and less dense heterogeneous opacities in right lower lobe (*white arrow*). There is also thickening and nodularity of the major fissure in between the two lobes.

DIFFERENTIAL DIAGNOSIS Multifocal pneumonia, multifocal invasive mucinous adenocarcinoma, aspiration pneumonitis, sarcoidosis.

DIAGNOSIS Multifocal invasive mucinous adenocarcinoma.

DISCUSSION Multifocal invasive mucinous adenocarcinoma of the lung was formerly known as multicentric bronchioalveolar carcinoma (BAC). Microscopically, these adenocarcinomas contain abundant mucinous tumor cells, often have a lepidic (sheetlike) growth pattern, and are often predominantly invasive. CT findings include consolidation with air bronchograms, and multifocal solid and semisolid nodules or masses. Lower lobe predominance is common.[1] Obviously, the radiographic appearance mimics bacterial pneumonia, but correlation with clinical symptoms is paramount; if patient does not have fever and chills suggestive of pneumonia, multifocal invasive adenocarcinoma should be moved higher on the differential.

Question for Further Thought

1. What is a symptom that is classically associated with multifocal invasive mucinous adenocarcinoma?

Reporting Responsibilities

The interpreting radiologist should strongly consider clinical history and use older images for comparison. The radiologist should give a differential, depending on clinical symptoms, and advise correlation with bronchoscopy if adenocarcinoma is suspected. If bacterial pneumonia is favored, a follow-up film after treatment should be obtained to confirm resolution.

What the Treating Physician Needs to Know

- Location, extent, and character of opacities.
- Chronicity (if old studies are available for comparison).
- Presence or absence of lymphadenopathy or effusions.

Answer

1. Bronchorrhea caused by copious mucin production by tumor cells.

CLINICAL HISTORY *50-year-old male with history of motor vehicle collision.*

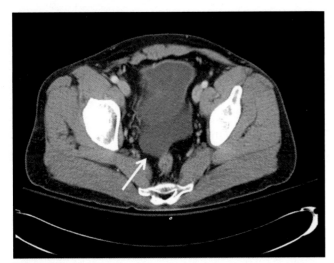

FIGURE 3A

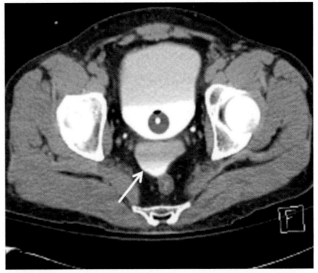

FIGURE 3B

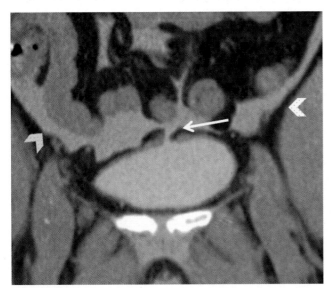

FIGURE 3C

FINDINGS Figure 3A: Axial contrast-enhanced CT image of the pelvis demonstrates simple free fluid posterior to the bladder (*arrow*). Figure 3B: Axial CT image of the pelvis from a CT cystogram demonstrates hyperdense intraperitoneal fluid with layering extravasated intravesicular contrast in the posterior pelvis (*arrow*). A Foley catheter and layering contrast are identified in the bladder. Figure 3C: Coronal reformatted image of the pelvis from a CT cystogram showing hyperdense fluid in the bladder and in the intraperitoneal space. A defect is visible at the bladder dome, indicating the site of the bladder rupture with extravasation of intravesicular contrast from the bladder (*arrow*) into the peritoneal spaces

along the mesentery, around bowel loops, and paracolic gutters (*arrowheads*).

DIFFERENTIAL DIAGNOSIS Intraperitoneal bladder rupture, extraperitoneal bladder rupture, combined bladder rupture, vascular injury.

DIAGNOSIS Intraperitoneal bladder rupture.

DISCUSSION Bladder rupture is a common injury with pelvic trauma, particularly in the presence of pelvic fractures. CT cystogram is the imaging test of choice to diagnose bladder rupture. Intraperitoneal bladder rupture is less common than extraperitoneal bladder rupture (80% to 85%) and commonly occurs as a result of blunt trauma with a full bladder (15% to 20% of bladder ruptures). Simultaneous or combined bladder rupture is less common, and both patterns of injury are seen.

Sandler et al. describes five types of bladder injuries according to degree of wall injury and anatomic location.[2]

- Type 1 is a bladder contusion with incomplete or partial tear of the bladder mucosa and normal findings on CT cystogram.

- Type 2 is an intraperitoneal rupture with a horizontal tear along the peritoneal portion of the bladder wall at the bladder dome and extravasation of contrast into the peritoneal spaces along the mesentery, around bowel loops, and in the paracolic gutters.

- Type 3 is an interstitial bladder injury with intramural hemorrhage and contrast material dissecting within the bladder wall without extravasation of contrast.

- Type 4 is an extraperitoneal rupture, which can be either simple or complex. In simple extraperitoneal rupture, the rupture is confined in the perivesical space. In complex extraperitoneal rupture, the contrast extends beyond the perivesical space and may dissect into a variety of fascial planes and spaces, such as the space of Retzius. Extravasated contrast can extend superiorly into the retroperitoneum involving the pararenal and perinephric spaces. This type of rupture is usually a result of laceration to the bladder wall from fracture fragments or direct stab wounds.

- Type 5 is combined intraperitoneal and extraperitoneal bladder injuries.

Defining the type of bladder rupture defines treatment management. Conservative management with Foley decompression is used for bladder contusions and interstitial injury. Intraperitoneal bladder rupture and combined bladder injuries require exploratory laparotomy with surgical repair. Extraperitoneal ruptures are usually treated with catheter decompression until hematuria clears and as long as the bladder neck is not injured. Surgery is reserved for refractory cases. Catheterization is performed only after urethral injury is excluded.

Questions for Further Thought

1. What sign is associated with extraperitoneal bladder rupture?

2. Why is a bladder rupture sometimes not seen on conventional trauma protocol CT scan of the abdomen and pelvis?

Reporting Responsibilities

Bladder injury or rupture requires immediate communication with the treating emergency and/or trauma physicians. If bladder injury is suspected or if there are pelvic trauma/fractures on conventional trauma protocol CT scan, further evaluation with CT cystography should be recommended.

What the Treating Physician Needs to Know

- Type of bladder rupture.
- Associated pelvic injuries and fractures.

Answers

1. "Molar tooth" sign is the typical appearance of the extravasated contrast within the perivesical space on CT cystogram after an extraperitoneal bladder rupture.

2. In order to visualize a bladder rupture on CT, the bladder must be filled with fluid and under pressure. This is achieved with a CT cystogram, but not necessarily with a conventional CT with varying degrees of bladder distention. If bladder rupture is suspected or there is pelvic trauma, a CT cystogram should be performed.

CLINICAL HISTORY *45-year-old male with history of motor vehicle collision with tree, prolonged extrication, and hypotension en route to ED.*

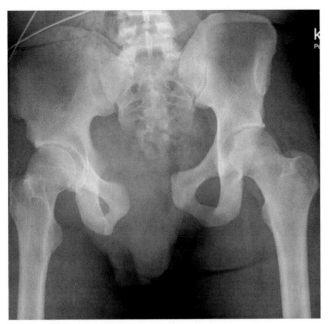

FIGURE 4A

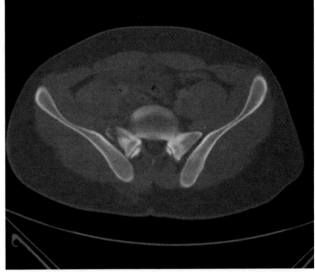

FIGURE 4B

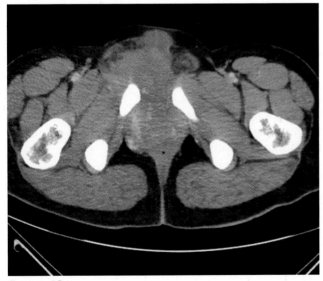

FIGURE 4C

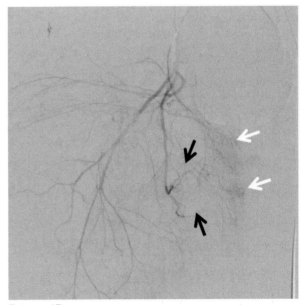

FIGURE 4D

FINDINGS Anteroposterior supine radiograph of the pelvis (Fig. 4A) demonstrates marked pubic symphysis diastasis to nearly 5 cm with marked right sacroiliac joint diastasis; likely right superior sacral ala fracture also noted. Axial CT image with bone window/level setting at the level of the superior right sacral ala (Fig. 4B) reveals a vertical sacral ala fracture. Axial CT image with soft tissue window/level setting (Fig. 4C) shows a large pelvic hematoma with areas of high density consistent with active extravasation. Selective right anterior iliac artery catheterization with angiogram

(Fig. 4D) reveals contrast blush associated with multiple distal branches (*white arrows*); additional contrast blush was noted a few frames later nearby (*black arrows*).

DIFFERENTIAL DIAGNOSIS Acetabulum fracture, pubic rami fractures, sacroiliac joint dislocation, open book pelvic fracture.

DIAGNOSIS Open book pelvic injury with active arterial extravasation.

DISCUSSION Open book pelvic fractures are associated with high-energy trauma, most commonly resulting from motor vehicle collisions (60%) or falls from heights (30%), and are associated with polytrauma (75%), more commonly in younger patients.[1] In the elderly demographic, open book pelvic fractures are often associated with lower-energy trauma. Fractures of the pelvic ring are relatively uncommon overall, making up approximately 1.5% of all fractures.[2] Open book fractures are a type of pelvic ring disruption in which an anteroposterior (AP) vector compressive force is applied to the pelvis. This compressive force results in a spectrum of injuries beginning with anterior arch injury (pubic symphysis disruption or pubic ramus fractures) and progressing in severity to include injuries of the posterior arch of the pelvis. Examples of such injuries include both ligamentous disruption and fractures: pubic symphysis diastasis with or without sacrotuberous and sacrospinous ligament disruption, widening of the anterior sacroiliac (SI) joints, complete SI joint diastasis, pubic ramus fractures, posterior ilium fractures, and sacral ala fractures. The open book pelvis, one of the most severe injuries resulting from an AP compressive force, occurs with pubic symphysis diastasis and anterior SI ligament disruption, resulting in external rotation of the hemipelvis, similar to that of opening a book. Open book fractures in the setting of high-energy trauma are unstable and are associated with life-threatening intrapelvic injuries; immediate recognition and management is essential to limit morbidity and mortality.

The pelvis is divided into the anterior arch, which includes the pubis and ischia, and the posterior arch, which includes the ilia, SI joints, and sacrum. Classification of the mechanism of injury helps predict treatment and prognosis of certain patterns of injury to the pelvic anterior and/or posterior arches. The Young and Burgess classification defines four types of pelvic ring injuries based on mechanism of injury forces: anteroposterior compression (described above), lateral compression, vertical shear, and combined. Lateral compression injuries occur when there is a squeezing-like force applied to the pelvis and result in transverse fractures of the pubic rami and posterior arch injuries. Vertical shear forces result in vertical oriented displacement at the pubic symphysis and SI joints, iliac wing, or sacrum. The combined mechanism involves any combination of lateral compression, anteroposterior compression, or vertical shear, the most common combined mechanism being lateral compression and vertical shear. This classification is useful to the treating clinicians because it provides treatment guidance and prediction of associated injuries.

Diagnosis of pelvic ring injuries is usually made clinically. Initial trauma evaluation includes an AP pelvic radiograph, which will often reveal initial clues to pelvic ring disruption. These include widening of the pubic symphysis and/or pubic ramus fractures. SI joint widening and posterior ilium fractures may also be seen, but posterior arch injuries are, in general, difficult to evaluate on radiographs. A notable pitfall in relying on the initial trauma radiograph is that the patient is likely already in an abdominal binder. If the patient is stable for further imaging, CT is obtained to assess for associated injuries and complications (i.e., vascular or solid organ injury). The patient has hopefully already been placed in pelvic stabilization at the time of CT. Stability of AP compression type injuries is characterized by the degree of pubic symphysis widening and whether or not the posterior arch is disrupted. An AP-type injury is considered stable if widening of the pubic symphysis is less than 2.5 cm without an associated posterior ring injury. Unstable AP mechanism injuries are those with greater than 2.5 cm of pubic diastasis and SI joint space widening or posterior arch fracture. Pubic symphysis diastasis of greater than 2.5 cm implies sacrotuberous and sacrospinous ligament disruption, which leads to some degree of rotational instability.

Management of open book fractures depends on initial hemodynamic resuscitation and rapid reduction of the fractures with temporary pelvic binding, traction, or external fixation, until more definitive surgical repair. An unstable pelvic injury with hemodynamic instability implies vascular injury and necessitates immediate resuscitation with fluids and/or transfusion. External fixation or pelvic binding may stabilize the pelvis, but catheter embolization or intrapelvic packing is often necessary for continued bleeding. If the patient remains hemodynamically stable following pelvic binding and CT shows active extravasation, catheter embolization can be considered.

Question for Further Thought

1. What are the associated complications/injuries not potentially seen on radiographs?

Reporting Responsibilities

Open book pelvis is a surgical emergency, which, hopefully, is already evident clinically; an immediate phone call should be made to the referring clinician.

What the Treating Physician Needs to Know

- Degree of pubic symphysis diastasis and SI joint involvement.
- Open or closed fracture.
- Associated injuries and fractures.

Answer

1. Soft tissue injuries associated with open book pelvis include retroperitoneal hemorrhage caused by venous or arterial injury, bladder or urethral rupture/injury, gastrointestinal injury, and lumbosacral plexus injury. Bladder and urethral injuries are reported in 4% to 25% of pelvic fractures, and even more commonly in straddle injuries (free-floating pubic symphysis).[2] CT can define bleeding or bladder injury. Retrograde urethrogram is helpful in assessing for urethral injury. Physical exam findings are helpful for determining lumbosacral plexus injury; MRI and nerve conduction studies may be needed to confirm.

CASE 5

CLINICAL HISTORY *6-year-old girl with spiking fevers, left ear swelling, and bilateral purulent ear drainage despite antibiotics and bilateral pressure equalization tube placement.*

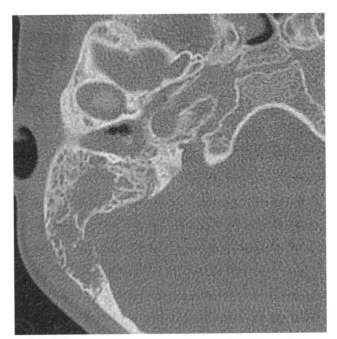

FIGURE 5A

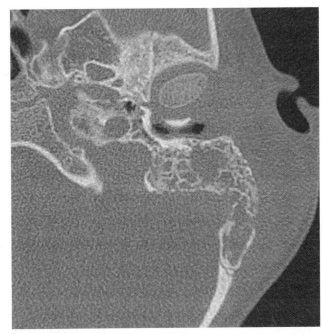

FIGURE 5B

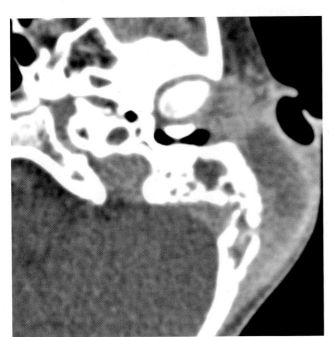

FIGURE 5C

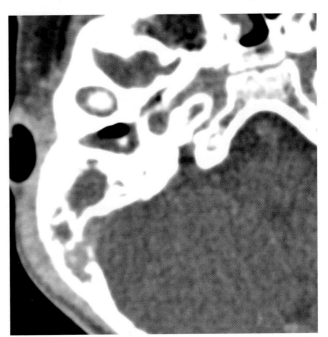

FIGURE 5D

FINDINGS Figures 5A and 5B: Axial contrast-enhanced CT through the temporal bones displayed in bone windows. There are diffuse permeative osseous changes through the bilateral mastoid air cells as well as complete opacification of both the mastoids and the middle ears. Notice the asymmetric fullness along the lateral margin of the left mastoid. Figures 5C and 5D: Soft tissue windowing at these same levels clearly depicts a peripherally enhancing subperiosteal fluid collection along the lateral margin of the left mastoids.

9

DIFFERENTIAL DIAGNOSIS The above imaging findings are pathognomonic of mastoiditis. No differential diagnosis should be provided. Benign or malignant bone tumors such as rhabdomyosarcoma, Langerhan cell hisiocytosis, or aneurysmal bone cysts could certainly cause destructive changes to the mastoids, but middle ear changes would be rare (tympanic membranes [TMs] would likely be clear on exam). Mumps or lymphadenopathy may cause preauricular swelling that may mimic mastoiditis clinically, but would not explain the above diffuse osseous changes and subperiosteal abscess.

DIAGNOSIS Coalescent mastoiditis and osteomyelitis with an associated subperiosteal abscess.

DISCUSSION Acute mastoiditis occurs most commonly in young children and is generally a complication of acute otitis media. The mastoid air cells communicate with the middle ear via the tympanic antrum. In turn, the middle ear communicates with the nasopharynx via the eustachian tubes. Untreated or incompletely treated acute otitis media can thus result in mastoiditis.

Acute otitis media is a clinical diagnosis that manifests with fever, otalgia, and erythema on otoscopy. If the TM appears normal on otoscopy, acute mastoiditis is unlikely. Most cases resolve without serious complications, and imaging plays no role. However, for those patients whose symptoms do not resolve despite appropriate antibiotics or who present with a clinical picture consistent with severe acute otitis media, CT is warranted to exclude acute mastoiditis. Severe acute otitis media and acute mastoiditis have similar clinical presentations, but acute mastoiditis tends to last longer and is often recurrent.

The mildest form of acute mastoiditis, incipient mastoiditis, is characterized by opacification of the mastoid air cells and a middle ear effusion, but demonstrates no evidence of osseous resorption or periostitis. Antibiotics alone are usually enough to cure incipient mastoiditis.

The more aggressive form of acute mastoiditis is known as coalescent mastoiditis, and is distinguished from incipient mastoiditis by the presence of osseous erosions through the pneumatic cell walls and coalescence into larger purulence-filled cavities. The distinction is critical because the treatment of coalescent mastoiditis requires myringotomy, surgical drainage, and oftentimes mastoidectomy in addition to the antibiotics.

Whenever a diagnosis of coalescent mastoiditis is made, pay particular attention to avoid missing an associated complication. If osseous erosion spreads laterally through the external mastoid cortex, a subperiosteal abscess can occur, as depicted in Figure 5D.

Additional complications associated with acute mastoiditis include petrous apicitis, epidural abscess, dural venous thrombophlebitis, or labyrinthitis. Other rare complications include meningitis, subdural abscesses, intraparyenchmal abscesses, carotid artery spasms, or deep neck abscesses.

If the CT findings do not explain the clinical picture or if there is concern for possible intracranial complication, an MRI of the brain should be ordered for further evaluation.

Question for Further Thought

1. What are the four main pathways by which infection spreads in acute mastoiditis?

Reporting Responsibilities

Just as important as reporting the findings of mastoiditis and visualized complications, be clear on the limitations of CT if an intracranial complication is suspected based on either the clinical or the CT findings. MRI is warranted for further evaluation in these cases.

What the Treating Physician Needs to Know

- Is there mastoiditis? If so, is it unilateral or bilateral? Does it look acute or chronic? If acute, does it look incipient or coalescent?
- If there is no mastoiditis, is there an alternative diagnosis to explain the patient's symptomology?
- Are there any obvious complications associated with the mastoiditis?
- Is any further imaging recommended? See above.

Answer

1. Preformed pathways, osseous erosion, thrombophlebitis, or hematogenous seeding.

CLINICAL HISTORY *67-year-old male with chest pain, hypotension, and elevated neutrophil count.*

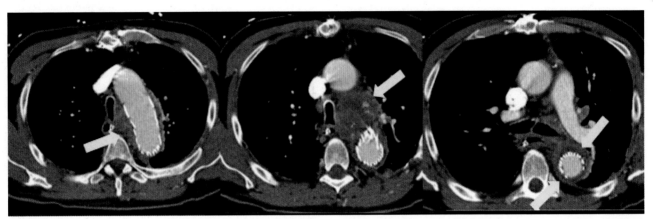

FIGURE 6A

FINDINGS Figure 6A: Serial axial contrast-enhanced CT images of the chest show the aorta with stent graft, and irregular enhancing soft tissue surrounding the arch and descending thoracic aorta (*yellow arrows*).

DIFFERENTIAL DIAGNOSIS Infected aortic stent graft with aortitis, acute mediastinal hematoma, small cell carcinoma.

DIAGNOSIS Infected aortic stent graft with aortitis.

DISCUSSION Contrast-enhanced computed tomography angiography (CTA) is the first-line imaging modality when acute abnormalities of the aorta are suspected. Findings of infectious aortitis are abnormal periaortic soft tissue with adjacent fat stranding or fluid, and, less commonly, periaortic gas collections. Noncontrast images are also useful, because the periaortic soft tissue enhances with contrast, differentiating it from acute hematoma.[1] Infectious aortitis typically occurs in a setting of an atherosclerotic aneurysm (mycotic aneurysm), but can also occur as a result of an infected stent graft, as in this case. Awareness and recognition of imaging findings associated with infected aneurysms are critical for early diagnosis and institution of adequate therapy, in view of the high risk of mortality. IV antibiotic therapy is critical, followed by possible stent removal and revascularization.[2,3]

Question for Further Thought

1. What is the most common pathogen found in infected vascular stents?

Reporting Responsibilities

The interpreting radiologist needs to report findings of abnormal enhancing periaortic soft tissue immediately so that IV antibiotic therapy can be initiated and ICU bed can be prepared. Presence of frank abscess should also be reported because drainage is sometimes a treatment option. Changes in aortic diameter and evidence of stent compromise are also important.

What the Treating Physician Needs to Know

- Location and extent of abnormal periaortic soft tissue.
- Chronicity (if old studies are available for comparison).
- Other findings described above.

Answer

1. Gram-negative salmonella bacilli and gram-positive streptococci.[3]

CLINICAL HISTORY *18-year-old female in a trauma—motor vehicle versus pedestrian.*

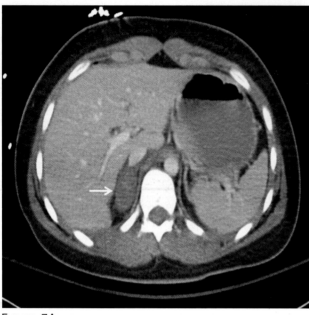

FIGURE 7A

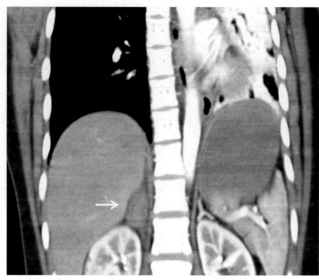

FIGURE 7B

FINDINGS Figures 7A and 7B: Axial and coronal contrast-enhanced CT images of the abdomen demonstrate an enlarged, dense hematoma in the right adrenal gland, measuring 56 HU, with mild adjacent stranding (*arrow*). Normal left adrenal gland. Left pneumothorax and collapse of the left lung identified on the coronal image.

DIFFERENTIAL DIAGNOSES Adrenal hemorrhage, adrenal adenoma, adrenal carcinoma, adrenal metastasis, adrenal lymphoma, infection of the adrenal gland (TB or fungal).

DIAGNOSIS Traumatic adrenal hemorrhage.

DISCUSSION Computed tomography (CT) is the modality of choice in evaluating the adrenal gland. The CT appearance of adrenal hemorrhage is asymmetric enlargement of the adrenal gland with a round or oval mass of high attenuation (usually ranging from 50 to 90 HU) and surrounding periadrenal mesenteric stranding. Thickening of the diaphragmatic crus can also be seen on CT. Adrenal hematomas will decrease in size and attenuation over time. Eventually, most resolve completely. Chronic hemorrhage demonstrates a thin-walled hemorrhagic pseudocyst with a hypoattenuating center or adrenal atrophy. Calcifications may develop up to 1 year in adults and within 1 to 2 weeks in neonates.

Blunt abdominal trauma is a common cause of unilateral adrenal hemorrhage. The right adrenal gland is most commonly involved. This may be caused by direct compression of the right adrenal gland between the liver and the spine or elevated venous pressures in the right adrenal gland caused by compression of the inferior vena cava. Right adrenal hemorrhage is usually seen with associated injuries to the liver, spleen, bilateral kidneys, and right pneumothorax. Left adrenal hemorrhage is usually associated with injuries to the spleen, left kidney, and left pneumothorax. Bilateral adrenal hemorrhage is rarely seen owing to trauma, but, if present, can lead to acute adrenal insufficiency.

Nontraumatic causes of adrenal hemorrhage in adults are usually seen in the setting of severe illness, such as sepsis, stress, tumor, procedures, and anticoagulation. Adrenal hemorrhage occurs most commonly in neonates owing to perinatal stress or injury related to birth trauma. The fetal adrenal is large and vascular and involutes rapidly within the first 6 weeks of life. As only the fetal adrenal tissue is typically involved, neonates do not normally develop adrenal insufficiency. Follow-up ultrasound is recommended to ensure that the hemorrhage is involuting, as an adrenal hematoma can mimic neuroblastoma.

The prognosis of adrenal hemorrhage depends on etiology rather than the extent of hemorrhage. Normal adrenal functioning is seen in unilateral adrenal hemorrhage, which usually resolves. Treatment is usually medical supportive therapy, and rarely surgical. Adrenalectomy is usually reserved for those with underlying tumors causing the hemorrhage.

Questions for Further Thought

1. What is Waterhouse–Friderichsen syndrome?
2. Acute intratumoral adrenal hemorrhage is most commonly seen in which entity?

Reporting Responsibilities

Adrenal hemorrhage should be emergently reported owing to its high occurrence in conjunction with other traumatic injuries or in cases of shock or sepsis. Especially in the case of bilateral adrenal hemorrhage, promptly starting the patient on steroid replacement therapy is critical.

What the Treating Physician Needs to Know

- Unilateral or bilateral involvement of the adrenal glands.
- Identification of other organ injuries in the setting of trauma.
- Follow-up of the adrenal hemorrhage is recommended to exclude underlying neoplasm.

Answers

1. Waterhouse–Friderichsen syndrome is nontraumatic adrenal hemorrhage caused by septicemia. Causative organisms include meningococcus, *Haemophilus influenzae*, *Pseudomonas aeruginosa*, *Escherichia coli*, and *Streptococcus pneumoniae*.
2. Pheochromocytoma is the most common tumor associated with adrenal hemorrhage.

CLINICAL HISTORY *41-year-old male with knee pain after a skiing injury.*

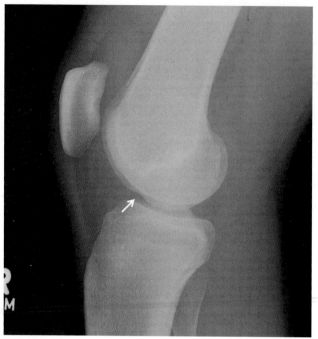

FIGURE 8A

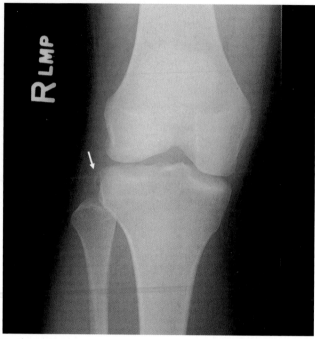

FIGURE 8B

FINDINGS Lateral radiograph of the right knee (Fig. 8A) reveals a moderate- to large-sized effusion and a deep lateral sulcus terminalis (*arrow*). Anteroposterior (AP) radiograph of the right knee in a different patient (Fig. 8B) reveals a vertically oriented curvilinear bone fragment (*arrow*) adjacent to the lateral aspect of the lateral tibial plateau.

DIFFERENTIAL DIAGNOSIS First case: normal variant, impaction fracture, impaction fracture with ligament injury. Second case: ligament avulsion fracture, fracture caused by direct trauma, osteophyte, accessory ossicle, heterotopic ossification.

DIAGNOSIS First case: deep lateral femoral condyle sulcus terminalis. Second case: Segond fracture.

DISCUSSION One of the more common injuries to the knee, especially in sports such as football, soccer, and skiing, is a tear of the anterior cruciate ligament (ACL). The ACL is an intercondylar ligament that attaches proximally at the medial posterior aspect of the lateral femoral condyle and distally at the medial aspect of the intercondylar eminence of the anterior tibia; its function is to prevent anterior translation of the tibia as well as to prevent hyperextension of the knee. Common mechanisms of ACL tear include valgus stress on the knee with the leg in relative extension, and a pivot shift. Pivot shift injury occurs when there is a valgus force applied to the flexed knee in combination with an external rotation

of the tibia or an internal rotation of the femur, which occurs when there is rapid deceleration with simultaneous direction change. The diagnosis of a deficient ACL is often missed on clinical and even radiographic grounds; in one study, the correct diagnosis was made in only 9.8% of patients on initial presentation.[1] The cost of missing the diagnosis is the potential for early onset osteoarthrosis resulting from loss of the stabilizing effect of the ACL.

Although this diagnosis is almost always made on the basis of physical examination and confirmed with MRI in indeterminate cases, there are radiographic findings that indicate ACL injury when seen: the Segond fracture and the deep sulcus sign. A Segond fracture is an avulsion fracture of the lateral tibial plateau. The exact pathology of the Segond fracture is a matter of debate; current thinking is that this fracture represents an avulsion of the very thin anterolateral ligament. Segond fractures are best appreciated on AP radiographs, seen as a small curvilinear bone fragment projecting parallel to the tibial plateau. CT increases sensitivity, although in most cases, will be passed in favor of MRI for its value in ligamentous evaluation. Segond fractures have been shown to be associated with ACL injury in 75% to 100% of cases.[2] This sign is also highly associated with meniscal tears.

The deep sulcus sign, also known as the lateral femoral notch sign, is suggestive of an osteochondral impaction fracture resulting from the impaction of the lateral femoral condyle on the posterior lateral tibial plateau during the relocation phase of the pivot-shift mechanism of injury. The sign describes a depression at the terminal sulcus, a feature of the lateral femoral condyle that represents the junction between the patellar articular surface and the tibial articular surface. Studies have shown mixed results, and the sensitivity appears to be quite low, but a depression of greater than 1.5 mm is suggestive of ACL injury. One study showed that for a depth greater than 2 mm, specificity of 100% and sensitivity of 3% were achieved; for a depth greater than 1.5 mm, specificity dropped to 78% and sensitivity increased to 37%.[3] The presence of two depressed notches—"the double notch sign"—has been shown to be 100% specific for ACL tear, though also with a low sensitivity of 17.2%.[4]

If a Segond fracture or the deep sulcus sign is seen on radiographs, further evaluation with MRI should be recommended, because the likelihood of concurrent ligamentous injury is high. Another radiographic finding that warrants mention is the arcuate sign, a name for the finding of proximal fibular avulsion fracture at the insertion of the arcuate ligament complex. The arcuate sign is an indication of posterolateral corner injury, which is often associated with ACL tear.

Question for Further Thought

1. What ligament is associated with the reverse Segond fracture?

Reporting Responsibilities

ACL rupture is not an emergency; a timely report is required.

What the Treating Physician Needs to Know

• The presence of either a Segond fracture or a deep sulcus sign is a highly specific sign of ACL tear. Nonemergent MRI will be needed to confirm the diagnosis.

Answer

1. The less common "Reverse Segond Fracture" is an avulsion fracture along the medial tibial rim, and raises suspicion for posterior cruciate ligament (PCL) injury, likely involving the deep fibers of the medial collateral ligament. Injury to the PCL may occur during falls with a flexed knee, and often during motor vehicle collisions (MVCs), in particular, when the knees are forced into the dashboard. The PCL attaches the anterior medial femoral condyle to the posterior intercondylar area of the tibia. The PCL is taut when the knee is flexed, and is therefore more prone to injury when the knee is in that position. The so-called "Dashboard Injury" to the PCL occurs when the tibia is forced backward by hitting the front dashboard during automobile accidents.

CASE 9

CLINICAL HISTORY *28-year-old patient with low back pain and lower extremity weakness following a motor vehicle collision.*

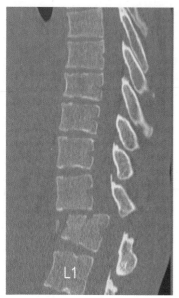

FIGURE 9A

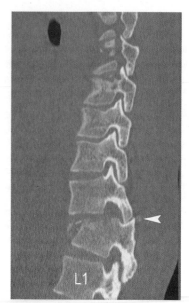

FIGURE 9B

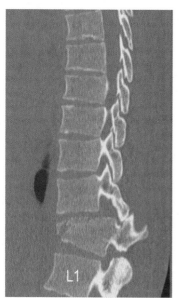

FIGURE 9C

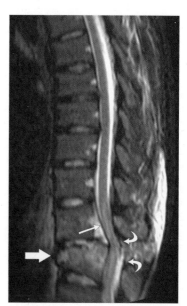

FIGURE 9D

FINDINGS Figure 9A: Sagittal CT of the thoracic spine at midline demonstrates anterior compression of T12 with displaced anterior fracture fragments and anterolisthesis of the T11 vertebral body relative to T12. There is resultant severe spinal canal stenosis. Figures 9B and 9C: Sagittal CT of thoracic spine to the left (Fig. 9B) and right of midline (Fig. 9C) demonstrate bilateral jumped facets, with a small displaced fracture of the left T12 superior articular process (*arrowhead* in Fig. 9B). Figure 9D: Sagittal STIR MR image demonstrates high signal intensity bone marrow edema throughout the T12 vertebral body caused by fracture. There is separation of the anterior longitudinal ligament (*thick arrow*) from the anterior aspect of T12, and lifting of the posterior longitudinal ligament (*thin arrow*) from the posterior T11 body with acute hemorrhage underlying the ligaments. There is widening of the interspinous space with signal abnormality within the interspinous and supraspinous ligaments as well as discontinuity of ligamentum flavum (*curved arrows*), indicating posterior ligamentous complex injuries. There is severe spinal stenosis and increased signal of the spinal cord as a result of acute compressive cord injury.

DIFFERENTIAL DIAGNOSIS The imaging findings are diagnostic of a *flexion–distraction injury with bilateral jumped facets*. Other injuries to consider would include a *Chance fracture* and *burst fracture*. Chance fractures are also flexion–distraction type injuries, but extend horizontally all the way through the vertebral body, pedicles, and spinous process. Burst fractures are compression injuries in which there is comminution of the vertebral body with retropulsion of the posterior vertebral body into the spinal canal. Facet dislocation is not a feature of burst fractures.

DIAGNOSIS Flexion–distraction injury to the thoracic spine with bilateral jumped facets (bilateral interfacetal dislocation).

DISCUSSION In the current case, the mechanism of injury corresponds to a severe flexion–distraction type of injury, with a superimposed axial load injury to the anterior column, tensile failure of the middle column, and posterior ligamentous injury with dislocation and locking of the facet joints. This pattern is likely the result of a high-force deceleration injury, and in this case, the cause was a motor vehicle collision (MVC). This is an unstable injury with osseous and ligamentous components, and it was subsequently treated with reduction after multilevel fusion from T9–L2 with bilateral pedicle screws, fixation rods, and interlaminar bone grafting.

Severe spinal injuries result in considerable patient morbidity, and in immense impact to the medical system. Over 10,000 patients annually suffer spinal cord injuries, with approximately one-third developing paraplegia or quadriplegia. Fractures to the thoracolumbar spine are usually the result of MVCs or falls, with approximately 60% occurring from T12–L2 levels.

Description of spinal fractures is frequently by the Denis classification system, which identifies three columns: anterior (anterior longitudinal ligament, anterior two-thirds of vertebral body/intervertebral disk), middle (posterior longitudinal ligament, posterior one-third of vertebral body/intervertebral disk), and posterior (articular processes, laminae, spinous processes, facet joint capsules, ligamentum flavum, interspinous and supraspinous ligaments). This allows for initial appraisal of acute spine injuries, with instability described in the setting of disruption of two of the three columns. In the setting of middle column disruption, it is often assumed that another column is also likely injured. Additional newer and more elaborate classification mechanisms exist, such as the Thoracolumbar Injury Classification Severity Score (TLICS), which incorporates newer imaging technologies and facilitates selection of treatment algorithms based upon injury morphology, posterior ligamentous complex integrity, and neurologic status of the patient.

CT with multiplanar reformatting is the optimal modality for identification of fractures and osseous landmarks. MRI can contribute to identification of radiographically occult vertebral fractures, and is indispensable for identification of ligamentous, intervertebral disk, and spinal cord injuries. The presence of significant edema or a large intramedullary cord hemorrhage is associated with poorer neurologic outcomes.

Question for Further Thought

1. Does a negative CT exclude an unstable spine injury?

Reporting Responsibilities

Findings of severe spine injury/fracture and findings of spinal stenosis should be communicated immediately to the referring clinician. Timing is essential to allow for identification and prompt treatment, which typically include immobilization, traction, and surgery. MRI should be suggested to further delineate occult findings on CT such as ligamentous, intervertebral disk, and spinal cord injuries.

What the Treating Physician Needs to Know
CT:

- What structures are fractured? What is the likely injury mechanism?
- Is this likely to represent an unstable injury?
    - Is there spinal malalignment or displacement of vertebral structures? Are the facets dislocated (perched or locked)? Is there a rotational component?
    - Is there widening of the intervertebral disk space, facet joints, or posterior elements, which may suggest the presence of ligamentous injury?
- Is there significant spinal stenosis? Are there bony fragments in the canal?
- Is there evidence for injury to the abdominal viscera?

MRI:

- Is there cord compression? Is there edema or hemorrhage in the cord?
- Are there findings of ligamentous disruption? If so, which ligaments are involved?
- Is there evidence of a significant epidural hematoma or traumatic disk herniation?

Answer

1. No, isolated ligamentous injury can lead to progressive and serious instability. MRI allows for improved visualization of ligamentous, intervertebral disk, and spinal cord injuries. Although the presence of some of these injuries may be inferred by the CT findings, MRI allows for identification of such injuries that may otherwise be radiographically occult.

CLINICAL HISTORY *71-year-old female with chest pain and chronic cough.*

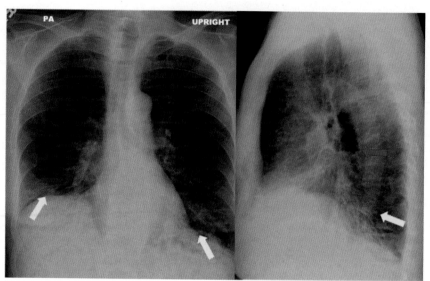

FIGURE 10A

FINDINGS Figure 10A: Posteroanterior and lateral chest films show bilateral basilar predominant linear opacities and basilar predominant bronchiectasis (*yellow arrows*), and an air–fluid level in the esophagus (*blue arrow*).

DIFFERENTIAL DIAGNOSIS Cystic fibrosis, COPD exacerbation, bronchiectasis caused by aspiration as a result of esophageal dysfunction.

DIAGNOSIS Bronchiectasis caused by aspiration as a result of esophageal dysfunction.

DISCUSSION Chronic or repeated bouts of aspiration may lead to basilar predominant bronchiectasis owing to chronic airway inflammation, and can eventually lead to fibrosis if untreated. On chest films, bronchiectasis appears as dilated airways, often with thickened or distorted walls that lack normal tapering, also called "tram-tracking." Perception of airways in the periphery of the lungs is abnormal, as normal small peripheral airways are not visible on chest films.[1] Aspiration has many causes, with swallow or esophageal dysfunction/reflux being most common. Normally, no or only a small amount of air is perceptible in the esophagus on chest films; an air–fluid level in the esophagus is abnormal. In this case, the patient presented with chest pain that was likely caused by reflux and/or esophageal dysmotility given

the abnormal air–fluid level in the midesophagus, and with cough caused by irritation of the cords by aspiration, poor clearance of secretions from bronchiectatic airways, or both.[2] Of course, in this age group, cardiac causes of chest pain were ruled out.

Question for Further Thought

1. What are other etiologies of basilar predominant bronchiectasis?

Reporting Responsibilities
The interpreting radiologist needs to report the constellation of findings and suggest a potential etiology so that further workup can be initiated. Presence of acute aspiration pneumonia (not seen in this case) should be reported because antibiotic coverage with anaerobic coverage is necessary.

What the Treating Physician Needs to Know
- Location and extent of abnormalities.
- Chronicity (if old studies are available for comparison).
- Presence of aspiration pneumonia.

Answer

1. Primary ciliary dyskinesia, immunoglobulin deficiency, α-1 antitrypsin deficiency.[3]

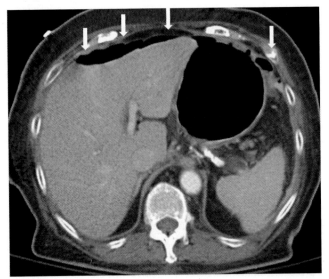

FIGURE 11A

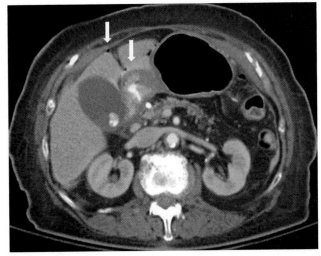

FIGURE 11B

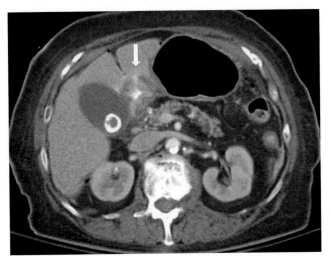

FIGURE 11C

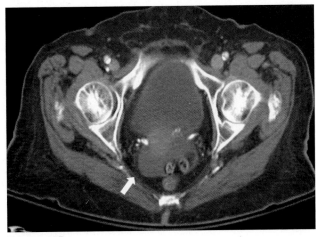

FIGURE 11D

FINDINGS Figure 11A: Axial contrast-enhanced CT image of the upper abdomen demonstrates pneumoperitoneum along the anterior abdomen (*arrows*). Figure 11B: Axial contrast-enhanced CT image of the upper abdomen demonstrates circumferential thickening of the duodenal bulb containing oral contrast. There is adjacent hyperdense fluid and a few tiny extraluminal air bubbles anterior to the duodenal bulb (*arrows*). Figure 11C: Axial contrast-enhanced CT image of the upper abdomen demonstrates a linear hyperdense tract extending from the lumen of the duodenal bulb through the wall, indicating oral contrast extravasation (*arrow*). Figure 11D: Axial contrast-enhanced CT of the pelvis demonstrates free fluid in the pelvic cul-de-sac (*arrow*).

DIFFERENTIAL DIAGNOSIS Iatrogenic duodenal perforation, perforated duodenal ulcer, duodenal Crohn's disease, duodenitis, duodenal adenocarcinoma, duodenal diverticulitis, traumatic injury to the duodenum, cholecystitis, and pancreatitis.

DIAGNOSIS Perforated duodenal ulcer.

DISCUSSION Duodenal ulcers commonly occur in the duodenal bulb. *Helicobacter pylori* (*H. pylori*) infection and NSAIDS are the most common causes of ulcer disease despite significant advances in diagnosis and treatment in the past few decades. Other more rare causes of ulcer disease

19

include Crohn's, other infectious agents, neoplasms, and a hypersecretory state from a gastrinoma (especially with multiple or postbulbar ulcers).

Signs and symptoms of peptic ulcer disease include burning epigastric pain occurring 2 to 4 hours after eating, which is relieved with eating or antacids. The symptoms often start days to weeks before presentation. Oftentimes, patients experience pain that may awaken them from sleep. *H. pylori* can be identified by a blood antibody test, stool antigen test, or carbon urea breath test. Risk factors for ulcers include nonsteriodal antiinflammatory drugs (NSAIDS), *H. pylori*, steroids, alcohol, and stressors, such as the ICU setting.

Upper gastrointestinal fluoroscopic exams are rarely performed as advances in upper gastrointestinal endoscopy allow a pathologic diagnosis and even treatment in the cases of bleeding ulcers. Abdominal radiographs can show free intraperitoneal or retroperitoneal air, depending on the portion of the duodenum that has perforated.

A nonperforated ulcer is rarely seen on CT. However, CT is great for identifying other findings that indicate ulcer disease or duodenitis. Findings on CT include duodenal wall thickening and edema, periduodenal fat stranding, luminal narrowing, and dilated stomach secondary to obstruction. CT findings of duodenal perforation include duodenal wall thickening, free intraperitoneal or retroperitoneal air and fluid, and possibly extravasation of oral contrast from the site of perforation. CT findings of a perforated duodenal ulcer may be subtle, with a few locules of intraperitoneal air and loss of a clear fat plane around the duodenum. Perforated duodenal ulcer remains one of the two most commonly missed surgical emergencies on abdominal CT, along with cholecystitis.

A duodenal diverticulum can sometimes be confused with a contained perforation. The duodenal diverticulum usually arises from the medial portion of the descending duodenum and demonstrates smooth, rounded borders and shows no fat stranding.

Besides iatrogenic free air, a perforated duodenal ulcer remains one of the most common causes of free intraperitoneal air along with perforated gastric ulcer and sigmoid diverticulitis. In the absence of a recent procedure or surgery, free intraperitoneal air found in the lesser sac is usually secondary to perforation of the posterior wall of the stomach or duodenum, and air in the right anterior pararenal space indicates perforated postbulbar duodenum. Free air in the sigmoid recess and left lower quadrant is usually secondary to perforated diverticulitis.

Treatment for a perforated duodenal ulcer is surgical. If the patient has *H. pylori*, treatment with antibiotics and antacids is indicated. Treatment for duodenal ulcer disease without *H. pylori* includes proton pump inhibitors or H_2 receptor antagonists.

Questions for Further Thought

1. Why are perforated duodenal ulcers commonly missed?
2. What would be the likely cause of a perforated postbulbar duodenal ulcer with prominent gastric wall hypertrophy?

Reporting Responsibilities

Perforated duodenal ulcer is a surgical emergency, and the ordering physician should be notified immediately.

What the Treating Physician Needs to Know

- Location of the perforated ulcer—is the ulcer intraperitoneal or retroperitoneal?
- Presence of free intraperitoneal air and source—identify subtle signs of fat stranding, bowel wall thickening, and abnormal air.

Answers

1. The findings of duodenitis and duodenal perforation can be very subtle, and extra care should be taken to carefully examine the duodenum.
2. Zollinger–Ellison syndrome with hypersecretion of gastrin from a gastrinoma.

CLINICAL HISTORY *Patient with hip arthroplasty presents with ipsilateral hip pain, swelling, erythema, and fever.*

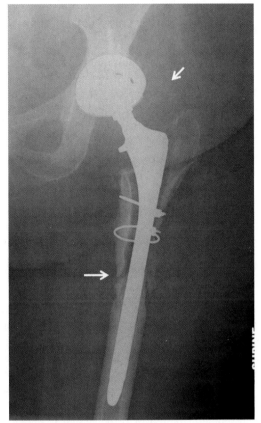

FIGURE **12A**

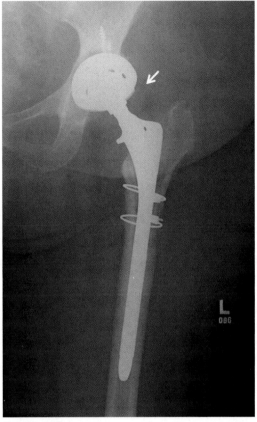

FIGURE **12B**

FINDINGS Anteroposterior (AP) view of the left hip (Fig. 12A) reveals a left total hip prosthesis with extensive lucency around the superior half of the femoral stem with an associated pathologic periprosthetic fracture (*long arrow*). AP view of the left hip from 1 year prior (Fig. 12B) reveals the same prosthesis with essentially normal supporting bone. Also note the large region of soft tissue density consistent with an effusion about the left hip in Figure 12A compared with Figure 12B (*short arrow*). (Images courtesy of Jordan Renner, MD, University of North Carolina, Chapel Hill, NC.)

DIFFERENTIAL DIAGNOSIS Particle disease, Prosthetic loosening, Osteomyelitis/septic joint, subchondral cyst, lytic tumor.

DIAGNOSIS Infected hip prosthesis.

DISCUSSION Instability, aseptic loosening, and infection are the most common reasons for hip pain after arthroplasty leading to revision. Infection occurs in approximately 1% to 2%[1] of first-time hip arthroplasties, and accounts for approximately 14.8%[2] of all revision arthroplasties. Infection may

occur through direct spread from adjacent soft tissue infection, surgical wound, or hematogenously from distant infection or transient bacteremia. Findings such as the presence of a sinus tract from the skin and elevated blood markers such as CRP, ESR, and WBC may aid the diagnosis. Patients most commonly present with pain in the hip region, including buttock, lateral hip, groin, or thigh pain. Fever, induration, or discharge may also be present. Infection around a hip arthroplasty is difficult to treat because the arthroplasty acts as a foreign body nidus upon which organisms can grow and disperse. In addition, prostheses have no blood supply and are impenetrable by antibiotics, as opposed to a native hip infection in which debridement/washout and intravenous antibiotics are able to contain an infection. It is therefore critical to recognize periprosthetic infection early to avoid undue bone loss and joint damage. Infection of a revision arthroplasty occurs at a higher rate, approximately 3.2% to 13%[3], and findings are less predictable postrevision.

An infected prosthesis can raise a diagnostic dilemma, because there is no specific study that provides a definite diagnosis. In the patient with hip pain, radiographs are often the first study obtained. In the setting of an infected prosthesis, a range of radiographic findings may be present from normal to overt periprosthetic osteolysis. Osteolysis is defined as greater than or equal to 2 mm at bone–cement interface, or bone–component interface. (Prostheses may be fixed with cement or with cementless techniques, with cementless types including ingrowth or on-growth methods; the acetabular component may be fixed with screws.) Distinguishing between osteolysis secondary to infection and aseptic loosening or particle disease (in polyethylene-containing prostheses) may also be a radiographic dilemma. Comparison with prior studies is essential, because temporal progression is important to raise suspicion for infection. Periprosthetic infection will often cause rapid osteolysis, whereas aseptic loosening results in more gradual development of periprosthetic lucency. Aseptic loosening may cause uniform periprosthetic lucency, whereas particle disease may cause patchy osteolysis, and infection may produce either pattern. New periosteal bone formation, adjacent soft tissue collection, or gas within the soft tissues also suggests infection. Cross-sectional imaging may be used as a problem-solving technique. CT may be used to demonstrate early osteolysis, or extent of osteolysis before revision. CT and MRI provide improved soft tissue differentiation, and collection, abscess, or joint distension may be identified within adjacent soft tissues. Despite beam hardening artifact on CT and susceptibility artifact on MRI, protocols are available to reduce these artifacts and increase diagnostic information from cross-sectional imaging. Microbiologic confirmation may be sought with blood culture, joint aspiration, and bone biopsy. In the end, however, joint aspiration is the most definitive method of diagnosing a septic joint.

Periprosthetic infection is usually treated with a two-stage revision procedure wherein the infected prosthesis is removed and the surrounding tissues debrided in the first step, and a new prosthesis is placed several weeks to months later in the second step. An antibiotic-impregnated spacer is often left in place. Intravenous antibiotics are also administered.

Questions for Further Thought

1. What role does nuclear medicine imaging play in evaluating joint prosthesis infection? What is the mechanism?
2. What are other causes of post-arthroplasty hip pain?

Reporting Responsibilities

An infected hip prosthesis is not an emergency requiring immediate intervention; a timely report is required. If soft tissue gas is present, the possibility of a necrotizing soft tissue infection, a surgical emergency, should be directly communicated to the referring clinician.

What the Treating Physician Needs to Know

- Presence and extent of osteolysis as well as presence of fluid collection or soft tissue gas.
- Joint aspiration is the gold standard for the diagnosis of an infected joint.

Answers

1. Nuclear medicine may provide a noninvasive method of distinguishing aseptic osteolysis from infective osteolysis, although this modality is not universally available. A combined Tc99m-sulfur colloid and tagged white blood cells (WBCs) provide information about the pathophysiology that will discern the two processes. Both sulfur colloid and tagged WBCs will accumulate within the bone marrow. Tagged WBCs will accumulate within infected tissue secondary to local neutrophil recruitment, but Tc99m-sulfur colloid will not. Therefore, if both tracers are present in a region of osteolysis, it is diagnosed as aseptic. If only tagged WBCs are present, then infection is diagnosed. This method is accurate in diagnosing infection in approximately 90% of cases.[2]
2. Iliopsoas bursitis, greater trochanter avulsion, gluteus medius/minimus tears, hematoma, dislocation/malposition, aseptic loosening.

CLINICAL HISTORY *57-year-old female with new onset of focal seizures. Medical history positive for breast cancer diagnosed and treated 3 years ago.*

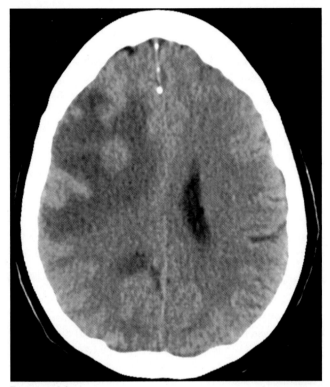

FIGURE 13A

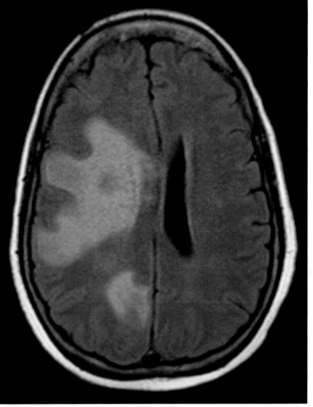

FIGURE 13B

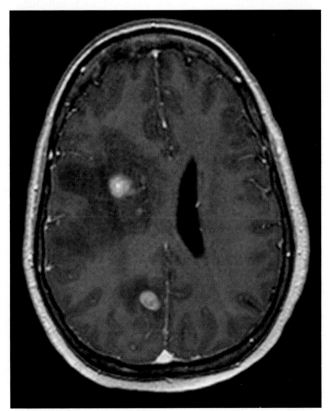

FIGURE 13C

FINDINGS Figure 13A: Axial noncontrast CT image through the brain at the level of the lateral ventricles demonstrates a mass that is isodense to gray matter within the right frontal corona radiata white matter with marked surrounding vasogenic edema. A second subtle area of vasogenic edema is seen posteriorly along the medial right occipital lobe. Figure 13B: Axial FLAIR image at approximately the same level as the CT demonstrates extensive hyperintense signal within the subcortical white matter of the right frontal and occipital lobes consistent with vasogenic edema. Figure 13C: Axial postcontrast T1 image demonstrates enhancement of the mass seen on CT as well as another enhancing lesions that was not delineated on CT imaging.

DIFFERENTIAL DIAGNOSIS There is a short list of common differentials for multifocal lesions in the brain. Primary among these considerations are *metastases* and multifocal *abscesses*. Multifocal metastases demonstrate enhancement on postcontrast CT and MRI in variable patterns from solid to nodular or peripheral and ringlike, while abscesses generally demonstrate a thin peripheral rim of enhancement. Additionally, pyogenic abscesses classically show central hyperintensity on diffusion-weighted imaging (DWI) and low signal intensity reflecting restricted diffusion on apparent diffusion coefficient (ADC) maps. Ring-enhancing metastases generally demonstrate facilitated diffusion (bright on DWI and ADC) centrally in the nonenhancing portions of the lesion. T2 imaging will also characteristically demonstrate hypointensity within an abscess capsule. *Multiple sclerosis (MS)* may also present with multiple, possibly incomplete, ring-enhancing parenchymal lesions corresponding to active demyelination plaques. Rarely, MS plaques can reach substantial size and exert mass effect in the tumefactive variant. MS lesions generally demonstrate T2 hyperintensity and are oriented perpendicular to the ventricles. Involvement of the corpus callosum is common in MS, whereas callosal involvement is distinctly uncommon in most other differentials, except this last differential diagnosis. *Glioblastoma* may present as multiple enhancing lesions within the brain. Necrosis and hemorrhage are very common in glioblastoma.

DIAGNOSIS Multifocal cerebral metastases from a primary breast cancer.

DISCUSSION Metastatic brain lesions occur in 15% to 40% of patients with cancer. Some of the most common primary malignancies in which brain metastases occur include lung cancer, breast cancer, and melanoma. Of those patients with imaging-detected brain metastases, up to 50% have two or more lesions. As in this case, metastatic brain lesions may be discovered on imaging after the onset of new neurologic signs or symptoms. Examples of such clinical presentations include seizures, syncope, persistent headaches, papilledema, or a focal neurologic deficit. However, brain metastases may be asymptomatic in up to 60% to 75% of patients. The presence of metastatic brain lesions may alter cancer staging and treatment. Therefore, imaging for brain metastases is often part of the initial staging workup for systemic malignancy.

Whether imaging is performed routinely for cancer staging or after the onset of neurologic symptoms, brain metastases demonstrate certain features on CT and MRI. Most metastatic lesions occur at the gray matter–white matter junction in the cerebral hemispheres. With lesser degrees of frequency respectively, lesions may also be found in the cerebellum (15%) and basal ganglia (3%). Certain primary neoplasms such as uterine and prostate cancer will preferentially metastasize to the posterior fossa. Occasionally, metastases may even be seen within the ventricles, choroid plexus, and pituitary gland. Certain primary neoplasms such as melanoma, choriocarcinoma, renal cell, and thyroid carcinoma also tend to give rise to hemorrhagic brain metastases. However, lung and breast cancer metastases may also hemorrhage and, given their high prevalence compared with other primaries, are the most likely causes of hemorrhagic metastases. When intra-axial lesions are detected, careful attention should also be paid to the meninges and calvarium for additional metastatic lesions.

Nonenhanced CT (NECT) is often the first-line imaging to be performed in a patient with acute neurologic symptoms. However, NECT alone is not recommended for screening for metastases because, as we have seen in this case, the sensitivity is relatively poor. On NECT, brain metastases may be single or multiple, ranging from hypodense to hyperdense. Varying degrees of vasogenic edema are detected by NECT, as well as the presence of hyperdense hemorrhage.

Screening for brain metastases is generally performed with contrast-enhanced MRI. Metastatic lesions generally demonstrate T2 hyperintensity with corresponding T1 iso- to hypointensity. An exception would be melanoma metastases, which may demonstrate T2 hypointensity/T1 hyperintensity secondary to the paramagnetic effects of melanin. Most metastases avidly enhance on postcontrast T1 images. As mentioned above, ring enhancing brain metastases may generally show high signal on DWI and ADC maps consistent with facilitated diffusion within the central nonenhancing region. T2 hyperintense vasogenic edema may range from nonexistent to exuberant. Small cortically based metastases are likely to demonstrate no edema. Hemorrhage, if present, may demonstrate T1 shortening (depending on age) and hypointense signal on gradient sequences.

Treatment of brain metastases may involve surgery, chemotherapy, and/or radiation. However, therapy is not uniform owing to the multitude of possible primary neoplasms, extent of systemic disease, extent of intracranial disease, and responsiveness of the particular tumor type to chemotherapy and radiation. The mainstay of treatment of multiple brain metastases is whole brain radiation therapy. Stereotactic radiosurgery is reserved for those patients with good performance status and limited disease. Surgery in the setting of multiple metastases is generally palliative, although studies have shown improved survival in patients with three or fewer lesions.

Question for Further Thought

1. Why do cerebral metastases have a proclivity for occurring at the gray matter–white matter junction?

Reporting Responsibilities

CT findings suggestive of a brain neoplasm should be communicated to the referring physician, and MRI should be suggested for further evaluation, given its greater degree of sensitivity. The official radiology report should detail the number of metastases, location (supratentorial/infratentorial, basal ganglia, etc.), presence and degree of mass effect, and the presence of any extra-axial lesions. In addition, the presence of other metastatic lesions in the skull base, calvarium, upper cervical spine, or extracranial soft tissues should be noted.

What the Treating Physician Needs to Know

- How many brain metastases are present, and where are they located?
- Is there extra-axial involvement, including pachymeninges, leptomeninges, ventricles, and choroid plexus? Are there metastases in the bones or extracranial soft tissues?

- Is there significant mass effect or midline shift? For lesions in the posterior fossa, is there significant compression of the 4th ventricle?

- Do any lesions demonstrate T1 shortening to suggest hemorrhage or melanoma?

Answer

1. Hematogenous spread of metastases to the brain generally tends to occur at the gray–white junction owing to the narrow caliber of blood vessels in this area, which leads to the entrapment of tumor emboli.

CLINICAL HISTORY *31-year-old woman with shortness of breath.*

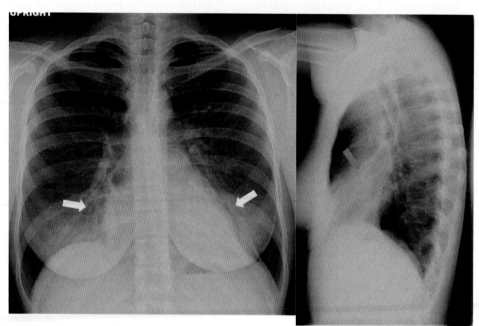

FIGURE 14A

FINDINGS Figure 14A: Posteroanterior and lateral chest films show mild hyperinflation of the lungs with attenuated vessels and prominent anterior clear space. Linear opacities in the right middle lobe and lingula (*yellow arrows*) correspond to opacities on the lateral film (*blue arrow*).

DIFFERENTIAL DIAGNOSIS Emphysema, pectus deformity, atypical mycobacterial infection.

DIAGNOSIS Acute asthma exacerbation.

DISCUSSION Individuals who present to the emergency department with a history of acute shortness of breath should be asked about a history of asthma or asthmalike symptoms. Common imaging findings in patients with acute exacerbation of asthma include hyperinflation, attenuation of lung markings, bronchial wall thickening, and atelectasis.[1] This patient had partial middle lobe and lingular atelectasis caused by mucus plugging. Emphysema usually presents in older

patients, and more marked changes in anteroposterior chest diameter and diaphragmatic flattening occur.

Question for Further Thought
1. Does a normal chest film exclude the diagnosis of asthma or asthma exacerbation?

Reporting Responsibility
Presence of the aforementioned imaging findings should be described in detail.

What the Treating Physician Needs to Know
- Mucus plugging or evidence of concomitant infection is necessary to report, because these may require more aggressive bronchodilator treatment or antibiotics, respectively.

Answer
1. No, many chest films in patients with asthma or asthma exacerbation may be normal.[2]

CLINICAL HISTORY *36-year-old female presenting to the emergency department with diffuse abdominal pain. Last menstrual period (LMP) was 9 weeks ago. She recently underwent dilation and curettage (D&C) for suspected ectopic pregnancy with no intrauterine chorionic villi detected during the procedure, and is currently on methotrexate. Transabdominal ultrasound was performed initially; the exam was terminated prior to an attempt at transvaginal ultrasound based on the preliminary findings.*

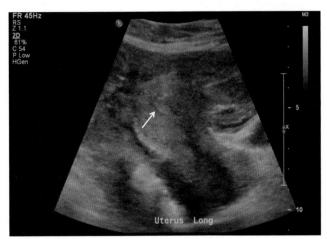

FIGURE 15A

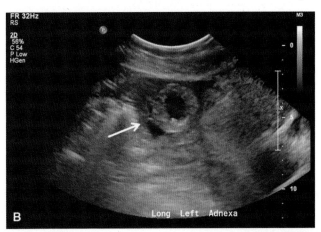

FIGURE 15B

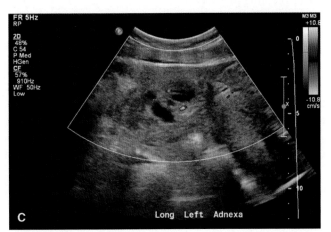

FIGURE 15C

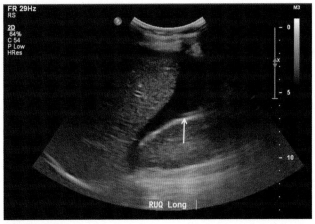

FIGURE 15D

FINDINGS Figure 15A: Transabdominal US longitudinal image of the uterus. The endometrial stripe is visualized (*arrow*). No intrauterine pregnancy is identified. Figures 15B and 15C: Transabdominal US longitudinal images of the left adnexa, with and without color Doppler. An echogenic ring with surrounding fluid is seen in the left adnexa (*arrow*). This is the "tubal ring sign," worrisome for tubal ectopic pregnancy. Mild vascularity is noted. Normal ovaries are not identified on imaging of the adnexae. Figure 15D: Transabdominal US longitudinal image of the right upper quadrant. Free fluid is seen in the upper abdomen (*arrow*), as well as the pelvis as seen in Figure 15B, which is worrisome for a ruptured ectopic pregnancy.

DIFFERENTIAL DIAGNOSIS
- Tubal ectopic pregnancy with rupture.
- Exophytic corpus luteum cyst with associated hemorrhage or rupture.

DIAGNOSIS Ruptured ectopic tubal pregnancy.

DISCUSSION Ectopic pregnancies account for 2% of all pregnancies.[1] Risk factors for ectopic pregnancy include previous ectopic pregnancy, a history of pelvic inflammatory disease, prior gynecologic surgery, use of assistive reproductive technology, endometriosis, use of an intrauterine device, congenital uterine anomalies, maternal smoking, advanced maternal age, and exposure to diethylstilbestrol.[2] Ectopic pregnancy is taught to classically present with the triad of pain, vaginal bleeding, and a palpable adnexal mass; however, these findings are nonspecific, and the most common symptom with which ectopic pregnancy presents is simply pain.[3] Pain and/or bleeding in the first trimester are common presenting symptoms that prompt evaluation with ultrasound to assess the status of the pregnancy.

Ultrasound signs of an intrauterine pregnancy typically can be visualized by 6 weeks after the last menstrual period.[4] If an intrauterine pregnancy is not seen on ultrasound, it may be too early in the pregnancy for ultrasound detection, there may be an abortion in progress, or there may be an ectopic pregnancy.

The findings of ectopic pregnancy on ultrasound are variable. Although ectopic pregnancies may implant within the ovary, the cervix, a C-section scar, or the abdominal cavity, they are most commonly tubal. Detection of a definitive extrauterine pregnancy (in other words, an extrauterine gestational sac in which an embryo or yolk sac is seen) is 100% specific for ectopic pregnancy, but is seen in less than half of ectopic pregnancies.[3]

The echogenic adnexal ringlike structure with internal fluid, or "tubal ring," seen in this case is the next most specific finding in ectopic pregnancy.[3] As mentioned above, the differential for such an appearance includes an exophytic corpus luteum cyst. To help differentiate between these two entities, one may try to determine whether the echogenic ring arises from or is separate from the ovary by applying transducer pressure to the interface between the ovary and the lesion. Movement of the lesion away from or in the opposite direction of the ovary suggests that it is separate from the ovary (and is thus more likely to be an ectopic pregnancy), whereas movement of the lesion with the ovary suggests that it is intraovarian.

Ectopic pregnancy may alternatively manifest on ultrasound as an extraovarian solid or complex adnexal mass owing to hematoma, with variable vascularity. This appearance is the most common sonographic finding of ectopic pregnancy, but the least specific.[3] Although an extraovarian solid mass has a broad differential including ovarian or adnexal mass or degenerating fibroid, such a mass must be considered worrisome for ectopic pregnancy in the setting of a positive pregnancy test without a documented intrauterine pregnancy.

Finally, many ectopic pregnancies do not demonstrate an extrauterine gestational sac or adnexal mass on ultrasound. The secondary finding of free fluid in the abdomen and pelvis is nonspecific, but hemorrhagic free fluid may be the only detected sign of a ruptured ectopic pregnancy, and thus a thorough evaluation for and reporting of free fluid is very important.

Although in the above case transabdominal ultrasound provided adequate imaging of the adnexal findings for diagnosis, transvaginal ultrasound generally provides better imaging of the adnexae, and both approaches are often performed during the same exam.

Ultimately, the diagnosis of ectopic pregnancy is made by a combination of ultrasound and clinical findings, including serial β-HCG levels, and, in some cases, laparoscopy. There are medical and surgical options for the management of ectopic pregnancy. Concern for rupture of an ectopic pregnancy will prompt urgent management.

Question for Further Thought

1. Methotrexate can be administered for medical management of ectopic pregnancy. What are the factors that influence the chance of successful management of ectopic pregnancy with methotrexate administration?

Reporting Responsibilities

A suspected ectopic pregnancy should be urgently reported to the ordering physician.

What the Treating Physician Needs to Know

- The size of the gestational sac or adnexal mass.
- The presence or absence of a detected embryo or yolk sac and of cardiac activity.
- The presence and estimated amount of free fluid or hemoperitoneum.

Answer

1. Factors that predict methotrexate treatment failure include higher initial beta-HCG levels (with some sources recommending surgical management with levels above 2,000 International Units/mL), high progesterone levels, gestational sac diameter greater than 3.5 cm, the presence of cardiac activity within a detected extrauterine embryo, and hemoperitoneum.[5] Additionally, methotrexate is contraindicated in a subset of patients, including those who are immunocompromised, have liver and kidney disease, and have certain medical conditions that may be exacerbated by methotrexate administration such as peptic ulcer disease.[5]

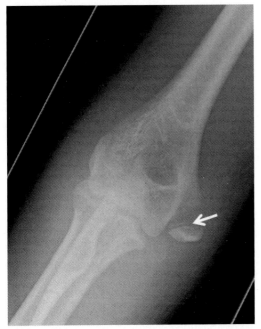

FIGURE 16A

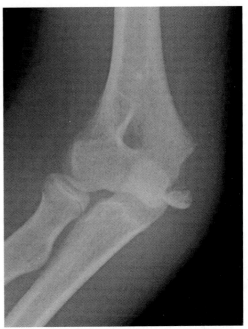

FIGURE 16B

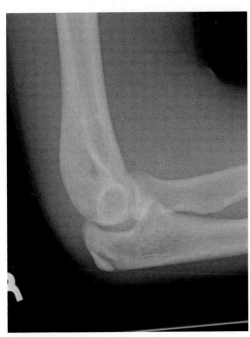

FIGURE 16C

FINDINGS Anteroposterior (Fig. 16A), oblique (Fig. 16B), and lateral (Fig. 16C) radiographs of the elbow demonstrate an ossified body medial and distal to the expected location of the medial epicondyle. An open growth plate (*arrow*) is noted associated with the ossified body. Marked soft tissue swelling is noted about the right elbow, greater along the medial aspect. No elbow effusion is seen.

DIFFERENTIAL DIAGNOSIS Medial epicondyle avulsion, fracture of the medial condyle.

DIAGNOSIS Medial epicondyle avulsion.

DISCUSSION The skeletally immature elbow can be a source of confusion owing to the multiple ossification centers, and the varying ages at which they appear. The well-known mnemonic CRITOE (capitellum, radial head, internal/medial epicondyle, trochlea, olecranon, and external/lateral epicondyle) is a helpful memory aid on which to rely. The medial epicondyle is typically seen at around 5 to 7 years of age. Although the exact timing of the appearance of the ossification centers is not important, the order in which they should appear is.

Avulsion of the medial epicondyle is the third most common elbow fracture in children, after supracondylar and lateral condylar fractures. This injury is most frequently seen in young adolescent males. The injury is most commonly caused by a fall on an outstretched arm with resultant valgus stress at the elbow. Because of this valgus stress, the common flexor tendon, which attaches to the medial epicondyle, produces traction on the apophysis. In approximately 50% of cases, it is associated with an elbow dislocation. This association is so great that one should be sure to locate the medial epicondyle whenever an elbow dislocation is seen, because it may become entrapped within the joint space between the trochlea and the proximal ulna.

Radiographic findings for a medial epicondyle fracture can range from subtle to overt. In more mild injuries, there may be subtle widening of the physis with minimal associated soft tissue swelling. As with many pediatric fractures, comparison with the contralateral appendage may be useful to assess the true presence of widening in these cases. With more profound injuries, there will typically be marked soft tissue swelling, and the epicondyle will be widely displaced. As already noted, the presence of concomitant elbow dislocation should be assessed. Alignment of the radiocapitellar line is useful for assessing the presence of a subtle elbow dislocation. Because the medial epicondyle apophysis is an extra-articular structure, the presence of an elbow effusion is variable, although one will typically be present when an elbow dislocation is also seen.

Therapy for the injury depends, in part, on the radiographic findings. If there is less than 5 mm of displacement, treatment is typically with casting and immobilization. If there is greater than 5 mm of displacement, displacement of the fragment into the joint space, or concomitant elbow dislocation, surgical intervention may be indicated.

This fracture can be confused with a fracture of the medial condyle, which is a much rarer entity. The condyles of the distal humerus represent the margins of both the distal humeral metaphysis and the epiphysis, whereas the *epi*condyles are strictly part of the *epi*physis. In a child younger than 5 years of age, an osseous fragment noted along the medial margin of the distal humerus is unlikely to represent a normal ossification center and instead will represent a fracture of the medial condyle. Alternatively, in a child with an ossified yet unfused medial epicondyle, particular attention should be paid to the medial metaphysis for evidence of a subtle fracture line or small bone flakes. MRI may be helpful in delineating the exact location of the injury. Differentiating these two fractures is important because the management of the two fractures is quite different.

Questions for Further Thought

1. When the medial epicondyle is entrapped within the joint space of the medial elbow, what ossification center can it be mistaken for?

2. What name is given to chronic injury to the medial epicondyle, and how might this manifest radiographically?

Reporting Responsibilities

Medial epicondyle avulsion is not an emergency; a timely report is needed.

What the Treating Physician Needs to Know

- Degree of displacement of the avulsed fragment.
- Presence of a concomitant elbow dislocation (or evidence that suggests dislocation may have occurred at the time of injury).
- Whether or not the avulsed epicondyle is entrapped within the joint space.

Answers

1. When the medial epicondyle becomes entrapped within the joint space, it will typically be interposed between the trochlea and the proximal ulna. In these instances, it can be mistaken for the ossification center of the trochlea, particularly if the trochlea is not yet ossified. This reinforces the importance of CRITOE and the order of appearance of the ossification centers. The ossification center of the trochlea will not be present if the medial epicondyle is not yet ossified.

2. Chronic injury to the medial epicondyle is known as Little Leaguer's elbow or medial apophysitis this condition classically presents in overhead throwing athletes (e.g., pitchers) in a subacute manner with weeks of medial elbow pain. On radiographs, the medial epicondyle can be somewhat osteopenic and fragmented with widening of the physis. MRI can be very helpful to make the diagnosis. The medial epicondyle will typically be edematous with widening and increased signal on T2-weighted images also noted in the physis. The presence of injury to the ulnar collateral ligament or common flexor tendon can also be assessed.

CASE 17

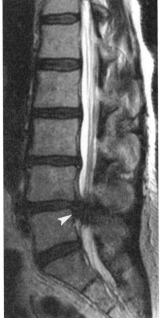

FIGURE 17A

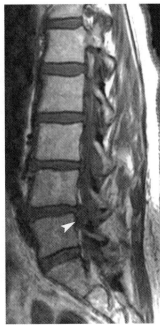

FIGURE 17B

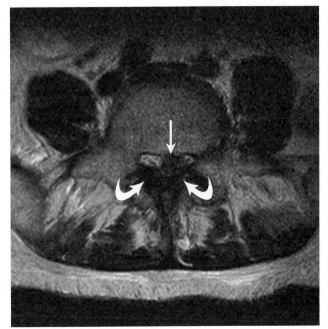

FIGURE 17C

FINDINGS Figures 17A and 17B: Sagittal T2-weighted (Fig. 17A) and T1-weighted (Fig. 17B) MR images through the lumbar spine demonstrating a globular, extradural soft tissue mass (*arrowheads*) posterior to the L4–L5 disk space, which appears contiguous with the intervertebral disk and of the same signal intensity as the disk on both pulse sequences. The mass extends slightly inferiorly relative to the disk level and completely obliterates the lumen of the spinal canal. Figure 17C: Axial T2WI just below the L4–L5 disk level again demonstrates the lesion (*arrow*), which on axial imaging has an ovoid shape and which, in combination with significant thickening of the ligamentum flavum (*curved arrows*), completely effaces the spinal canal. Note the complete absence of any visible CSF.

DIFFERENTIAL DIAGNOSIS In this case, there are, clearly, findings worrisome for a spinal block at the L4–L5 level, and the differential becomes one of what is causing the stenosis. The primary diagnostic consideration in this case is an *extruded (herniated) intervertebral disk fragment*. When a disk herniation is suspected, efforts should be made to determine whether the disk fragment has become separated from its parent disk (*sequestered disk*). Alternative considerations for extradural mass lesions in the lumbar spine include a *schwannoma*, *metastasis*, *epidural abscess*, or *epidural hematoma*. Schwannomas generally arise from the spinal nerve roots and are therefore usually located more laterally in the neural foramina. Metastases usually spread into the epidural

space from the adjacent vertebral bodies. In this case, the nearby L4 and L5 vertebrae demonstrate normal marrow signal. Epidural abscesses usually develop in the setting diskitis or septic arthritis. In this case, there are no findings to suggest an infectious etiology. Finally, epidural hematomas tend to be more longitudinally extensive, although they can be focal when associated with a fracture or acute disk herniation.

DIAGNOSIS Cauda equina syndrome secondary to an L4–L5 disk extrusion.

DISCUSSION Back pain accounts for 7.3 million emergency department (ED) visits annually, and an average of 20,000 ED visits per day. A definitive cause of symptoms is not identifiable in roughly 85% of patients with low back pain, and it is presumed that most of these instances are caused by soft tissue pathology in the muscles or ligaments. In these cases of nonspecific back pain and in cases of uncomplicated radiculopathy presumed to result from a disk herniation, conservative treatment is advocated, and routine imaging is generally not warranted in the acute setting.

There are, however, situations in which urgent imaging for back pain may be warranted. Specifically, early imaging should be considered in patients who have back pain associated with one or more clinical "red flags" that raise concern for a serious underlying condition such as cauda equina syndrome, vertebral infection, or cancer with impending spinal cord compression. Early detection of these conditions is critical because a significant delay in diagnosis in these patients may be associated with a poorer overall outcome. "Red flag" findings elicited on patient history or physical examination include bowel or bladder dysfunction, saddle anesthesia, immunosuppression, history of IV drug abuse, unexplained fever, chronic steroid use, osteoporosis, significant trauma, a history of cancer or unexplained weight loss, a focal neurologic deficit, or the presence of progressive or disabling symptoms.

Cauda equina syndrome is a neurologic syndrome caused by compression of the conus medullaris or the spinal nerve roots of the cauda equina. It is characterized by the triad of saddle anesthesia, loss of bowel or bladder function, and lower extremity weakness. In addition to saddle anesthesia, rectal examination will show decreased or absent rectal tone in 80% of patients. Urinary retention, usually diagnosed by determining a postvoid residual, is evident in 90% of patients. Occasionally, patients may present with urinary incontinence secondary to overflow incontinence from underlying urinary retention. Cauda equina syndrome can be classified into incomplete and complete forms. The incomplete form includes the presence of saddle anesthesia without urinary retention or incontinence, whereas in the complete form, both saddle anesthesia and urinary retention or incontinence are present.

Patients with suspected cauda equina syndrome should undergo urgent MRI of the spine to confirm the presence of conus or cauda equina compression and to localize the causative lesion. Although most of the cases are a result of lumbar spine pathology, lesions higher in the spine causing similar symptoms are occasionally encountered. In patients who are unable to undergo MRI, a CT myelogram should be performed. Large midline disk herniations—most commonly at L4–L5, followed by L5–S1 and L3–L4—are responsible for most instances of cauda equina syndrome, and the condition has been reported to be associated with between 1% and 6% of lumbar disk herniations requiring surgical treatment. Cauda equina syndrome can also be the result of trauma, spinal tumors, spinal hematomas or abscesses, acute transverse myelitis, and inflammatory conditions such as ankylosing spondylitis.

Early surgical decompression (within 48 hours of symptom onset) is generally considered the ideal treatment approach in order to reduce the likelihood of long-term neurologic disability.

Question for Further Thought

1. Why do patients with cauda equina syndrome develop urinary retention?

Reporting Responsibilities

Spinal imaging suggestive of a complete spinal block should be communicated promptly, because a significant delay in diagnosis could lead to poorer outcomes and long-term neurologic disability. If cauda equina syndrome is clinically suspected and lumbar spine imaging is negative, imaging of the remainder of the spine should be suggested, because spinal lesions located more cephalad may rarely present with similar symptoms.

What the Treating Physician Needs to Know

- Is there evidence of a lesion compressing the conus medullaris or cauda equina? If so, where is the lesion, and what is its craniocaudal extent?
- What is the cause of canal compression (e.g., herniated disk, spinal tumor, hematoma, abscess)?
- If there is no evidence of spinal stenosis or compression, is there an alternative finding to explain the patient's symptoms?

Answer

1. The innervation of the bladder is complex and includes parasympathetic, sympathetic, and somatic components. The parasympathetic innervation to the bladder is supplied by the second through fourth sacral nerve roots, and the sympathetic innervation is via the hypogastric plexus (supplied by T11–L3). The parasympathetic system promotes bladder emptying by causing contraction of the detrusor urinae muscle and relaxation of the internal sphincter, whereas the sympathetic system promotes urinary storage by relaxing the detrusor urinae and contracting the internal sphincter. In addition, the external sphincter muscle, a striated muscle, is controlled by the pudendal nerve, which also arises from the second through fourth sacral nerves. Lesions compressing the cauda equina would, therefore, most likely compromise parasympathetic innervation to the bladder and innervation to the external sphincter, while sparing sympathetic innervation, leading to inability to contract the detrusor urinae and sphincter muscles to allow bladder emptying.

CLINICAL HISTORY *22-year-old male after high-speed motor vehicle collision with continuous air leak from right chest tube and lack of right lung reinflation.*

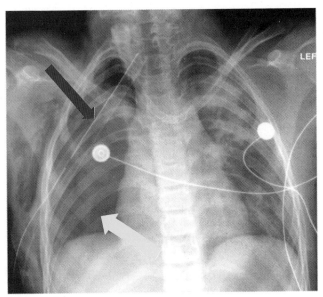

FIGURE 18A

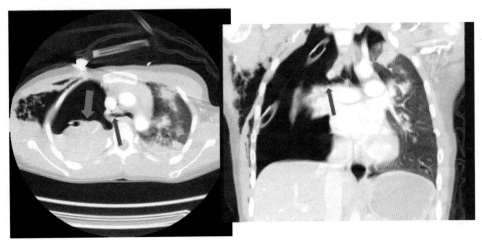

FIGURE 18B

FINDINGS Figure 18A: Anteroposterior (AP) supine film of the chest. Right chest tube (*blue arrow*) is in place. No normal right lung markings are present, and lung is not inflated (*yellow arrow*). Figure 18B: Axial contrast-enhanced CT image of the chest. The right lung (*blue arrow*) is completely collapsed, and has "fallen" into the dependent right hemithorax. Air fills the remainder of the right hemithorax. A right mainstem bronchial stump (*red arrow*) confirms complete bronchial laceration. Left-sided opacity is a pulmonary contusion.

DIFFERENTIAL DIAGNOSIS Bronchial injury, esophageal injury, pulmonary laceration.

DIAGNOSIS Bronchial injury.

DISCUSSION Most bronchial injuries occur within 2.5 cm of the carina and tend to affect the right mainstem bronchus more commonly. These patients typically present with dyspnea and hemoptysis. Radiographically, the presence of rib fractures (which can cause bronchial injury) and soft tissue emphysema are common.[1] The appearance of a collapsed lung in a dependent position (posterior in a supine patient undergoing CT) is indicative of bronchial injury and represents the fallen lung sign (*blue arrow*, Fig. 18B). On the chest radiograph (Fig. 18A) of this patient, there is a refractory pneumothorax despite proper insertion of a functioning chest tube. This should raise suspicion for a bronchial tear. Additionally, mislocation of an endotracheal tube could provide a clue to this diagnosis.[2]

Question for Further Thought

1. What is the utility of the fallen lung sign for imaging studies in the trauma setting?

Reporting Responsibilities

A bronchial rupture must be surgically repaired, so it is critical for the radiologist to report any suspicion of this injury as well as location, and to notify the care team. Severe blunt force trauma is required for this injury, so the radiologist should look for other serious findings such as possible esophageal rupture, pneumomediastinum, pneumothorax, and associated rib fractures. Timely reporting is essential because approximately 80% of these trauma patients die within 2 hours of presentation.[3]

What the Treating Physician Needs to Know

- Presence of tracheobronchial injury with location.
- Associated rib fractures or evidence of other osseous injury.
- Associated esophageal injury or rupture.
- Presence of pneumothorax, pneumomediastinum, or subcutaneous emphysema.[4]

Answer

1. Approximately 1% to 3% of patients that experienced blunt chest trauma have an airway injury. Tracheobronchial rupture is seen in <1% of patients with blunt trauma. The fallen lung sign is not always seen in these patients; however, it is highly specific and essentially pathognomonic of tracheobronchial rupture when present.[5]

CLINICAL HISTORY *73-year-old man with a history of heterozygous factor V Leiden deficiency and a recent history of deep vein thrombosis treated with anticoagulation, presented with an enlarging abdominal mass.*

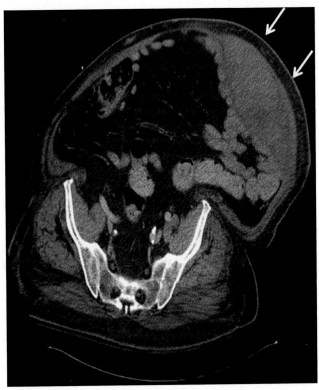

FIGURE 19A

FINDINGS Figure 19A: Axial contrast-enhanced CT through the pelvis shows marked thickening of the left rectus abdominis muscle with a biconvex lentiform shape and heterogeneous contents that are slightly hyperattenuated, compatible with rectus sheath hematoma (*arrows*).

DIFFERENTIAL DIAGNOSIS Solitary fibrous tumor, desmoid, neurofibroma, metastases, lymphoma, sarcoma, abdominal wall abscess, rectus sheath hematoma.

DIAGNOSIS Rectus sheath hematoma.

DISCUSSION A hematoma in the sheath of the rectus abdominis muscle results from injury to the superior or inferior epigastric arteries or rectus muscle. Causes of rectus sheath hematoma include trauma, abdominal surgery, and vigorous abdominal muscle contractions. Spontaneous nontraumatic hematoma occurs most commonly because of anticoagulation. Signs of rectus sheath hematoma include ecchymosis in the periumbilical region or the flanks, and a tender abdominal mass on examination, which remains or becomes more conspicuous (Fothergill sign) or tender (Camett sign) on tensing the abdominal wall.

Rectus sheath hematoma is most commonly located in the lower abdomen. Inferior to the arcuate ligament, the posterior wall of the rectus sheath and the aponeurosis from the three lateral abdominal muscles are absent, allowing the hematoma in this region to be more extensive. A hematoma seen superior to the arcuate ligament is a result of bleeding from the superior epigastric artery or its branches, whereas that inferior to the arcuate ligament is caused by the inferior epigastric artery or its branches.

Contrast-enhanced CT is the modality of choice in most acute trauma cases. Rectus sheath hematoma is easy to detect and diagnose on CT and typically appears as a biconvex lentiform configuration on cross-sectional imaging. This can be uniform in appearance or heterogeneous. An acute hematoma is typically hyperdense. A fluid hematocrit level can sometimes be seen. Active extravasation may occur in severe cases. The hematoma is typically nonenhancing. A noncontrast CT would suffice in the confirmation of the presence and size of the hematoma and also for follow-up.

Ultrasound can be used as the initial test for pediatric and pregnant patients, and to follow up rectus sheath hematoma. Similar to CT, a rectus sheath hematoma appears as a heterogeneous ovoid lesion on transverse images, and biconvex on longitudinal images.

Rectus sheath hematomas are treated conservatively in hemodynamically stable patients. If the hematoma is related to coagulopathy, antiplatelet/anticoagulant therapy may require adjustment or cessation with volume resuscitation, supporting measures, and correction of the anticoagulation state. A traumatic nonexpanding hematoma is typically self-limiting, taking months to resolve, and is mostly treated conservatively. In rare situations, percutaneous arterial embolization or surgery may be required if persistent bleeding and hemodynamic instability occur.

Follow-up to resolution is usually performed to exclude underlying abnormality. If a nontender abdominal wall mass is identified in the absence of trauma or bleeding diatheses and with worrisome features, such as irregular margins, enhancement, and invasive features, malignancy should be considered.

Question for Further Thought

1. Should ultrasound or MRI be performed instead of CT?

Reporting Responsibilities

A large rectus sheath hematoma may cause a drop in hemoglobin or may indicate further loss. The treating physician should be notified for closer follow-up. If there is coagulopathy or antiplatelet/anticoagulant therapy, more urgent notification should be made for timely reversal. Any signs of active bleeding should be urgently reported to the ordering physician.

What the Treating Physician Needs to Know

- Size, location, and extent of the rectus sheath hematoma.
- Any signs of active bleeding.
- Presence of concomitant trauma to the other viscera, or other sites of spontaneous hematoma (e.g., psoas muscle).

Answer

1. Ultrasound or MRI is not the preferred modality at initial presentation for trauma or active hemorrhage. CT is a fast exam, and has superior spatial resolution in assessing the muscle and fat planes of the anterior abdominal wall. Ultrasound can be used as an initial test for pediatric and pregnant patients, and to follow up rectus sheath hematoma. Availability of MRI resources and long scanning time limits its application in acute settings.

CLINICAL HISTORY *25-year-old male with pain following a snowboarding incident.*

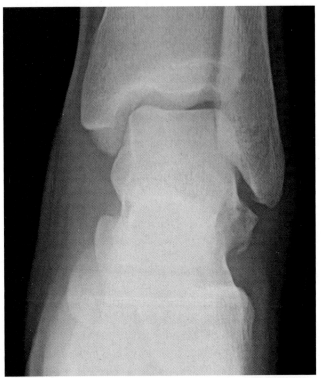

FIGURE 20A

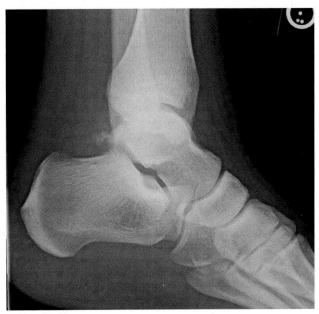

FIGURE 20B

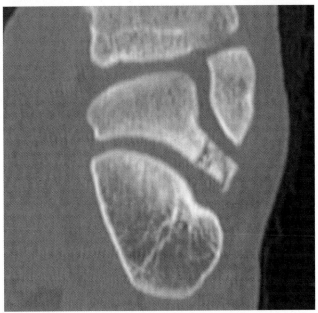

FIGURE 20C

FINDINGS On the anteroposterior (AP) view of the ankle (Fig. 20A), a thin linear fragment is present along the lateral margin of talus, inferior to the lateral process of the talus. The fragment is displaced less than 2 mm. The fragment is difficult to visualize on the lateral projection (Fig. 20B) because of the overlying calcaneus. Incidental note is made of an os trigonum. Coronal CT image of the same patient (Fig. 20C) demonstrates a minimally displaced, comminuted fracture through the lateral process of the talus, which extends to the talofibular and subtalar joints.

DIFFERENTIAL DIAGNOSIS Lateral process of the talus fracture, talar neck fracture.

DIAGNOSIS Lateral process of the talus fracture.

DISCUSSION Lateral process of the talus fractures are fractures of active individuals that are often misdiagnosed as an ankle sprain. They are classically referred to as "snowboarder fractures" because the injury often results from forced dorsiflexion and inversion, which reflects the orientation of the foot while strapped into snowboard bindings. In fact, it has a 15-fold greater incidence in snowboarders than in the general population.[1] Radiographs can underestimate the extent of injury or even miss the fracture 40% to 50% of the time.[2] Knowledge of this entity is important because fractures that are missed or treated inappropriately have a significant risk of poor outcome, including nonunion, early osteoarthrosis, and in some cases the eventual need for subtalar fusion.

Two processes project from the body of the talus—the lateral and posterior process. The lateral process originates from the posterior aspect of the lateral talar body and has two articular surfaces. Dorsolaterally, there is an articulation with the fibula (lateral malleolus). Inferomedially, there is an articulation with the anterior aspect of the posterior facet of the calcaneus at the subtalar joint. Despite its small size, numerous ligaments originate from the lateral process of the talus, including the lateral talocalcaneal, cervical, bifurcate, and anterior talofibular ligaments. As such, it is an important structure in stabilizing both the talofibular and the subtalar joints.

In addition to his general classification of talus fractures, Hawkins described three fracture patterns specific to the lateral process of the talus. A grade I fracture is a simple fracture that extends to both the talofibular and the talocalcaneal articular surfaces. A grade II fracture is a comminuted fracture that involves the entire lateral process and also both articular surfaces. A grade III fracture is a chip fracture that involves only the subtalar joint.

Lateral process of talus fractures are best seen on the AP view, which is included in the standard radiographic ankle series (AP, lateral, and mortise views). The fracture fragments may be small and obscured by overlapping adjacent bony structures. If suspected, Broden's views may be obtained (foot internally rotated, centered at lateral malleolus, and with varying degrees of cephalic tilt). Harris views (axial projection, angled approximately 35 to 45 degrees) can also be obtained to better assess extension into the subtalar joint. In the absence of a visualized fracture, a posterior subtalar effusion is highly suggestive of occult fracture. Clinical suspicion should be raised in the setting of an ankle injury with point tenderness approximately 1 cm distal to the lateral malleolus. CT is often obtained to confirm and further characterize lateral process of talus fractures.

Complete evaluation of the extent of injury is important because the size of the fracture, involvement of the subtalar joint, and displacement of the fracture fragments are all taken into consideration when determining the need for operative management. Management is directly guided by the above described grading system. A grade I fracture requires internal fixation if it is displaced more than 2 mm. If less than 2 mm, casting may be performed without operative management. A grade II fracture requires excision of the comminution fragments (and casting). A grade III fracture requires casting, with closed reduction attempted if possible. Follow-up imaging is recommended to exclude interval increased displacement or the development of avascular necrosis.

Questions for Further Thought

1. What is the differential diagnosis for a lateral process of talus fracture?
2. How are talar neck fractures classified?

Reporting Responsibilities

A lateral process of talus fracture is not an emergency; a timely report is needed.

What the Treating Physician Needs to Know

- Which articular surface is involved.
- Accurate measurement of displacement; >2 mm of displacement needs operative management.
- Presence of comminution fragments requires excision.

Answers

1. One differential consideration is a fragment from a talar neck or body fracture. Differentiation is important because this may indicate a more extensive injury that requires a greater extent of fixation, a different approach (combined lateral and medial approach as opposed to just a lateral approach), or even the need for malleolar osteotomies for complete stabilization of the subtalar joint. Another important differential consideration would include an inferiorly displaced lateral malleolus fracture—closely evaluate the tip of the lateral malleolus to confirm that the cortical margins appear intact. Finally, a potential pitfall is the presence of an os trigonum, an accessory ossicle of the talus that can project over the region of the lateral process on AP radiographs. This can be evaluated on the lateral radiograph where the anterior margin of the os trigonum is posterior to the talus and the margins appear corticated. Contralateral radiographs may be helpful if there is question.

2. In addition to lateral process of the talus classification, Hawkins also developed a classification system for talar neck fractures. Type I fractures are nondisplaced fractures of the talar neck without dislocation. Type II fractures are displaced, with subluxation or dislocation of the subtalar joint. Type III fractures are similar to type II fractures with the additional involvement of the tibiotalar joint. Type IV fractures involve the subtalar, tibiotalar, and talonavicular joints. Type III/IV and some type II fractures require operative treatment. This classification system serves as a guide to management and also as a prognostic indicator, specifically for the development of avascular necrosis (AVN); the risk approximates 10% in type I fractures and up to 90% in type III fractures.

CLINICAL HISTORY *29-year-old male involved in a motor vehicle accident. The patient does not recall striking his head, but complains of tenderness over the right zygomatic arch and maxilla.*

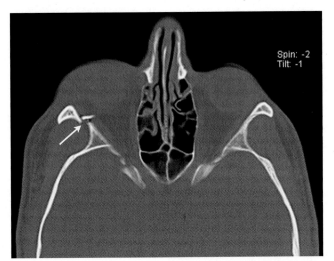

FIGURE 21A

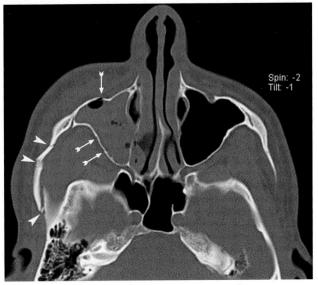

FIGURE 21B

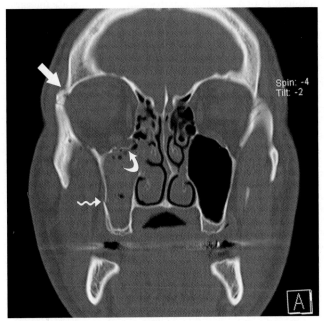

FIGURE 21C

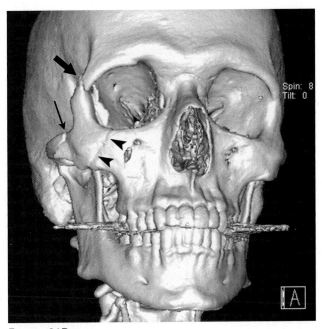

FIGURE 21D

FINDINGS Figures 21A and 21B: Axial noncontrast maxillofacial CT images. Figure 21A demonstrates a comminuted fracture (*thin white arrow*) through the right lateral orbital wall involving the sphenozygomatic suture, with posterolateral displacement of the lateral orbital rim, and a medially displaced and laterally angulated comminution fragment encroaching on the orbit. In Figure 21B, there is a comminuted fracture of the right zygomatic arch (*white arrowheads*), including a more posterior fracture through the base of the zygomatic process of the temporal bone. There are also nondisplaced fractures through the anterior and posterolateral walls of the right maxillary sinus (*hatched arrows*). Figure 21C: Coronal reformatted CT image demonstrates an additional fracture of the right superolateral orbital rim (*thick white arrow*), just above the frontozygomatic suture. There is a comminuted, inferiorly displaced fracture through the right orbital floor (*curved arrow*) involving the infraorbital nerve canal, and a minimally displaced fracture of the lateral wall of the right maxillary sinus (*wavy arrow*). Figure 21D: Right anterior oblique projection of a 3D surface shaded rendering demonstrates fractures of the right lateral (*thick black arrow*) and inferior orbital rims (*black arrowheads*) and right zygomatic arch (*thin black arrow*).

DIFFERENTIAL DIAGNOSIS The above imaging findings are pathognomonic of *zygomaticomaxillary complex (ZMC) fracture*. However, it is useful to distinguish this fracture from an isolated *zygomatic arch fracture*, which does not involve the orbital rims or maxillary sinus. Distinguishing a ZMC fracture from a LeFort III fracture is also important because the management differs for the two. Like the ZMC complex fracture, the LeFort III involves the zygomatic arch, but in contradistinction to ZMC fractures, also has associated pterygoid plate involvement. Lefort I and II fractures do not involve the zygomatic arch. *Naso-orbitoethmoid* fractures occur in the midface in the region of the medial canthus. In some patients, the fracture pattern is difficult to classify and may demonstrate multiple overlapping features. Such fractures are termed *complex midfacial fractures*.

DIAGNOSIS ZMC fracture.

DISCUSSION The imaging findings in this case are typical for a ZMC fracture. Most instances of ZMC fractures are a result of direct trauma to the malar region. These fractures are second only to nasal bone injuries in terms of facial bone injury frequency, with approximately 40% of midface fractures falling under the category of ZMC fractures. The zygomatic bone articulates with the maxillary, frontal, temporal, and sphenoid bones. All four of these anchors of the zygomatic arch are damaged in ZMC fractures, and therefore the term quadrapod or quadramalar fracture is also used to describe these injuries. The components of ZMC fracture include fractures through the: (1) zygomatic arch; (2) inferior and lateral orbital rims; (3) orbital floor; and (4) anterior and posterior maxillary walls. Therefore, ZMC fractures disrupt the upper transverse maxillary and lateral maxillary midface buttresses.

ZMC fractures most commonly occur in teenagers and young adults. Patients often present after trauma with increased facial width and abnormal sensation of the cheek and upper lip. Up to 90% of patients may have abnormal sensation of the cheek secondary to involvement of the infraorbital

nerve canal and subsequent injury to the infraorbital nerve. Impingement of the temporalis muscle may also lead to trismus.

Treatment of ZMC fractures depends on the degree of comminution and displacement. One of the primary goals of treatment is to restore orbital volume and reestablish facial symmetry. In order to achieve cosmesis, the facial widths need to be symmetric. Correct alignment of the zygoma and sphenoid are essential in reestablishing facial symmetry and rotational balance. The rotational deformity can be assessed by the degree of angulation of the sphenozygomatic suture (lateral orbital wall), and the amount of zygoma displacement can be quantified by the degree of impaction of the malar eminence in the axial plane.

Questions for Further Thought

1. Why is it important to correct angular deformities of the lateral orbital wall in ZMC fractures?
2. Why is it important to correct angular deformities of the temporal process of the zygomatic arch in ZMC fractures?

Reporting Responsibilities

The official radiology report should specify the fractures of the ZMC that are involved. Angulation, comminution, and displacement should also be communicated clearly. In addition, it is important to identify and communicate intracranial and globe injures that may be unexpected and should be communicated promptly.

What the Treating Physician Needs to Know

- What is the degree of angulation of the sphenozygomatic suture?
- What is the degree of comminution and displacement of the fracture components?
- Is there an orbital or brain injury?

Answers

1. Correcting angular deformity at the sphenozygomatic suture is important for reestablishing normal intraorbital volume. If significant lateral rotational deformity is not corrected, there may be a resultant residual increase in orbital volume, leading to facial asymmetry.
2. Failure to reduce the angulation of the temporal bone before the remaining fractures are addressed will lead to increase in facial width and cheek underprojection.

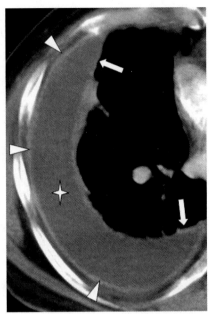

FIGURE 22A

FINDINGS Figure 22A: Axial contrast-enhanced CT of right hemithorax shows thickened enhancing visceral pleura (*arrows*) and thickened enhancing parietal pleura (*arrowheads*), surrounding a fluid collection (*star*) that is higher in attenuation than simple fluid.

DIFFERENTIAL DIAGNOSIS Empyema, simple pleural effusion, hydropneumothorax, pulmonary abscess, chylothorax.

DIAGNOSIS Empyema.

DISCUSSION An empyema is a collection of purulent fluid in the pleural space.[1] Empyemas are loculated, as opposed to a simple transudative effusion, which most often layers dependently in the pleural space. On CT, the purulent fluid is surrounded by thickened and enhancing pleura, known as the "split pleura sign," also illustrated in the Figure 22A. Findings of chronic empyema include increased thickness of adjacent extrapleural fat.[1] Diagnosis of empyema can be confirmed with thoracentesis and return of purulent fluid. Analysis of fluid typically reveals elevated neutrophil count, pH below 7.0, or glucose below 40 mg/dL. *Streptococcus pneumoniae* and *Staphylococcus aureus* are commonly causative agents.[2]

Question for Further Thought

1. What radiographic features differentiate an empyema from a lung abscess?

Reporting Responsibilities

If an empyema is suspected, early reporting is required as thoracotomy and tube drainage along with antibiotic treatment are indicated should the diagnosis be confirmed. Early treatment is important to prevent complications such as a formation of a fibrothorax, sepsis, or permanently impaired lung function.

What the Treating Physician Needs to Know

- Location and size of the empyema.
- Presence or absence of associated lung infection.
- Proximity to or mass effect the empyema has on other structures (lungs, bronchi).
- Chest wall involvement.

Answer

1. Differentiating empyema from lung abscess is important, because the treatment of the conditions is not identical. Chest films are useful in initial analysis, but CT may be necessary to distinguish between the two or make refinements in diagnosis. Empyemas generally have sharper borders between the fluid collection and the lung parenchyma, with displacement of vessels and bronchi away from the collection[5], whereas lung abscesses may lack this discrete boundary between fluid and parenchyma. Empyemas tend to be more elliptical or crescentic, and are most often peripheral, whereas lung abscesses are more spherical, and may be in the center of the lung.[1,5] Empyemas generally have smoother walls because they are bound by pleura, whereas abscesses have thick or irregular walls.[5]

First-line treatment for empyema is IV antibiotics and drainage by percutaneous tube thoracostomy. Chronic or multilocated empyemas often require decortication, either by video-assisted thoracoscopic surgery (VATS) or open thoracotomy.[3] First-line treatment of lung abscess is IV antibiotics and postural drainage[4], followed by tube thoracostomy only if antibiotic treatment fails.

CLINICAL HISTORY *48-year-old female with acute abdominal pain and bloating.*

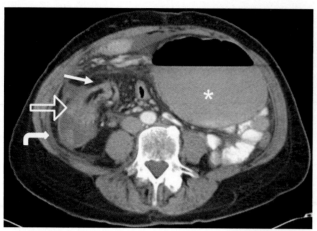

FIGURE 23A

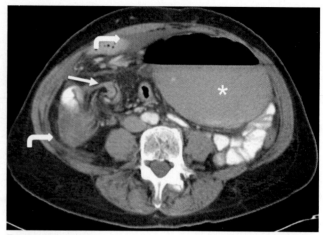

FIGURE 23B

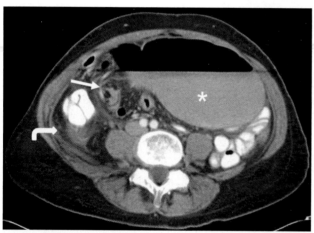

FIGURE 23C

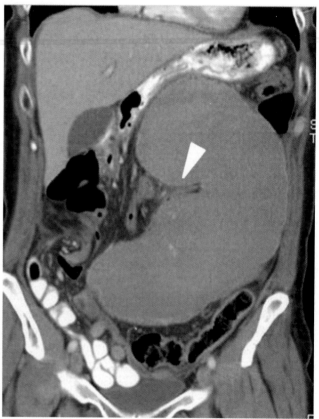

FIGURE 23E

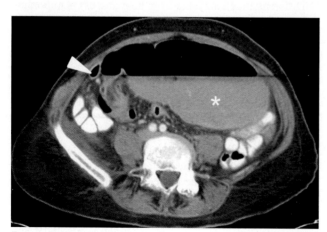

FIGURE 23D

FINDINGS Figures 23A, 23B, 23C, and 23D: Axial contrast-enhanced CT images of the abdomen demonstrate a dilated volvulated cecum (*asterisk*) with a long air–fluid level and whirling/twisting of the mesenteric vessels and colon in the right lower quadrant (*arrow*). The right colon is decompressed (*open arrow* in Fig. 23A). Small volume of free fluid is noted on the axial images (*curved arrow*). Figure 23D best shows the beaking of the cecum as it begins twisting on itself (*arrowhead*). Figure 23E: Coronal CT image of the abdomen shows the kidney bean shape of the dilated volvulated cecum, which points to the left upper quadrant. The dilated cecum bends on itself at the level of the terminal ileum and ileocecal valve (*arrowhead*).

DIFFERENTIAL DIAGNOSIS Cecal volvulus, sigmoid volvulus, distended stomach from high-grade obstruction and large bowel obstruction caused by mass.

DIAGNOSIS Cecal volvulus.

DISCUSSION Cecal volvulus is a rotational twist of the right hemicolon on its axis. It occurs when there is developmental failure of peritoneal fixation, which allows the cecum to be mobile and twist around a fixed point. There are three pathophysiologic types of cecal volvulus: the axial torsion type, where the cecum twists along its longitudinal axis; the loop type, where the cecum twists along its longitudinal axis and then inverts upward; and cecal bascule, where the cecum folds anteriorly upon itself without torsion. The axial torsion and loop types of cecal volvulus usually involve the distal ileum.

The imaging findings are characteristic of cecal volvulus. On abdominal radiographs, there is a large kidney bean–shaped dilated large bowel, usually extending from the right lower quadrant to the left upper quadrant.

CT images show a markedly dilated cecum with a long air–fluid level and a beaked appearance of the dilated bowel entering into the volvulated segment. The whirl sign is the twisting appearance of the mesenteric vessels and collapsed cecum at the site of the torsion. The distal colon is relatively decompressed. Potential complications include bowel perforation, bowel ischemia, and proximal small bowel obstruction (which may or may not be present, depending on the acuity).

Of note, the location of the cecum can differ, depending on the type of cecal volvulus. Axial torsion of cecum usually results in the cecum in the right lower abdomen, whereas the loop type results in the cecum in the left upper quadrant. In cecal bascule, the cecum usually folds upward into the midabdomen.

Treatment typically includes surgery with detorsion and cecopexy or colectomy, depending on the viability of the bowel. Prognosis is excellent without complications, but can be poor with bowel infarction.

Question for Further Thought
1. What other organs can torse?

Reporting Responsibilities
Cecal volvulus is a surgical emergency and should be communicated to the ordering physician immediately.

What the Treating Physician Needs to Know
- Signs of bowel ischemia, infarction, or perforation, including pneumatosis, free intraperitoneal air, and venous gas.
- Whether a mass is present, serving as a fulcrum for the volvulus.
- The diameter of the cecum.

Answer
1. Almost any organ can torse and cause a medical emergency. Sigmoid volvulus is common and arises from the pelvis. Other commonly torsed organs include small bowel, ovary, and testicle. More rare entities include splenic torsion, lung torsion, and hepatic torsion.

CLINICAL HISTORY *Patient presents with shoulder pain and limited motion after direct trauma.*

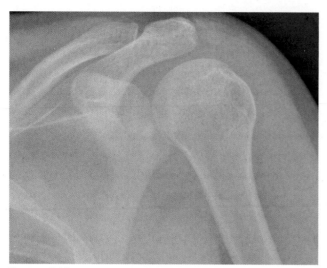

FIGURE 24A

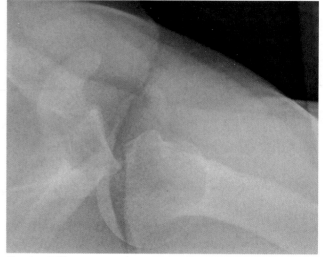

FIGURE 24B

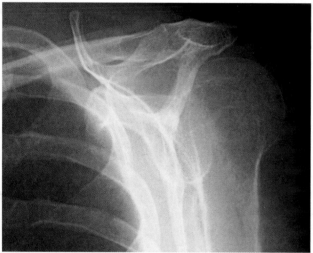

FIGURE 24C

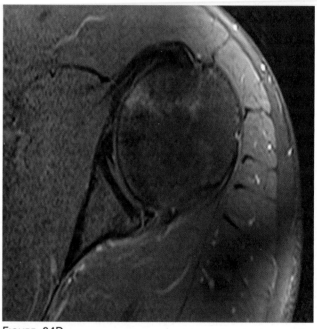

FIGURE 24D

FINDINGS An anteroposterior (AP) view of the left shoulder (Fig. 24A) with the proximal humerus in internal rotation demonstrates less than the usual amount of overlap between the humeral head and the glenoid expected for this view, sometimes described as a loss of the "half-moon overlap sign." The axillary view (Fig. 24B) demonstrates posterior dislocation of the humeral head and a large triangular defect of the anterior aspect of the articular surface that is "engaged" with the posterior glenoid rim. A scapular-Y view in another patient (Fig. 24C) demonstrates posterior displacement of

the humeral head in relation to the glenoid, also indicating a posterior dislocation. An axial T2-weighted fat-suppressed MR image in a third patient (Fig. 24D) demonstrates a posterior labral tear and a small contusion of the anterior humeral head articular surface, a reverse soft tissue Bankart and reverse Hill–Sachs lesion.

DIFFERENTIAL DIAGNOSIS Posterior shoulder dislocation (On the AP view alone: Normal, posterior shoulder dislocation, pseudosubluxation).

DIAGNOSIS Posterior shoulder dislocation.

DISCUSSION The shoulder is the most unstable joint and is prone to the most frequent rate of dislocations, with most dislocations being anterior. Approximately 2% to 5% of shoulder dislocations are posterior. The most common etiology of posterior shoulder dislocation is direct, forceful trauma (responsible for approximately 67%), which may occur from axial force applied to an upper extremity in an adducted, internally rotated position, and with forward elevation. Seizure and electrocution are less common causes, with seizure resulting from powerful contraction of the internal rotators, which overcome the posterior stabilizers. At physical exam, the patient may present with the shoulder in internal rotation and a prominent coracoid anteriorly and prominence of the humeral head posteriorly. The arm will be held in internal rotation, flexion, and adduction with limited range of motion. Fifteen percent of posterior glenohumeral dislocations are bilateral. Posterior glenohumeral joint dislocations may be subtle both on physical exam and radiographically. Approximately 60% to 79% are missed initially.[1] Another reason that this injury may be overlooked is presence of concomitant fracture, which may confound the clinical picture. Therefore, patients may present in the acute, chronic, or recurrent phases. Soft tissue injuries include posterior capsule injury, labral injury, and tears of the teres minor and infraspinatus tendons. Posterior glenoid rim fracture may also occur. Associated neurovascular injury is unusual, and less common than that seen with anterior dislocation.

Radiographs are often the initial study performed when there is suspicion for shoulder dislocation. The humeral head will be located posterior to the glenoid on the scapular-Y view and the axillary view. It is essential to obtain an axillary or scapular-Y view of the shoulder, because findings can be quite subtle on the AP views. On the AP views, the humerus is fixed in internal rotation with the lesser tuberosity oriented medially and the greater tuberosity oriented laterally, creating the "lightbulb sign." Dislocation is often in a straight posterior (subacromial) direction. Loss of the "half-moon overlap sign" or of the normal overlay between the glenoid and the humeral head is also seen in the AP view, and appears as widening of the glenohumeral interval (also known as the "rim sign"). Images should be carefully evaluated for associated osseous injuries, most commonly the reverse Hill–Sachs lesion and the reverse Bankart fracture. The reverse Hill–Sachs lesion is an impaction fracture of the anteromedial surface of the humeral head resulting from the impact of anteromedial humeral head on the posterior surface of the glenoid during dislocation. This may appear as the "trough line" on the AP radiograph. The reverse Bankart fracture is a fracture of the posterior glenoid rim resulting from impact with the humeral head. Surgical neck as well as greater and lesser tuberosity

fractures may be present; careful inspection of these sites is warranted. In the setting of a reverse Hill–Sachs lesion, CT is helpful for characterizing the degree of humeral head impaction because increasing size results in greater glenohumeral instability, and predisposes to recurrent dislocation. CT may be acquired prior to closed reduction for detection of nondisplaced fracture to avoid displacement of the fracture upon reduction. If posterior shoulder dislocation goes unrecognized, the glenohumeral joint remains dislocated, and the greater the resorption of subchondral bone about a reverse Hill–Sachs defect, causing the defect to enlarge. In addition, this defect may serve as a propagation point for fracture of the anatomic neck, and the resulting deformity of the articular surface predisposes to articular cartilage damage, osteoarthrosis, and avascular necrosis. Recognition on initial presentation decreases the chance that the patient will progress to needing an arthroplasty.

Management is situational, and depends upon factors such as size of humeral head defect, presence of additional fracture, vascularity of the humeral head, and duration of dislocation. If a reverse Hill–Sachs defect is present, the size of the defect is important for management, categorized as <20%, 20% to 45%, or >45% to 50% of the articular surface. Treatment options range from closed reduction alone, open reduction, or surgical repair/arthroplasty based on the location and extent of injury. Many with a defect >20% of the articular surface will require surgical repair. As a general principle, repair of osseous defects (reverse Hill–Sachs or Bankart) requires an open procedure, and repair of soft tissue structures may be done arthroscopically. Recurrent instability and impaired shoulder function are complications after treatment.

Questions for Further Thought

1. What activities are particularly associated with posterior shoulder dislocation?
2. What specific types of soft tissue injury may occur from posterior shoulder dislocation and how can they be evaluated?

Reporting Responsibilities

Posterior shoulder dislocation is not an emergency; a timely report is needed. Given the frequency with which this diagnosis is overlooked clinically and radiographically, a phone call may be warranted.

What the Treating Physician Needs to Know

- Presence of dislocation as well as osseous injuries or fractures associated with posterior dislocation.
- Size (percentage of articular surface) of reverse Hill-Sachs lesion if cross-sectional imaging obtained.

Answers

1. Any sport in which an athlete may experience direct force to the anterior shoulder or force transmitted through the arm. For example, American football players, in particular, are prone to posterior traumatic glenohumeral dislocation, especially in the defensive lineman position. Wrestlers are also at risk. As a confounding factor, the shoulder becomes more prone to instability/posterior dislocation during competition as the stabilizer muscles become fatigued.

2. Posterior labral tear (reverse Bankart lesion), posterior capsulolabral periosteal sleeve avulsion, tear of posterior band of inferior glenohumeral ligament, or posterosuperior capsular tears may occur. Evaluate with MRI, and frequently, MR arthrogram, where necessary. MR arthrography has greater sensitivity for subtle injuries owing to distension of the joint.

CLINICAL HISTORY *5-year old girl with panhypopituitarism and a recent history of viral illness was found unresponsive by parents, with wet vomitus around her mouth. Paramedics initiated cardiopulmonary resuscitation at the scene.*

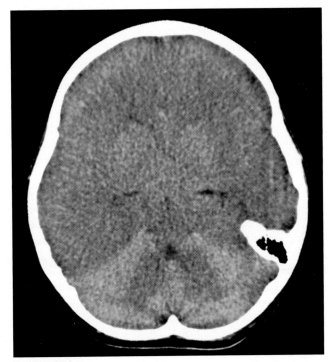

FIGURE 25A

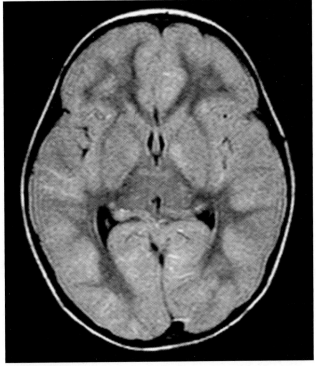

FIGURE 25B

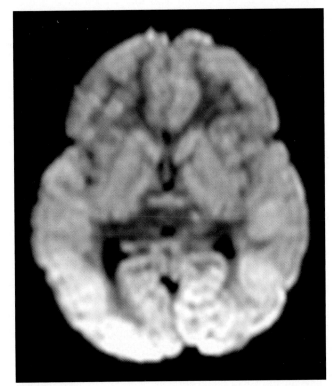

FIGURE 25C

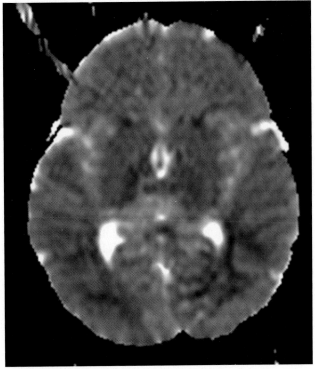

FIGURE 25D

FINDINGS Figure 25A: Axial noncontrast CT images through the brain at the level of the foramen of Monro demonstrates diffuse cerebral edema with loss of the normal gray matter–white matter discrimination. There is relative hyperintensity of the cerebellum juxtaposed against the low-density edematous cerebral hemispheres, the so-called "white cerebellum sign." Figure 25B: Axial FLAIR image obtained 4 days later at the level of the foramen of Monro demonstrates bilateral hyperintensity of the lentiform nuclei and diffuse cortical hyperintensity, particularly at the occipital lobes. Additionally, there is diffuse thickening of the cortex and effacement of the sulci. Figures 25C and 25D: Axial diffusion-weighted imaging (DWI) (Fig. 25C) and corresponding apparent diffusion coefficient (ADC) map (Fig. 25D) images at the level of the foramen of Monro demonstrate symmetric restricted diffusion throughout the cortex and basal ganglia. The ADC map demonstrates hypointensity in the regions of high signal intensity on DWI, consistent with diffusion restriction.

DIFFERENTIAL DIAGNOSIS In the appropriate clinical setting, the above findings are pathognomonic of *anoxic brain injury with diffuse cerebral edema.* Diffuse cerebral edema related to trauma would most closely mimic findings of hypoxic–ischemic encephalopathy, with significant overlap in findings. These entities share common defining features, including diffuse cortical edema and effacement of CSF-containing spaces caused by parenchymal swelling. However, traumatic cerebral edema is often accompanied by intracranial hemorrhage and, at times, skull fractures. The main differentiating feature between traumatic and hypoxic–ischemic cerebral edema is patient history. Cerebral hypoxia related to *carbon monoxide poisoning* may appear similar to anoxic brain injury on nonenhanced CT, with symmetric cerebral edema and involvement of the basal ganglia, and diffusion restriction in these areas on DWI. Carbon monoxide poisoning may also result in a delayed encephalopathy 2 to 3 weeks after insult, at which time MR imaging may demonstrate restricted diffusion predominantly in the subcortical white matter and residual symmetric T2 hyperintensity of the globi pallidi. *Cerebral infarctions* may demonstrate hyperintensity on DWI, sometimes involving large areas of the brain; however, the findings are generally wedge-shaped in appearance and localized to a vascular territory. *Creutzfeldt–Jakob disease (CJD)* is another condition that may mimic the findings of HII on imaging. The clinical pictures of these two entities could not be more different, but MRI imaging will demonstrate restricted diffusion on DWI sequences in a diffuse, symmetric cortical and basal ganglia pattern. T2 imaging sequences in CJD will also demonstrate hyperintensity in the cortical gray matter and basal ganglia.

DIAGNOSIS Hypoxic–ischemic brain injury with diffuse cerebral edema secondary to prolonged respiratory arrest.

DISCUSSION Hypoxic–ischemic brain injury (HII) is a common cause of significant morbidity and mortality across all age groups. In children, likely etiologies include choking, drowning and nonaccidental trauma. In adults, HII is most commonly caused by cardiopulmonary arrest. Although there are different causes of HII across age groups, the pathophysiology remains largely the same. Reduced cerebral blood flow and blood oxygenation lead to a cascade of cellular injury and death secondary to breakdown of intracellular metabolism. Injured and dying neurons may release excitatory neurotransmitters into the already oxygen-depleted local environment that cause a series of destructive events in adjacent neurons, leading to cell injury and death. Generally speaking, the most metabolically active portions of the brain—typically the cortex and deep gray matter—are the most susceptible to HII.

CT imaging is usually the first-line imaging study performed, because it is widely available and can be performed with relative rapidity. Expected findings on CT include diffusely decreased attenuation of the deep and cortical gray matter and loss of gray–white matter discrimination secondary to diffuse cerebral edema. Global edema will also lead to effacement of the CSF-containing spaces, and if sufficiently severe, may lead to herniation. Within the first 24 hours, CT may demonstrate the "reversal sign," where gray matter appears less dense than white matter. This finding is thought to be because of distension of deep medullary veins as a function of reduced venous outflow from elevated intracranial pressure secondary to diffuse edema. The "white cerebellum sign"—which is evident in Figure 25A—is a variant or component of the reversal sign where the cerebellum appears high in attenuation relative to the edematous cerebral hemispheres. The etiology of this finding is thought to be maintained perfusion of the brain stem and cerebellum secondary to posterior redistribution of blood flow.

MR imaging is generally more sensitive to HII, particularly in the first few hours after insult when CT finding may lag behind actual extent of injury. Diffusion-weighted imaging may be positive as early as 3 hours after insult. The structures most likely to demonstrate high intensity on DWI include the deep gray matter, thalami, brain stem, cerebellar hemispheres, hippocampi, and cortical gray matter (particularly the occipital and perirolandic cortices). Diffusion abnormalities will "pseudonormalize" over a week. Pseudonormalization occurs when the diffusion imaging and ADC maps appear normal and falsely represent improvement in the disease process. T2-weighted images become positive after DWI changes are evident, and demonstrate hyperintensity and swelling of affected gray matter structures. T2 hyperintensity may persist in the basal ganglia into chronicity. In chronic HII, the cortex may demonstrate T1 hyperintensity corresponding to cortical necrosis.

Treatment of hypoxic–ischemic encephalopathy is largely supportive. Given successful cardiopulmonary resuscitation according to Advanced Cardiac Life Support (ACLS) guidelines, patients are maintained with mechanical ventilation, and hemodynamic stability is monitored. Current guidelines advocate the use of therapeutic hypothermia in those patients who do not regain consciousness after CPR. Patients are cooled to 32°C to 34°C for 12 to 24 hours after presentation.

Although current studies have failed to show definite benefit for those patients suffering from global hypoxic–ischemic encephalopathy, induced hypothermia has also not shown to be of harm. Additionally, therapeutic hypothermia has demonstrated improved survival and quality of life in those patients who have experienced only mild to moderate cerebral hypoxia/ischemia.

Question for Further Thought

1. When might hypertonic saline and osmotherapy (mannitol) be considered in patients suffering from hypoxic–ischemic encephalopathy?

Reporting Responsibilities

Findings of hypoxic–ischemic encephalopathy should be communicated promptly to the referring clinician. The referring clinician should be made aware of the severity of injury as well as any evidence of cerebral herniation. If the patient history strongly indicates an event leading to HII, but the initial imaging is normal or minimally abnormal, MRI should be recommended for further evaluation. MRI is often more sensitive to early changes related to HII given that diffusion imaging can be positive as early as 3 hours after injury. The official radiology report should include the severity of injury as gauged by cerebral edema and effacement of CSF-containing spaces. Involvement of basal ganglia and cerebellum should also specifically be included. Finally, the presence of evidence of cerebral herniation should be made clear.

What the Treating Physician Needs to Know

- Does the imaging reasonably reflect a patient history of hypoxic–ischemic injury? If not, should a repeat or additional study be ordered?
- If the patient is a child, is there evidence to suggest nonaccidental trauma?
- Does the patient have imaging signs to suggest cerebral herniation?

Answer

1. Hypertonic saline and osmotherapy should be considered in patients suffering from hypoxic–ischemic encephalopathy when imaging demonstrates signs of cerebral herniation in addition to diffuse cerebral edema.

CLINICAL HISTORY *29-year-old female in rollover motor vehicle accident with paradoxical respiratory movement of a portion of right chest wall.*

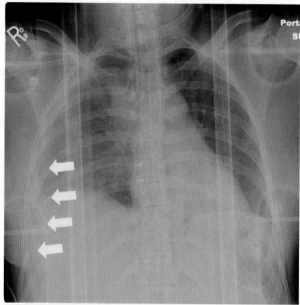

FIGURE 26A

FINDINGS Figure 26A: Anteroposterior supine chest film with patient on a backboard shows displaced fractures of right 5th, 6th, 7th, and 8th posterolateral ribs (*yellow arrows*), with each rib being fractured in more than one place. Endotracheal tube and nasogastric tube are in place.

DIFFERENTIAL DIAGNOSIS Simple rib fracture, flail chest, lung herniation.

DIAGNOSIS Flail chest.

DISCUSSION Flail chest is a condition that occurs after blunt chest wall trauma. Multiple fractures of three or more contiguous ribs or simple fractures of four or more contiguous ribs result in a segment of the chest wall that moves independently of the rest of the chest wall (a flail segment). This results in paradoxical movement of this segment, resulting in decreased ventilation, increased risk of atelectasis, and impaired pulmonary drainage. Flail chest is often evident on physical exam, and plain film radiography is conformational. Findings can include multiple fractures of three or more contiguous ribs, or single fracture of four or more contiguous ribs. Associated findings can include extrapleural hematoma (presenting as focal, peripheral, lobulated areas of abnormal opacity on plain film), pulmonary contusion (patchy air space opacities that do not follow anatomic boundaries), and pulmonary laceration.[2,4] Another possible complication of flail chest is herniation of the lung through the flail segment. The risk of this complication is increased if the patient is on positive pressure ventilation, and is best visualized with CT if suspected. The herniated segment can strangulate, requiring surgical correction.

Question for Further Thought

1. What factors affect morbidity and mortality in patients with flail chest?

Reporting Responsibilities

Timely reporting of the diagnosis of flail chest is necessary, given the high morbidity and mortality associated with it and that rapid mechanical ventilation is often key. Suspected findings of pulmonary contusion, laceration, hematoma, pneumothorax, or other injuries should also be reported.

What the Treating Physician Needs to Know

- Number and location of rib fractures.
- Presence or absence of pulmonary contusion, laceration, pneumothorax, hematoma.
- Whether further diagnostic evaluation would be useful.

Answer

1. Mortality in patients with isolated flail chest is 16%. Several factors can have an impact on outcomes in patients with flail chest. Patients with bilateral anterior costochondral separation have a higher need for mechanical ventilation support, higher injury severity score, and mortality than patients with a single-sided posterolateral flail chest. The presence of associated head trauma and of pulmonary contusion also both independently increase mortality (19% and 42%, respectively). Injury score and mortality are worse in patients older than 55, with presence of shock increasing mortality.[1,3]

CLINICAL HISTORY *30-year-old female with neck pain following high-speed motor vehicle collision.*

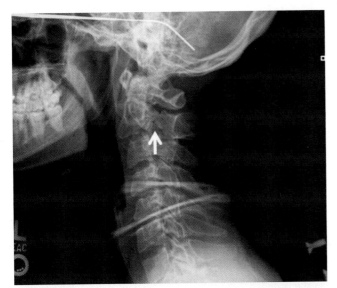

FIGURE 27A

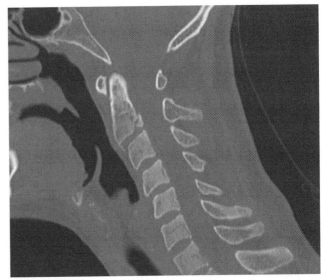

FIGURE 27B

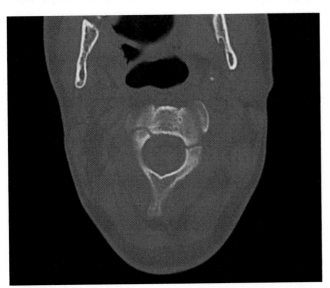

FIGURE 27C

FINDINGS Lateral radiograph (Fig. 27A) of the cervical spine demonstrates a fracture through the pars interarticularis (*arrow*) of C2 with anterolisthesis of C2 on C3 and mild posterior angulation. Sagittal CT image through the right lateral aspect of C2 (Fig. 27B) and transverse (Fig. 27C) CT image at the level of the C2 vertebral body confirm bilateral pars interarticularis fractures with anterolisthesis of C2 on C3. The overall degree of anterolisthesis is often best seen on the radiographs.

DIFFERENTIAL DIAGNOSIS Traumatic spondylolisthesis of the axis (TSA), congenital spondylolisthesis of the axis, odontoid fracture.

DIAGNOSIS TSA ("Hangman Fracture").

DISCUSSION TSA is the second most common fracture of the C2 vertebral body, after fractures of the dens, accounting for 22% of axis fractures and 4% of cervical spine fractures overall.[1] Although colloquially named "hangman's fracture" in reference to trauma incurred by judicial hangings, modern day TSA is most commonly a result of motor vehicle collisions, followed in incidence by falls and diving accidents. Although classically considered a hyperextension injury because of its association with the injury incurred in judicial hanging with a submental knot, the more severe forms of TSA are associated with a greater component of flexion, whether as a type of rebound injury or as a purely flexion injury. The posterior element fractures associated with TSA were originally described as bilateral pars interarticularis fractures, but any of the posterior elements may be involved, and fracture location may be different on either side. In both the hyperextension and hyperflexion forms, the rotational stress applied to the C2 body and dens is transmitted to the weaker posterior elements, which have no room to accommodate the rotational stress and subsequently fracture. Continued rotation results in soft tissue injury to the longitudinal ligaments and the C2–3 disk. The spectrum of TSA-type injuries includes both stable and unstable forms; early recognition of the injury and the type is essential to early initiation of appropriate management and prevention of complications. Fortunately, patients who survive the initial trauma rarely suffer neurologic deficits because the diameter of the cervical spinal canal is greatest at C2, and spondylolisthesis generally results in further expansion of the canal.

The goal of a classification system is to determine treatment and prognosis. For TSA, the goal is to predict fracture stability. The status of the anterior longitudinal ligament (ALL), the posterior longitudinal ligament (PLL), and the C2–3 disk is central to this determination. Unfortunately, no one classification system can accurately predict stability; additional clinical and imaging evaluation may be needed to determine degree of stability. The classification system developed by Effendi et al., modified by Levine and Edwards, based on static radiographic and CT appearance, is widely used to describe these fractures.[2,3] Four variants are described, all associated with bilateral posterior element fractures. The mechanism, radiographic findings, and associated soft tissue injuries are listed by type:

- Type I—Hyperextension with axial loading; less than 3 mm of displacement, no angulation; more accurately termed "traumatic spondylolysis."

- Type II—Hyperextension followed by hyperflexion, both with axial compression; anterior C2 vertebral body displacement (>3 mm), significant (undefined, other classifications use 11° for a cutoff) angulation; ALL, PLL, and C2–3 disruption.

- Type IIA—Hyperflexion with distraction; C2 vertebral body angulation without displacement; PLL and C2–3 disruption, ALL intact.

- Type III—Hyperflexion with compression; anterior C2 vertebral body displacement, significant angulation, and unilateral or bilateral locked facets; ALL, PLL, and C2–3 disruption.

Type I and II fractures are the most common. Type I injuries are generally considered stable, whereas type II, IIA, and III are generally considered unstable.

Before the ubiquitous use of CT in the evaluation of cervical spine trauma, the lateral radiograph was the initial imaging study to demonstrate features of TSA. Fractures through the C2 posterior elements and dislocation or angulation of the C2 vertebral body are the main radiographic findings. Angulation is best measured between the inferior endplates of C2 and C3. Associated prevertebral soft tissue swelling is common. Avulsion of the anterior inferior corner of the C2 vertebral body may be present, suggestive of injury of the ALL. TSA with a flexion component may be associated with anterosuperior endplate compression deformities of C3. However, the sensitivity of radiographs for TSA is as low as 40%.[4] In modern day emergency departments, CT can be performed rapidly and offers higher sensitivity and specificity for cervical spine injury over radiography. Consequently, CT has largely replaced radiography in the evaluation of patients at high risk for cervical spine injury. Features of TSA detected on radiography are readily evident on CT. However, CT may reveal subtle findings including nondisplaced fractures of the posterior elements or injury to the transverse foramina that may not be apparent on radiographs. CT angiography can be rapidly obtained in the setting of transverse foramen involvement to evaluate for vertebral artery injury. The determination of stability is of utmost importance because this guides management. Radiographs and CT are static examinations of the cervical spine; although there may be overt signs of instability (marked angulation or displacement), reduced but unstable lesions will be missed. Documentation of the status of the longitudinal ligaments and the intervertebral disk is best determined on MRI. If MRI is unavailable, physician-performed flexion–extension fluoroscopy can help to differentiate stable from unstable injuries: for example, widening of the posterior C2–3 disk space in flexion in an apparent type I TSA changes the classification to a type IIA injury.[2] Patients demonstrating neurologic deficits, with or without injuries identified on CT, should undergo further evaluation with MRI. MRI is superior to CT for detection of blood in the spinal canal, spinal cord compression, and spinal cord edema as well as disk and ligamentous injury. MR angiography may be obtained with MRI if vascular injury is a suspected cause of the patient's neurologic deficits and CT angiography has not been performed.

Acute complications of TSA include neurologic injury and vertebral artery injury. Permanent neurologic injury is on the order of 2% to 3%, and transient neural deficits may occur in up to 25% of patients.[4] Although vertebral artery injury may present with acute vertebrobasilar symptoms, the onset of neurologic symptoms may be delayed up to a few days. Vertebral artery injury has been reported to occur in nearly 28% of cases in one series.[5]

Treatment options for TSA vary according to the initial classification and stability of the lesion. Type I fractures respond well to conservative management using traction followed by stabilization with a cervical collar or cervicothoracic brace. Type II fractures are managed similarly, but over a longer duration of time. Some type II fractures fail to reduce appropriately with conservative management and require open reduction and internal fixation. Type IIA and III injuries are generally treated surgically. Few complications are seen in patients who are managed appropriately. The primary complications are malunion or nonunion in conservatively managed patients.

Question for Further Thought

1. How does TSA differ from the injury seen in judicial hanging?

Reporting Responsibilities

Given the potential for instability, TSA should be reported emergently; direct communication with the referring clinician is required.

What the Treating Physician Needs to Know

- Radiographs have low sensitivity for TSA, and CT should be obtained in all suspected cases.

- Position of fracture fragments including displacement and angulation.

- Fracture stability is determined on the basis of clinical data and soft tissue evaluation: nondisplaced, nonangulated fractures do not exclude instability; MRI is needed in these cases.

- Involvement of the transverse foramina: CTA or MRA should be obtained.
- Involvement of the spinal canal.
- Additional cervical spine fractures.

Answer

1. Traumatic hyperextension fractures of the axis are reminiscent of the injury caused by judicial hangings making use of a submental knot. However, the mechanism of injury is different. The judicial hanging resulted in hyperextension and distraction, which results in tearing of the spinal cord. The hyperextension form of TSA sustained in motor vehicle trauma, falls, and diving accidents is typically a result of hyperextension with axial compression; trauma to the cord is uncommon.

CLINICAL HISTORY *21-year-old man who fell on the ice after jumping off a ledge.*

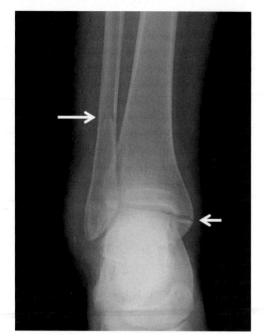

FIGURE 28A

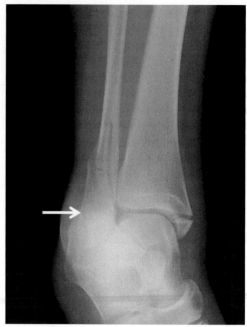

FIGURE 28B

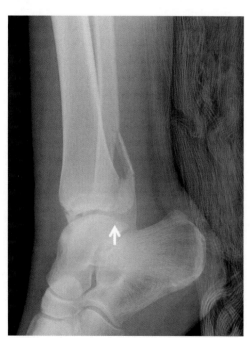

FIGURE 28C

FINDINGS Supine anteroposterior (AP) radiograph of the ankle (Fig. 28A) demonstrates a transverse fracture through the medial malleolus (*short arrow*), and a fracture of the distal fibula above the level of the syndesmosis (*long arrow*). There is surrounding soft tissue swelling, greatest laterally. The ankle mortise view (Fig. 28B) reveals that the fracture of the distal fibula obliquely extends into the ankle mortise

(*arrow*). The ankle mortise remains grossly approximated. The cross-table lateral view of the ankle (Fig. 28C) reveals a nondisplaced fracture of the posterior malleolus (*arrow*). Also demonstrated on the lateral view is mild posterior displacement and overriding of the oblique lateral malleolus fracture (*arrow*).

DIFFERENTIAL DIAGNOSIS Inversion ankle injury, eversion ankle injury.

DIAGNOSIS Trimalleolar ankle fracture secondary to eversion injury.

DISCUSSION Ankle fractures are, along with hip fractures, one of the most common fractures of the lower extremity. One study from the United Kingdom found them to be ~22% of all lower extremity fractures.[1] Although most mechanisms result only in soft tissue injury, a percentage may also result in fractures that require more aggressive therapy. Published guidelines are available to help the clinician discern whether radiologic evaluation is warranted. These "Ottawa ankle rules" have been shown to demonstrate nearly 100% sensitivity in detecting fractures.[2] According to these guidelines, imaging should be pursued only if there is tenderness over the malleolar areas or if there is pain significant enough to restrict weight bearing immediately after injury and also at the time of evaluation.

Initial imaging of the ankle consists of a standard radiographic series of AP, mortise, and lateral views. History is important in the assessment of these images because the mechanism of injury can help identify fractures as well as possible ligamentous injuries. However, when the history is not forthcoming, assessment of the fracture pattern on these images can suggest a mechanism of injury and help guide evaluation of the soft tissues.

Multiple classification schemes have been proposed and utilized. One system (Lauge-Hansen) approaches the classification of fractures on the basis of a two-part description of the mechanism. The first part is described in terms of pronation or supination, whereas the second part is described in terms of dorsiflexion, eversion, abduction, or adduction. This system was designed with the idea that surgery should follow a reversal of the injury mechanism in order to optimize reduction and outcomes. This system, however, has given way to the Weber system.

The Weber system classifies fractures into A, B, or C, with each category implying a certain mechanism and increasing possibility of distal tibiofibular syndesmotic involvement. The Weber A fracture is usually a result of a supination–adduction injury; the Weber B fracture is a result of supination, external rotation; and the Weber C fracture can occur with any of the pronation mechanisms. The key in evaluation of the fracture patterns with this system is in recognizing the site of avulsion injury. Avulsion fractures are a result of tensile, distracting forces on the bone; the presence of such fractures should alert the interpreter to assess other side of the ankle for associated impaction-type injuries. The Weber A injury is an avulsion fracture of the lateral malleolus, usually distal to the tibial plafond; forces are extending from lateral to medial. Although there can be involvement of the medial malleolus, there is no risk of syndesmotic injury. Weber B and C fractures are avulsion fractures of the medial malleolus that have a lateral component owing to the associated impaction injuries of the talus on the lateral malleolus; both result in a vertically oriented oblique fracture of the distal fibula. However, Weber B fractures occur at the level of the tibiotalar joint line, whereas Weber C fractures are above the joint. These types of fractures are associated with a risk of syndesmotic injury (Weber C greater than Weber B) because forces extend from medial to lateral.

The syndesmosis is an important structure to assess because it plays a significant role in ankle stability. Involvement usually requires internal fixation. Evaluation for integrity of the syndesmosis is performed by assessing the interosseous clear space between the distal tibia and fibula, 1 cm from the joint line. Widening of the interosseous clear space by >10 mm is abnormal and raises concern for such injury. However, the assessment must be made on a properly positioned radiograph because dorsiflexion, external rotation, and nonorthogonal views may falsely widen the distance.

In addition, an avulsion fracture may not always be present. In these cases, a ligament tear is an equivalent injury that needs to be ruled out. The most concerning of these types of injuries are the Weber B and C fractures that may be associated with a deltoid ligament tear. Deltoid ligament injury will be suggested by marked soft tissue swelling centered over the medial malleolus. The ankle mortise may also be widened. The medial clear space of the mortise should not exceed 4 mm. If it is ≥6 mm, or wider than the distance between the tibial plafond and talus, then there is likely injury to the ligament. Caution is advised to make sure properly positioned radiographs are used when assessing these measurements.

Treatment options depend on the ability of the fractured ankle to maintain tibiotalar congruence and stability until osseous union. Conservative treatment is usually in the form of a boot or cast with decreased weight bearing for ~6 weeks. Unstable injuries are either treated with open reduction and internal fixation, or occasionally with conservative management and close follow-up. Bimalleolar and trimalleolar fractures are treated the same. As alluded to above, syndesmotic involvement results in instability and is treated with a screw that traverses the distal tibiofibular joint. Outcomes are usually good, although posttraumatic arthritis has been estimated to occur ~14% of the time.[3] In addition, ankle fractures, particularly, fracture-dislocations, can result in intra-articular loose bodies that relocate into the joint space after reduction. It is important to identify any such abnormalities in view of their implications for therapy. The soft tissues should also be evaluated for pockets of gas, because these would suggest an open injury and require more acute surgical management.

Questions for Further Thought

1. Other than the malleoli, which other bony structures should be scrutinized for fracture when evaluating ankle radiographs?

2. What should the radiologist suggest as the next step in evaluation of an isolated medial malleolus avulsion fracture sustained during an ankle eversion injury?

Reporting Responsibilities
Ankle fractures are not emergencies; a timely report is required.

What the Treating Physician Needs to Know
- Fracture location and orientation.
- Distal tibiofibular syndesmosis involvement.
- Integrity of the ankle mortise.
- Intra-articular loose bodies.
- Signs suggestive of open injury.

Answers

1. The base of the fifth metatarsal, anterior process of the calcaneus, and the lateral talus should be evaluated. A base of fifth metatarsal fracture is a type of avulsion fracture

that results from an inversion injury. However, unlike the fractures described above, the anterior process of the calcaneus and the lateral process of the talus fractures result from abnormal flexion of the foot. The anterior process of the calcaneus can be fractured during forced adduction and plantar flexion, whereas a lateral talus fracture results from forced dorsiflexion and inversion.

2. A full-length radiograph of the lower leg should be suggested because of the concern for a high fibula (Maisonneuve) fracture. The impaction of the talus onto the fibula can result in a fracture anywhere along the fibula. This fracture would be missed on conventional ankle radiographs.

CLINICAL HISTORY *27-year-old male with a 1-week history of sore throat, fever, and neck pain.*

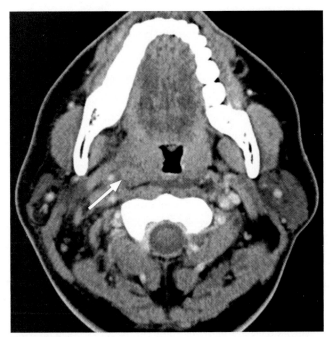

FIGURE 29A

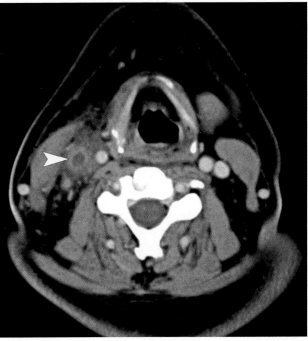

FIGURE 29B

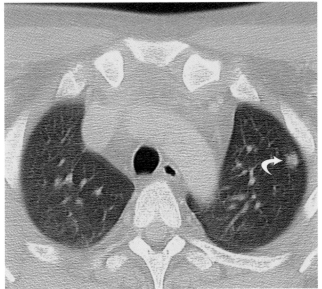

FIGURE 29C

FINDINGS Figure 29A: Contrast enhanced neck CT demonstrating Asymmetric enlargement of the right palatine tonsil (*arrow*) with adjacent parapharyngeal and carotid space fat stranding, and a small retropharyngeal effusion. Figure 29B: An oval, rim-enhancing, centrally hypodense lesion (*arrowhead*) with surrounding fat stranding is noted lateral to and displacing the right internal carotid artery. Note the absence of a normal contrast–filled internal jugular vein on this side.

Figure 29C: There is a left upper lobe peripheral nodule with hazy margins (*curved arrow*). Although not shown, there were several additional similar-appearing mostly subpleural lung nodules present bilaterally.

DIFFERENTIAL DIAGNOSIS None. Although jugular vein thrombosis can occur in many settings, the combination of imaging and clinical findings is compatible with septic thrombophlebitis.

DIAGNOSIS Lemierre's syndrome (postpharyngitis venous thrombosis) with septic thrombophlebitis of the internal jugular vein and septic emboli to the lungs.

DISCUSSION Septic thrombophlebitis of the neck usually occurs after an episode of pharyngitis, but may also occur from other head and neck infections such as otitis media/mastoiditis or odontogenic infection. The infection spreads directly to the draining veins and lymph nodes and then into the jugular veins, from where it can then gain access to the rest of the body via the bloodstream. The classic causal organism in cases of Lemierre's syndrome is *Fusobacterium necrophorum*—an anaerobic oral cavity bacillus—usually combined with other oral cavity anaerobes. In this case, the patient's blood cultures were positive for Fusobacterium.

Lemierre's syndrome was more common in the preantibiotic era, but is not uncommonly seen today. It usually occurs in previously healthy teenagers and young adults and is more common among males than females. Signs and symptoms include those of pharyngitis and systemic infection (tender swollen neck, sore throat, fever, myalgias). The classic picture is sepsis about a week after "resolved" pharyngitis.

The imaging triad of pharyngeal fullness, neck vein thrombosis, and peripheral pulmonary nodules is classic. The thrombosis may be in a small draining vein or involve the internal or external jugular vein. Air may be seen in the vein. The pharynx, teeth and middle ear/mastoid should be inspected as possible primary sources of infection. One may also see fat stranding, reactive adenopathy, and retropharyngeal effusion. The lungs are by far the most common site of distant spread of infection, where one will see septic emboli evidenced by peripheral nodules, some of which may cavitate or demonstrate a central feeding vessel sign. The next most common site of spread is to the joints, causing a septic arthritis. Other distant sites of spread are rare. If intracranial extension of infection is suspected, MRI is helpful, and magnetic resonance venography (MRV) can be considered to assess the cephalad extent of thrombus.

A correct diagnosis is important for the patient to receive appropriate treatment. Initiation of appropriate antibiotics to cover anaerobes along with anticoagulation for venous thrombosis is the treatment of choice. Development of septic arthritis may require arthrocentesis and surgery. The prognosis for Lemierre's syndrome is guarded, with a mortality rate of about 8%.

Question for Further Thought

1. How does treatment for typical pharyngitis differ from that for Lemierre's syndrome?

Reporting Responsibilities

This is an emergency and should be discussed with the ordering physician.

What the Treating Physician Needs to Know

- The presence of venous thrombosis.
- Is there a likely source of infection other than the pharynx?
- Are there any associated abscesses that may require drainage?
- Is there evidence of intracranial spread of infection that would require a brain MRI?
- Is there evidence of septic emboli to the lungs?

Answer

1. Pharyngitis is typically caused by group A beta-hemolytic streptococcus and is routinely treated with penicillin or amoxicillin, frequently on an empiric basis without a culture diagnosis. Lemierre's syndrome is treated with antibiotics directed toward anaerobes and anticoagulants. The differences in treatment highlight the importance of arriving at the correct diagnosis.

CLINICAL HISTORY *30-year-old male with shortness of breath after thoracentesis.*

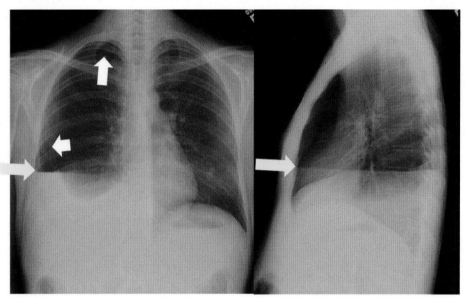

FIGURE 30A

FINDINGS Figure 30A: Upright posteroanterior (PA) chest film shows the visceral pleura (*white arrows*) of the right lung against a background of black air in the pleural space. An air–fluid level (*yellow arrows*) in the right pleural space is visible on both PA and lateral films. Note obscuration of right hemidiaphragm.

DIFFERENTIAL DIAGNOSIS Pneumothorax, pleural effusion, hydropneumothorax, lobar collapse, pneumonia.

DIAGNOSIS Hydropneumothorax (iatrogenic).

DISCUSSION Hydropneumothorax occurs when there is both air and fluid in the pleural space. Presenting symptoms include chest pain and shortness of breath, and physical exam reveals decreased breath sounds on the affected side and an audible succession splash. Diagnosis is made with chest X-ray, preferably upright or decubitus. Presence of pleural fluid alone will not result in an air–fluid level; air must also be present in the pleural space to observe an air–fluid level, which should be perfectly horizontal on an upright film. Simple fluid, blood, and pus all have the same density on plain film, so the character of the fluid must be surmised by history or other radiographic findings.

Trauma is the most common cause, and the fluid observed is often blood (hemopneumothorax). Spontaneous pneumothorax may be accompanied by a reactive pleural effusion or blood. Other causes include rupture of necrotic pneumonia, lung abscess, or cavitary lung lesion into the pleural space, and iatrogenic causes include thoracentesis complicated by

lung injury, or endoscopy complicated by perforation.[1] Complications include formation of a tension hydropneumothorax and pyopneumothorax. Management nearly always includes tube thoracostomy (chest tube).

Question for Further Thought

1. Is the air in the pleural space in pyopneumothorax the result of a gas-forming organism?

Reporting Responsibilities

Hydropneumothorax can be caused by a variety of conditions, many of which are life threatening and require immediate action. Immediate reporting is therefore necessary so that the treating physician can initiate drainage with a chest tube.

What the Treating Physician Needs to Know

- Laterality and presence or absence of mediastinal shift.
- Presence or absence of loculations.
- Presence or absence of associated findings suggestive of specific pathology (fractures, pneumonia, pneumomediastinum).

Answer

1. Pyopneumothorax is a condition similar to a hydropneumothorax, except that the fluid collection in the former is pus or frankly infected. In contrast to infections elsewhere in the body that present with gas in soft tissue, such infections in the pleural space are rarely caused by gas-forming

organisms such as *Clostridium perfringens* in the absence of penetrating injury.[5] Pyopneumothorax most often occurs as a complication of necrotic bacterial pneumonia or lung abscess,[2,3] with visceral pleural compromise and subsequent air leakage from the lung into the pleural space. Patients with pyopneumothorax often present with cough, fever, as well as dyspnea and chest pain. In endemic regions, *Mycobacterium tuberculosis* is a common cause of pyopneumothorax.[4] Treatment involves placement of a chest tube for continued drainage of the infected fluid collection as well as antibiotic treatment to address underlying infection.

CLINICAL HISTORY *16-year-old male with a history of acute onset of scrotal pain.*

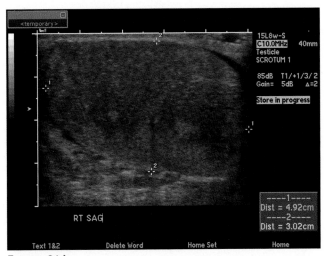

FIGURE 31A

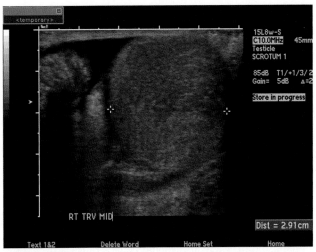

FIGURE 31B

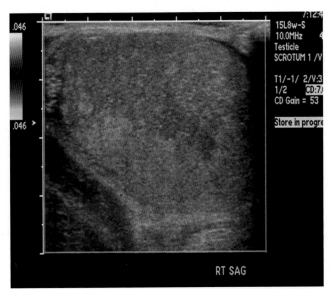

FIGURE 31C

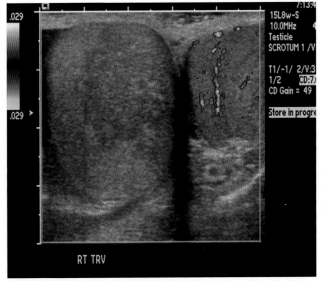

FIGURE 31D

FINDINGS Figures 31A and 31B: Longitudinal and transverse grayscale US images show heterogeneous echotexture of the abnormal right testicle (*between cursors*). Figure 31C: Color Doppler sonogram of the right testicle shows absence of blood flow. Figure 31D: Color Doppler image of the right and left testicles on the same image for comparison demonstrates absence of flow in the right testicle and flow in the left testicle. At surgery, bilateral bell-clapper deformities were identified. The right testicle was detorsed and viable. Bilateral orchiopexies were performed.

DIFFERENTIAL DIAGNOSIS Epididymo-orchitis, testicular torsion, torsion of the appendix testis, testicular abscess, testicular tumor, testicular trauma.

DIAGNOSIS Testicular torsion.

DISCUSSION Testicular torsion occurs when a testicle twists on the spermatic cord, resulting in compromised blood flow to the affected testis. The most common symptom is acute onset of testicular pain. There are two types of testicular torsion, extravaginal and intravaginal. Intravaginal torsion is overwhelmingly the most common form, typically occurring in adolescents and young adults. Bell-clapper deformity, or inadequate fixation of the testis to the tunica vaginalis, leaves the testis free to rotate and predisposes to intravaginal torsion. Extravaginal torsion most commonly occurs in neonates, and the torsion occurs at the level of the external inguinal ring, with both the testis and the tunica vaginalis twisting. Differentiating between these two entities is not needed because they are treated identically.

As the testis twists along the spermatic cord, there is initially obstruction of venous flow from the testicle with subsequent arterial compromise. The degree of ischemia depends on the number of twists in the spermatic cord and duration of the torsion. Most testes can be salvaged within 4 to 6 hours after the onset of acute scrotal pain. Most cases of testicular torsion are spontaneous; however, in 5% to 8% of cases, significant trauma has been reported.[1] Clinically, the onset of pain should be sudden with lack of pain relief on elevation of the scrotum. There also should be lack of fever or urethral discharge, which would indicate infectious etiologies. Additionally, intermittent testicular torsion can occur in which there may be periods of acute groin pain and emesis punctuated by subsequent pain relief resulting from spontaneous detorsion.

Ultrasound is the modality of choice in imaging testicular torsion. Ultrasound allows for the assessment of testis without subjecting the gonads to ionizing radiation. Both testicles should be imaged in order to compare with the normal testis, ideally on the same image. On grayscale imaging, an enlarged testis with homogeneous, hypoechoic echotexture is an early sign of testicular torsion. With later presentations, the echotexture of the testis will become progressively more heterogeneous. With color Doppler imaging, there will frequently be diminished blood flow, although in cases of intermittent torsion, the testis may actually be hyperemic. As with ovarian torsion, the absence of venous and/or arterial waveforms can be a useful adjunct to the grayscale images, but the presence of flow should not provide false reassurance. The whirlpool sign is seen with twisting of the spermatic cord at the external inguinal canal. Reactive hydrocele, reactive scrotal thickening, and reactive scrotal hyperemia can also be seen.

It is important to recognize epididymo-orchitis, which closely mimics torsion. Epididymo-orchitis usually presents with scrotal pain, swelling, redness, tenderness, fever, and/or discharge. Epididymo-orchitis usually demonstrates an enlarged testis and epididymis with heterogeneous echotexture; however, there is normally increased flow on color Doppler.

Torsion of the appendix testis is also a mimicker of testicular torsion. The clinical presentation of these two entities is virtually identical, although classically, torsion of the appendix testis will present with a "blue dot sign." Torsion of the appendix testis occurs when a small soft tissue excrescence arising from either the epididymal head or the testis twists on its pedicle. On ultrasound, this torsed excrescence will appear as an ovoid, hypovascular, heterogeneous structure near the superior aspect of the testis. There may be surrounding hyperemia, thickening of the scrotal skin, and a reactive hydrocele.

The treatment for testicular torsion is surgical detorsion. If surgery is performed within 6 hours of onset of symptoms, the testicle has a high likelihood of being salvaged. If the testicle is no longer viable, orchiectomy is usually performed. In confirmed testicular torsion, the contralateral testicle on the nonaffected side is at risk for torsion, and orchiopexy is performed during surgery as a preventative measure.

Questions for Further Thought

1. What are the salvage rates after the acute onset of pain and subsequent detorsion?
2. Does the presence of flow on color Doppler provide reassurance that the testis is not torsed?

Reporting Responsibilities

Testicular torsion is a surgical emergency, and the referring physician should be notified immediately. Early recognition and restoration of blood flow is important in salvaging the testicle. Surgical repair must occur within 6 hours of onset of symptoms in order to salvage the testicle.

What the Treating Physician Needs to Know

- Evidence of torsion in the setting of acute scrotal pain.
- Suggestion of necrosis or infarction based on the ultrasound, indicating decreased salvageability.

Answers

1. If the onset of pain to detorsion is less than 6 hours, then there is near 100% salvage rate. If the time is between 6 and 12 hours, then the salvage rate is about 50% and approximately 20% between 12 and 24 hours.[2]
2. Although the absence of flow is highly suspicious for torsion, the presence of flow on Doppler does not exclude the diagnosis of testicular torsion. In fact, in the setting of intermittent torsion, there may actually be increased flow.

CLINICAL HISTORY *28-year-old female with a history of motor vehicle collision (MVC) who presents with wrist pain.*

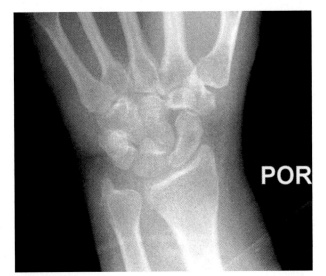

FIGURE 32A

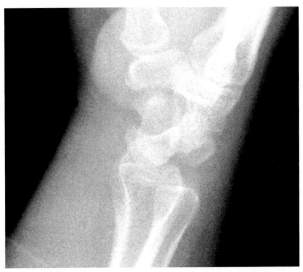

FIGURE 32B

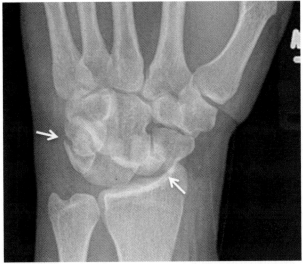

FIGURE 32C

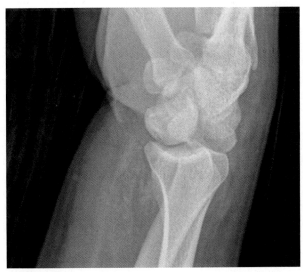

FIGURE 32D

FINDINGS Portable posteroanterior (PA) radiograph of the left wrist (Fig. 32A) shows a triangular lunate with abnormal overlap of the lunate and capitate ("piece of pie" sign). The middle carpal arc (distal concave curve of the scaphoid, lunate, and triquetrum) is disrupted. Subtle contour abnormality of the proximal carpal arc (proximal convex curve of the scaphoid, lunate, and triquetrum) at the scapholunate joint is also noted. The portable lateral radiograph of the wrist (Fig. 32B) shows, with the exception of the lunate, dislocation of the entire carpus dorsal to the radius; only the lunate maintains its normal relationship with the radius. PA (Fig. 32C) and lateral (Fig. 32D) radiographs of the wrist from a different patient show similar findings with additional scaphoid waist and triquetral fractures (*arrows*).

DIFFERENTIAL DIAGNOSIS Lunate dislocation, perilunate dislocation, lunate fracture-dislocation, perilunate fracture-dislocation.

DIAGNOSIS Dorsal perilunate dislocation (Figs. 32A and 32B), dorsal transscaphoid transtriquetral perilunate fracture-dislocation (Figs. 32C and 32D).

DISCUSSION Perilunate dislocations and perilunate fracture-dislocations are usually the result of high-energy trauma (i.e., falls, motor vehicle collisions, or sports-related injuries) with wrist hyperextension, ulnar deviation, and intercarpal supination (achieved with a fixed carpus and a pronating forearm).[1] Injuries may be purely ligamentous or a combination of ligament tears and fractures; the transscaphoid perilunate fracture-dislocation comprises up to 60% of these injuries. Prompt recognition and treatment are needed to minimize the long-term effects of a potentially severely debilitating injury. Unfortunately, 25% of injuries are unrecognized at presentation[2], some possibly because of spontaneous reduction.

Perilunate dislocations represent a spectrum of perilunate instability based on the degree of disruption of the ligamentous and bony structures supporting the lunate. Mayfield described four stages of perilunate instability, which begins with disruption of the supporting structures on the radial side of the lunate and progresses ulnarly about the lunate.[1]

- Stage I: Scapholunate dissociation; scapholunate widening, rotary subluxation of the scaphoid.
- Stage II: Stage I plus capitolunate dissociation; radiographically subtle, possible dorsal subluxation of the capitate.
- Stage III: Perilunate dislocation (Stage II plus lunotriquetral dissociation); dorsal dislocation of the carpus, lunate maintains relationship with distal radius.
- Stage IV: Lunate dislocation (Stage III plus radiolunate dissociation); volar dislocation and rotation of the lunate, remainder of carpus maintains near anatomic alignment with the carpus.

In perilunate fracture-dislocations, some of the ligament tears may be replaced with an equivalent carpal bone fracture: for example, the scaphoid may be fractured instead of the scapholunate ligament, and the triquetrum may be fractured instead of the lunotriquetral ligament.

Imaging diagnosis begins with analysis of the PA and lateral radiographs of the wrist. The lateral radiograph is the most specific view for making the diagnosis of a perilunate dislocation. Identification of dorsal dislocation of the capitate (along with the remainder of the carpus) at the capitolunate joint, which disrupts the normal collinear alignment of the radius, lunate, and capitate, is the key to diagnosis. The lunate remains in normal anatomic alignment with the distal radius. The PA radiograph can suggest a perilunate injury by revealing disruption of Gilula's first and second carpal arcs and a triangular tilted lunate ("piece of pie" sign) that overlaps with the capitate, both signs of a perilunate or lunate dislocation.[3] (Gilula's first carpal arc is the smooth proximal convex curve formed by the scaphoid, lunate, and triquetrum; the second carpal arc is the smooth distal concave curve of these same bones; and the third arc is the smooth proximal convex curve formed by the capitate and the hamate.[4]) Fractures associated with perilunate dislocations are generally displaced, but cross-sectional imaging (CT and/or MRI) can be used for problem solving subtle cases and surgical planning. Sonography can also be used to assess the status of the carpal tunnel.

The most important radiographic distinction is differentiating a perilunate dislocation from the more severe lunate dislocation. In a perilunate dislocation, the radiolunate joint is preserved with dorsal displacement of the carpus. In a lunate dislocation, the radiolunate joint is disrupted, and the lunate is displaced volarly relative to the radius and

remaining carpal bones; the remaining carpus maintains (or nearly maintains) its normal alignment with the radius. In other words, in a lunate dislocation, only the lunate appears malaligned. In a perilunate dislocation, all the carpal bones except the lunate are displaced.

Management involves immediate closed reduction to reduce pressure on the median nerve and articular cartilage. Median nerve injury occurs in 24% to 45% of cases of perilunate and lunate dislocations combined[5]; the rate for perilunate dislocation is likely on the lower end of the spectrum. Acute carpal tunnel syndrome may develop, necessitating an immediate open procedure. Closed reduction is followed by early internal fixation/stabilization. Even with optimal surgical management, loss of wrist flexion–extension, loss of grip strength, and early posttraumatic osteoarthrosis occurs.[5] Delayed intervention leads to worse outcomes.

Questions for Further Thought

1. Which ligaments are torn in a perilunate dislocation?
2. What are the lesser and greater carpal arcs?
3. What are the limitations of the Mayfield perilunate instability model?

Reporting Responsibilities

Perilunate dislocation is an emergent finding; direct communication with the referring clinician is required.

What the Treating Physician Needs to Know

- Direction of the perilunate dislocation and presence of any associated fractures.
- Additional fractures not associated with the perilunate dislocation or fracture-dislocation.
- Open versus closed injury.
- The risk of associated neurovascular injury requires urgent reduction.

Answers

1. In order to dissociate the carpus from the lunate, the scapholunate, radioscaphoid, radiocapitate, radial collateral, lunotriquetral, long radiolunate, and volar ulnotriquetral ligaments must be torn. The dorsal radiocarpal ligament remains intact.

2. The lesser arc describes a line following the radioscaphoid, scapholunate, capitolunate, lunotriquetral, and radioulnar joints; lesser arc injuries are purely ligamentous. The greater arc describes a line through the short axes of the scaphoid, capitate, hamate, and triquetrum; fracture of any one of these greater arc components serves as an equivalent injury to the associated ligament tears. A pure greater arc perilunate fracture-dislocation is incredibly rare.

3. The Mayfield model for perilunate instability is predicated on a path of ligament or bone failure beginning on the radial side of the wrist and progressing ulnarly around the lunate. Dislocations can also occur from forces beginning on the ulnar side of the wrist or even from direct trauma.

CLINICAL HISTORY *8-year-old female involved in a head-on motor vehicle collision. The patient was a restrained rear-seat passenger. She currently complains of pain in her midback.*

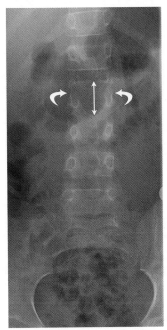

FIGURE 33A

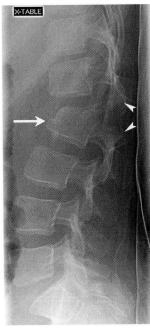

FIGURE 33B

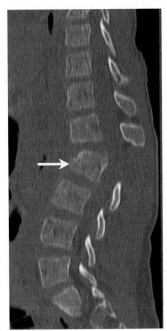

FIGURE 33C

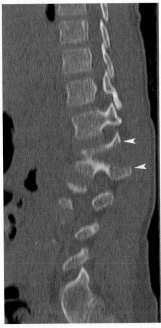

FIGURE 33D

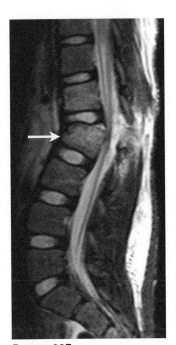

FIGURE 33E

FINDINGS Figure 33A: Anteroposterior (AP) radiograph of the lumbar spine demonstrates splitting of the bilateral L2 pedicles (*curved arrows*) as well as widening of the L1–L2 interspinous space. Figure 33B: Cross-table lateral lumbar spine radiograph demonstrates anterior wedging of the L2 vertebral body (*arrow*). There are markedly distracted, horizontally oriented fractures that extend through the pedicles and interarticular processes of L2 (*arrowheads*). There is also anterolisthesis of L1 on L2 with widening of the posterior disk space, causing focal kyphosis. Figures 33C and 33D: Sagittal reformatted CT images of the lumbar spine again demonstrate wedging of the L2 vertebral body (*arrow* in Fig. 33C) and widening of the interspinous space. The parasagittal CT image (Fig. 33D) demonstrates the distracted fracture line extending through and vertically splitting the left posterior vertebral arch (*arrowheads*). Figure 33E: Midsagittal STIR image of the lumbar spine demonstrates anterior compression of the L2 vertebral body (*arrow*). There is edema within the vertebral body as well as in the L1 vertebra above. More posteriorly, there is disruption of the posterior longitudinal ligament at its attachment to the posterior-superior aspect of L2 and of ligamentum flavum. There is extensive edema in the paraspinous soft tissues.

DIFFERENTIAL DIAGNOSIS The findings of this case are diagnostic of a *Chance fracture,* and no differential is necessary. Other thoracolumbar spine injuries include *compression fractures*, *burst fractures, translational and rotational injuries* such as unilateral and bilateral interfacetal dislocations and fracture dislocations, and *hyperextension injuries*. Although there is clear evidence of vertebral body compression in this case, typical injuries caused by pure axial loading (compression and burst fractures) should not cause distraction of the posterior vertebral arch. Similarly, although cases of interfacetal dislocations involve some distractive force to produce jumping of facets, these injuries would also not produce a distracted horizontal fracture plane through the pedicle and intra-articular process. Hyperextension injuries usually produce widening of the anterior disk space or a distracted fracture of the anterior vertebral body.

DIAGNOSIS L2 Chance (flexion–distraction) fracture.

DISCUSSION Chance-type fractures are unstable flexion–distraction injuries of the spine characterized by distraction of the posterior elements. They usually occur in the region of the thoracolumbar junction (most frequently, between the T12 and L2 levels) and account for between 5% and 15% of thoracolumbar spine fractures. Most Chance-type fractures occur in association with head-on motor vehicle collisions in which the victim is restrained, classically using a 2-point restraint. With sudden vehicular decelerations, the lap belt serves as a fulcrum that subjects the spine at the belt level to both flexion and tensile forces. The classic Chance fracture that was first described in 1948 is characterized by horizontally oriented fracture extending through and splitting the vertebral body and neural arch with minimal or no anterior compression. However, up to 48% of patients may demonstrate an associated burst-type fracture at the involved level (the so-called Chance-burst fracture). These Chance-burst fractures are more likely to be seen in patients wearing a 3-point restraint (lap and shoulder belt). Recognizing this variant of flexion–distraction injury is important because it may significantly impact management of the spinal injury. Application of an extension cast in a patient with a retropulsed bone fragment may produce further retropulsion and consequent injury to the spinal cord.

Variations of Chance-type injuries that involve splitting of both bone and soft tissue elements are common, and in some cases, the injury may involve only soft tissue without bone injury, with the plane of distraction running through the intervertebral disk and ligamentous structures (the so-called soft tissue Chance injury). Soft tissue Chance injuries are associated with anterior vertebral body subluxation as well as unilateral or bilateral interfacetal dislocation. These purely soft tissue injuries may be difficult to diagnose on plain radiography and even CT. Any widening of the facet joints or interspinous space in the setting of major trauma should trigger the performance of an MRI to assess for ligamentous injury.

In addition to the fact that these are unstable spinal injuries, Chance-type fractures are also important to recognize because of the high likelihood of associated abdominal injuries (up to 40%), with injuries to the bowel and mesentery being the most common. Therefore, if a flexion–distraction injury of the thoracolumbar spine is suspected, abdominal imaging with CT should be performed to evaluate the abdominal viscera. Associated abdominal injuries are more commonly seen in victims wearing only a 2-point restraint than in those wearing a 3-point restraint. Neurologic injury caused by Chance fractures is uncommon in adults, and complete paraplegia in adults has seldom been reported. However, the incidence of paraplegia in pediatric Chance fractures is quite a bit higher, at 15%.

Most Chance-type fractures are treated with posterior spinal fusion; however, purely osseous injuries with minimal deformity can be successfully treated nonoperatively with closed reduction in a hyperextension brace and immobilization in a cast. The Thoracolumbar Injury Classification and Severity Score (TLICS) is now frequently used to classify the severity of thoracolumbar spine fractures and to help guide management. This system evaluates three characteristics, with points being assigned for each based on the degree of severity. Specific characteristics evaluated include injury morphology/mechanism (1 to 4 points); neurologic status (0 to 3 points); and posterior ligamentous complex (PLC) integrity (0 to 2 points). Points are summed, and a TLICSS >4 typically indicates that surgical management is warranted, whereas a score <4 supports nonsurgical management.

Question for Further Thought

1. Why are burst fractures associated with flexion–distraction injuries more common among patients wearing 3-point restraints than those wearing 2-point restraints?

Reporting Responsibilities

Any findings suggestive of spinal instability should be promptly reported to the clinical team to ensure that appropriate spine precautions are being followed. For all thoracolumbar spine injuries, important features to report include the suspected mechanism of injury (compression, burst, translation/rotation, or distraction) as well as the status of the posterior ligamentous complex (intact, suspected/indeterminate, or disrupted). Significant distraction of the posterior elements on plain radiography or CT implies disruption of the posterior ligamentous complex. In equivocal cases, in which injury to the posterior ligamentous complex is still suspected, further investigation with MRI should be recommended to confirm or rule out ligamentous disruption as well as to evaluate the spinal cord. Furthermore, an abdominal CT should be recommended and closely scrutinized for evidence of visceral injury for patients with Chance-type fractures.

What the Treating Physician Needs to Know

- What is the presumed mechanism of thoracolumbar spine injury, and what is the status of the posterior ligamentous complex? Is the pattern of injury suggestive of a flexion–distraction injury (i.e., is there evidence of distraction of the posterior elements)?
- Is there evidence of associated abdominal visceral injury?
- Is there an associated burst fracture? If so, is there retropulsion of bone fragments into the spinal canal?
- Is there anterolisthesis or evidence of facet dislocation?
- Is there evidence of injury to or compression of the spinal cord or cauda equina on MRI?

Answer

1. The shoulder strap in a 3-point restraint functions to hold the chest back, thus limiting the degree of flexion occurring at the waist. It is hypothesized that in flexion–distraction–type injuries, the amount of compression experienced by the vertebral body is dependent upon the degree of flexion and the location of the axis of rotation when the compressive force is applied. With increasing flexion, the fulcrum about which compression is applied moves progressively anteriorly from within the vertebral body to within the abdomen. Therefore, compression without flexion would produce a burst fracture, compression with moderate flexion would produce a flexion–distraction injury with anterior compression, and compression with a large amount of flexion (as occurs with use of a 2-point restraint) would produce an entirely distractive injury. This may also explain why abdominal visceral injuries are more commonly associated with Chance fractures than with burst fractures.

CLINICAL HISTORY *69-year-old female with chest pain.*

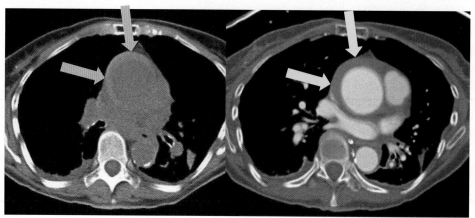

FIGURE 34A

FINDINGS Figure 34A: Axial noncontrast CT image shows near-circumferential high attenuation soft tissue (*blue arrows*) in the wall of a dilated ascending aorta; note that the blood in the lumen of the aorta is lower in attenuation than in the wall. Axial contrast-enhanced CT image at the same level shows contrast in the aortic lumen, and persistence of the abnormal soft tissue in the aortic wall (*yellow arrows*).

DIFFERENTIAL DIAGNOSIS Acute intramural hematoma, atheromatous plaque, penetrating ulcer, chronic thrombus.

DIAGNOSIS Acute aortic intramural hematoma.

DISCUSSION Noncontrast CT images are sensitive in the detection of acute intramural hematomas, because the attenuation of acute hemorrhage in the wall of the aorta is higher than that of intraluminal blood. The rim may be crescentic, or may involve the entire circumference of the aorta, and represents acute blood within the wall of the aorta. The appearance of acute intramural hematoma on contrast-enhanced CT images alone may be mistaken for atheromatous plaque or circumferential thrombus. Acute hematomas do not enhance or enhance minimally, differentiating them from enhancing periaortic soft tissue seen in infectious or inflammatory aortitis.[1]

Question for Further Thought

1. How are acute intramural hematomas treated?

Reporting Responsibilities

The findings need to be promptly reported to the referring clinician because untreated acute intramural hematoma in the ascending aorta can be rapidly fatal. The most important elements to report are (1) the involvement of the ascending aorta, (2) presence or absence of coronary artery ostial compromise, (3) presence of pericardial effusion, (4) extension into great vessels, arch, or descending thoracic aorta.

What the Treating Physician Needs to Know

- Location and extent of acute intramural hematoma (ascending vs. descending or both).
- Presence or absence of coronary artery ostial compromise.
- Presence or absence of pericardial effusion.
- Extension into great vessels, arch, or descending thoracic aorta.
- Size of aorta.

Answer

1. Acute aortic hematomas are treated in much the same way as aortic dissections. Those that involve the ascending aorta are typically surgical emergencies, because of the risk of coronary artery compromise and the risk of tamponade from rupture into pericardium.[1] Those that involve only the descending thoracic aorta may be medically managed.

CLINICAL HISTORY *36-year-old inmate with a psychiatric disorder ingested eight razor blades and a pen. On a different occasion, the patient ingested six batteries.*

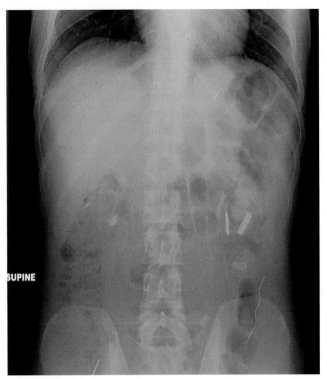

FIGURE 35A

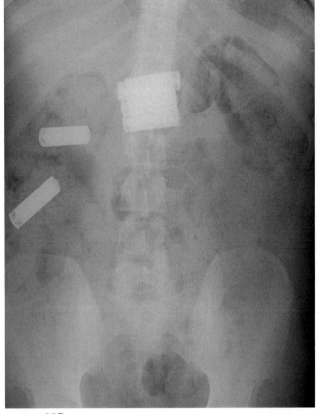

FIGURE 35B

FINDINGS Figure 35A: Radiograph of the abdomen demonstrates multiple foreign bodies that correlated with the given history, and identifies additional foreign bodies not revealed in the history. Straightened paper clips are identified in the lower quadrants. Objects made of plastic are not seen in the plain radiograph. Figure 35B: Radiograph of the abdomen of the same patient at a different time point demonstrates multiple ingested batteries in the stomach and duodenum. Four double AA batteries were removed from the stomach, with gastric ulcers and slight burns from the batteries identified at endoscopy.

DIFFERENTIAL DIAGNOSIS Ingested foreign body, ingested tablets, inserted foreign material, surgical material.

DIAGNOSIS Ingested foreign bodies.

DISCUSSION Orally ingested foreign bodies can occur accidentally or voluntarily. These are most commonly caused by accidentally ingested nondigestible components of food during meals in adults, such as fish bones, poultry bones, meat bolus, and toothpicks. Other commonly ingested foreign bodies are coins, batteries, and narcotic packets. Groups that are at increased risk for accidental ingestions of foreign

bodies include children, the elderly, mentally handicapped persons, those with psychiatric conditions, and those of certain professions that hold small objects in their mouths, such as a carpenter or seamstress. Voluntary foreign body ingestions are commonly seen in penitentiary inmates, psychiatric patients, and drug dealers. An accurate history from patients can be difficult, and imaging is often required to assess the presence and location of these foreign bodies.

Most of the swallowed objects have an uneventful passage through the gastrointestinal tract, but some of these may become lodged and cause local inflammation or bowel obstruction. Sites of obstruction are often where the bowel loops are narrower or tortuous, which include the pylorus, duodenal loop, and ileocecal junction. Bowel perforation is not common, but can be seen owing to sharp pointed objects, such as toothpicks, needles, and small bones. Sites of bowel perforation are most commonly located at the terminal ileum, sigmoid colon, and rectum. Other complications include severe hemorrhage, abscess formation, and peritonitis.

Preliminary studies often include plain radiographs, such as a lateral neck radiograph, frontal chest radiograph, and abdominal radiograph. If an unusual opacity is identified on a frontal radiograph, an orthogonal view is needed to localize the object within or external to the body. Secondary features on radiographs of thickened soft tissue, such as in the prevertebral space of the neck, or abnormal locations of air pockets indicating subcutaneous emphysema, pneumomediastinum, or pneumoperitoneum, may raise concern for foreign bodies. Computed tomography (CT) is used to further evaluate abnormal findings on radiographs, and to evaluate for bowel obstruction, perforation, and abscess formation.

Foreign bodies in the oral cavity and esophagus are typically removed endoscopically. Alkaline batteries may result in corrosion and heavy metal poisoning, and sharp objects can cause perforation. Wherever possible, hazardous objects should be removed endoscopically. Other objects are managed conservatively, if there is satisfactory migration on serial radiographs or CT. Nonmigration of the foreign bodies on serial radiographs may prompt endoscopic intervention. Once embedded in the bowel wall, these objects may proceed to cause ulceration, perforation, and abscess formation. In cases of bowel perforation, surgical intervention is necessary.

Question for Further Thought

1. What are the radiographic findings to look out for in a patient suspected of smuggling drugs?

Reporting Responsibilities

Ingested foreign bodies should be immediately reported to the referring clinician, including the number, locations, and the likelihood of batteries and sharp objects.

What the Treating Physician Needs to Know

- Description of the foreign bodies, including the number and location.
- Presence of batteries and sharp objects. Alkaline batteries may result in corrosion and heavy metal poisoning. Sharp objects can cause perforation.
- Presence of bowel obstruction or perforation with free air adjacent to the esophagus or free air in the abdomen and pelvis.

Answer

1. Drug mule is someone who smuggles drugs by ingesting drug-filled packets, usually condoms or balloons filled with cocaine or heroin. If there is a high clinical suspicion of a drug mule, careful surveillance of plain radiographs for multiple well-demarcated opacities with a surrounding crescent of air may help in diagnosis. This can be confirmed on CT. Rupture of these packages can lead to acute drug toxicity.

CLINICAL HISTORY *20-year-old female who was transported to the ED by EMS after a restrained motor vehicle collision. She is complaining of left leg and hip pain.*

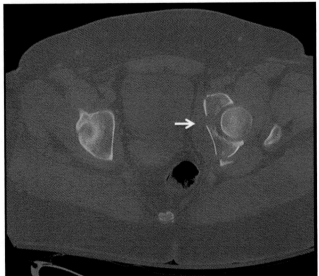
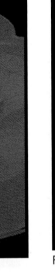

FIGURE 36A

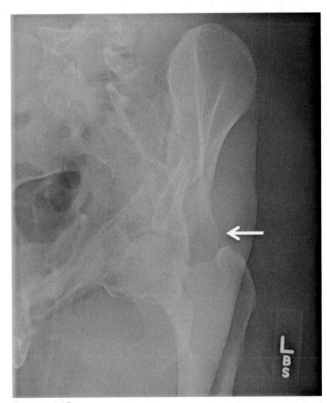

FIGURE 36B

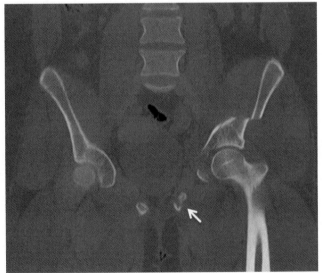

FIGURE 36C

FIGURE 36D

FINDINGS Axial CT image (Fig. 36A) depicts a comminuted fracture with a dominant coronal plane fracture line (*arrow*) dividing the acetabulum into anterior and posterior portions. Sagittal CT image (Fig. 36B) demonstrates a comminuted fracture involving the acetabular roof; there is posterolateral displacement of the ilium relative to the acetabulum and a nondisplaced posterior wall fracture fragment (*arrow*).

Coronal CT image (Fig. 36C) shows a minimally displaced inferior pubic ramus fracture (*arrow*) and the medially impacted comminuted left acetabular fracture. An obturator oblique radiograph (Fig. 36D) shows a comminuted left acetabular fracture with disruption of both the iliopectineal and ilioischial lines. The unsupported left ilium fragment comes to a point inferiorly and laterally, the "spur" sign (*arrow*).

DIFFERENTIAL DIAGNOSIS Anterior column acetabular fracture, posterior column acetabular fracture, T-type acetabular fracture, both column acetabular fracture.

DIAGNOSIS Both column acetabular fracture.

DISCUSSION Acetabular fractures are most often seen in patients in their third to fifth decades that have experienced high-energy trauma.[1] They can also occur in patients of advanced age owing to low-energy trauma, such as a fall; however, this is seen much less often and is caused by osteoporotic changes. Because of the many types of acetabular fracture patterns with disparate management implications, the ability to accurately describe an acetabular fracture is essential. Both column fractures are most often associated with high-energy trauma, regardless of patient age, and are always unstable. Both column fractures are the most common type of acetabular fracture, making up approximately 27% of all diagnosed acetabular fractures.[1]

Acetabular fractures are classified by the Judet–Letournel classification. In this classification, acetabular fractures are divided into two main categories: elementary fractures and associated patterns. Elementary fractures are solitary fractures including wall fractures (anterior and posterior), column fractures (anterior and posterior), and transverse fractures. The anterior column is composed of the superior pubic ramus (iliopubis), anterior acetabulum, and anterior ilium through to the anterior iliac crest. The posterior column is composed of the inferior pubic ramus (ischiopubis), the posterior acetabular wall, and posterior ilium through the posterior superior iliac spine. Associated pattern fractures incorporate at least two elementary forms; both column fractures are an associated pattern fracture because they combine the elementary anterior column and posterior column fractures.

Both column acetabular fractures run coronally through both the anterior and posterior columns separating them from each other and from the axial skeleton. Identifying disruption of specific pelvic landmarks is key to the diagnosis of acetabular fractures. Both column acetabular fractures involve disruption of all acetabular landmarks (iliopectineal and ilioischial lines, acetabular roof, anterior and posterior acetabular rims) as well as an associated ischiopubic/inferior pubic ramus fracture (obturator foramen disruption). Inward displacement of the posterior column and central dislocation of the femoral head are both common with this fracture type. Both column acetabular fractures are inherently unstable because there is a complete separation of the acetabular weight-bearing surface from the axial skeleton.

Both column acetabular fractures are commonly identified on anteroposterior (AP) and Judet (45° oblique views) radiographs initially, but advanced imaging such as CT is often then utilized for further fracture characterization and/or surgical planning. Radiographic and CT findings specific to both column fractures include a coronal plane fracture running through the acetabulum with inferior extension into the ischiopubis (inferior ramus). As with other isolated column fractures, the fracture line divides the acetabular roof into anterior and posterior components. There is disruption of all acetabular landmarks and complete dissociation of the anterior and posterior columns from each other and from the axial skeleton. The "spur" sign is pathognomonic of a both column fracture. The "spur" sign is best seen on the obturator oblique view, and represents an iliac bone fragment that remains attached to the sacroiliac joint, but is no longer attached to the fractured acetabulum (Fig. 36D).

Because of their unstable nature, both column fractures are almost universally treated with open reduction and internal fixation. Associated intrapelvic injuries are common and require rapid evaluation. They include injury to traversing neurovascular structures, the bladder/urethra, as well as the bowel/rectum.

Questions for Further Thought

1. What is a common measurement used to characterize the stability of an acetabular fracture, and how is this measurement assessed?
2. What are the most common long-term complications of acetabular fractures?

Reporting Responsibilities

Acetabular fractures themselves are not necessarily emergencies, but are markers of high-energy trauma that may be associated with severe neurovascular and intrapelvic organ damage; a timely report is required. Identification of active extravasation on CT is a potential emergency; direct communication with the referring clinician is required.

What the Treating Physician Needs to Know

- Anatomic location, classification, and characterization of acetabular fractures are extremely important in that the treatment varies considerably with the fracture type. Characterization involves amount of displacement/distraction, presence/absence of intra-articular loose bodies, and comments about comminution.
- Both column fractures are inherently unstable and require operative management.
- CT is generally needed for complete fracture characterization. Intrapelvic injury is common with both column fractures; this CT can also be helpful in ruling out potentially devastating vascular or viscus injury.

Answers

1. The roof arc measurement is often used to determine whether the remaining intact acetabular dome is sufficient for stability and weight bearing. The roof arc is measured as the angle between a vertical line drawn through the center of the femoral head and an intersecting line drawn through the fracture site. The medial roof arc is measured on the AP pelvis, the anterior arc is measured on the obturator oblique, and the posterior arc is measured on the iliac oblique. In order for the hip to be considered stable, the medial arc must be >45°, the anterior arc must be >25°, and the posterior arc must be >70°.

2. The common long-term complications of acetabular fractures are very important to consider because many of them can be seen on routine follow-up imaging. The most common complication seen after these fractures is posttraumatic osteoarthrosis. Anatomic reduction of an acetabular fracture is essential to minimize the possibility of this complication. The next most common complication is heterotopic ossification. Heterotopic ossification can lead to pain and decreased functional range of motion, especially if it progresses without intervention. Given the relatively tenuous blood supply to the femoral head, the patient may develop osteonecrosis of the femoral head, especially if there is associated femoral head dislocation for a prolonged period of time. Osteonecrosis may first be identified on follow-up imaging prior to the development of pain and functional limitations. Finally, as with any major orthopedic injury, one should always maintain a high index of suspicion for deep vein thrombosis and/or pulmonary embolism.

CLINICAL HISTORY *63-year-old female who presents to the emergency room with headache and nausea following a syncopal episode.*

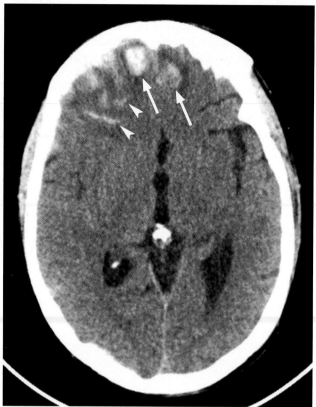

FIGURE 37A

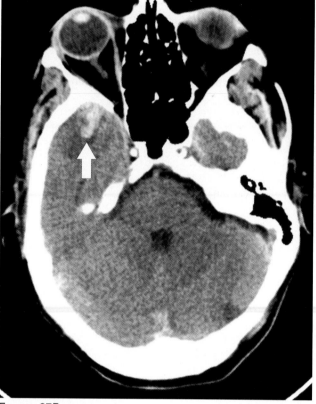

FIGURE 37B

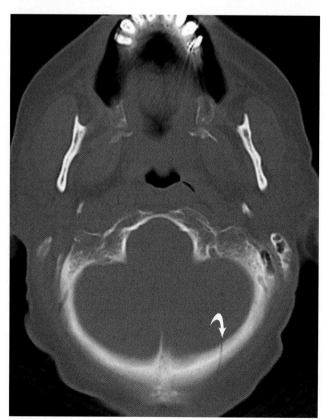

FIGURE 37C

FINDINGS Figures 37A and 37B: Axial noncontrast head CT images displayed in brain windows demonstrate hyperdense, hemorrhagic intra-axial lesions involving cortex and subcortical white matter with mild surrounding edema, situated immediately subjacent to the inner cortex of the calvarium in the most anterior portions of the bilateral frontal lobes (*arrows* in Fig. 37A) and right temporal lobe (*wide arrow* in Fig. 37B). There is also evidence of subarachnoid hemorrhage in the right frontal lobe sulci (*arrowhead* in Fig. 37A). Image through the posterior fossa displayed with a bone window (Fig. 37C) demonstrates a nondisplaced left occipital bone fracture (*curved arrow*).

DIFFERENTIAL DIAGNOSIS In the setting of trauma, the differential for hemorrhagic brain lesions would include *hemorrhagic contusions* and *hemorrhagic shear injury*. Hemorrhages from shear injury tend to be small and usually occur in the lobar white matter at the gray–white matter interfaces or in the corpus callosum. Other differential considerations for peripherally located parenchymal brain hemorrhages, when the history of trauma is unknown, include *amyloid angiopathy, hemorrhagic metastases, hypertensive hemorrhage, hemorrhagic venous infarction*, and *hemorrhagic transformation of an ischemic stroke*. Hemorrhages caused by amyloid may be multiple and are often of varying ages, whereas hemorrhagic metastases will usually demonstrate some contrast enhancement. Hypertensive hemorrhage, venous infarction, and hemorrhagic transformation of stroke generally do not present with simultaneous hemorrhages in remote locations.

DIAGNOSIS Hemorrhagic cortical contusions.

DISCUSSION Cortical contusions represent bruises of the brain's surface that are characterized histologically by necrosis and hemorrhage of the cortex and leptomeninges. They result from either a forceful impact or translational movement between the brain and the overlying skull or skull base, and therefore typically involve the superficial gray matter with relative sparing of the adjacent white matter. Cortical contusions are the most common parenchymal brain injuries, accounting for over 40% of traumatic brain lesions, and are identified in 5% to 10% of patients with moderate to severe head trauma.

The pattern of injury varies, depending upon whether the patient's head is stationary or moving at the moment of impact, and the terms "coup" and "contrecoup" are traditionally used to describe brain contusions. Coup injuries occur when a motionless head is struck by a moving object and are found at the site of cranial impact. Contrecoup injuries typically occur when the head is accelerating and impacts against an unyielding surface; these contusions are located on the side of the brain opposite the site of initial impact, with the anterior and inferior frontal lobes and temporal poles being particularly vulnerable to such injuries, as was the case here, in which the patient's occiput likely struck the ground during her syncopal episode (suggested by the occipital bone fracture). In addition to coup and contrecoup lesions, contusions also occur commonly along the inferior surfaces of the frontal and temporal lobes, presumably because of translational movement of the brain along the rough bony contours of the bones along the floors of the anterior and middle cranial fossae, respectively. Rarely, closed head injuries may result in so-called intermediary hemorrhages of the basal ganglia and thalami, which are presumed to be because of shearing of the perforating vessels supplying the deep gray matter structures. Frontal and temporal impacts at low accelerations are more likely to result in injury than are similar occipital impacts. Contusions that are not accompanied by brain stem injury or significant mass effect typically result in better outcomes than diffuse axonal injury (DAI) (although the two often coexist).

Roughly half of cortical contusions are hemorrhagic on CT and appear as ovoid hyperdensities centered at a gyral surface with a thin halo of surrounding edema. Nonhemorrhagic contusions can be difficult to see on early CT, but will generally become conspicuous on scans performed days later, when significant edema develops in the area. Large hemorrhagic contusions often increase in size within the first 48 hours, and initially nonhemorrhagic contusions can develop hemorrhage in a delayed fashion. As hemorrhage and edema resolve over the course of several weeks, contusions become less conspicuous on CT, but may leave a region of encephalomalacia.

Question for Further Thought

1. Why are contusions of the occipital lobes and cerebellum relatively uncommon?

Reporting Responsibilities

In any patient presenting with a history of head trauma, it is important to look for and describe the presence, type, and location of intracranial hemorrhage. Parenchymal hemorrhages may be the result of contusion or shearing injury, and it is important to try to distinguish between the two, because the latter is more likely to be accompanied by DAI and to portend a worse prognosis. In addition, it is critical to identify and alert the team to findings suggesting significant brain edema or mass effect, because these may necessitate urgent neurosurgical intervention. In instances in which the patient's clinical status appears worse than the CT would suggest, recommending further evaluation with MRI may be warranted because it is more sensitive to the findings of DAI.

What the Treating Physician Needs to Know

- Is the parenchymal hemorrhage more likely to represent contusion, hemorrhagic shearing injury, or both?
- Are there associated traumatic findings, such as skull fractures, subdural or epidural hematomas, or subarachnoid hemorrhage?
- Is there evidence of significant edema or mass effect that may necessitate surgical intervention?

Answer

1. Contusions of the occipital lobes and cerebellum are uncommon because the inner aspect of the occipital bone is very smooth, unlike the bones making up the anterior and middle cranial fossae, which have a rougher contour.

CLINICAL HISTORY *41-year-old female with malaise and cough.*

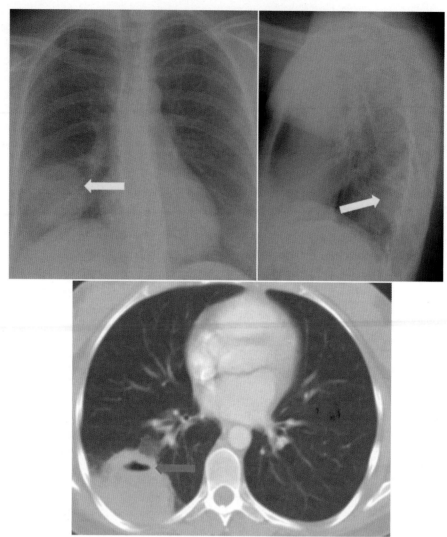

FIGURE 38A

FINDINGS Figure 38A: Posteroanterior (PA) plain film of the chest (*left*). There is a dense round opacity (*yellow arrow*) in the right lung base containing a small air–fluid level. Axial CT image of the chest (*right*). The spherical opacity is in the right lower lobe, and the air–fluid level (*blue arrow*) is again noted.

DIFFERENTIAL DIAGNOSIS Lung abscess, empyema, bronchogenic carcinoma, pulmonary metastasis, diaphragmatic hernia.

DIAGNOSIS Lung abscess.

DISCUSSION Lung abscesses are confined pockets of infection classified as either primary (from aspiration or pneumonia) or secondary (from another disease process such as

bronchogenic carcinoma or inhaled foreign body).[1,2] Radiographically, abscesses are round and cavitary with air–fluid levels present. The margins of the abscess are thick and well defined, differentiating it from an empyema. There is usually pulmonary consolidation surrounding the abscess, which resolves with treatment before the central cavity clears.

Question for Further Thought

1. What is the most common location for pulmonary abscess and why?

Reporting Responsibilities

The radiologist should characterize the abscess by size, location, presence of air–fluid levels, necrosis, and any signs of extension into the pleura (empyema). As always, a comparison with previous imaging studies is recommended.

What the Treating Physician Needs to Know

- Is this an empyema or abscess?
- Could this be a result of a neoplastic process (secondary abscess)?

Answer

1. Aspiration is the leading cause of pulmonary abscesses, which is why the superior portion of the right lower lobe is commonly affected.[3]

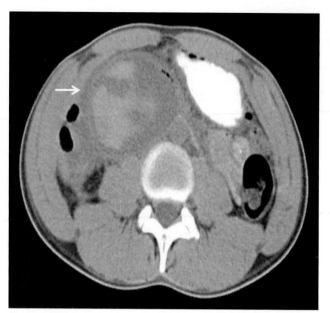

FIGURE 39A

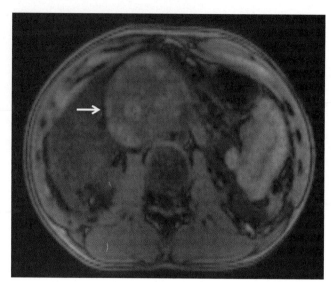

FIGURE 39B

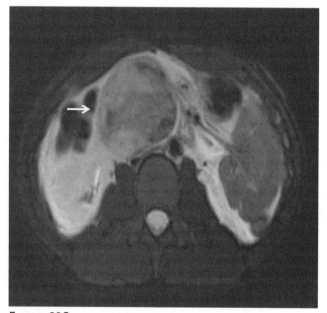

FIGURE 39C

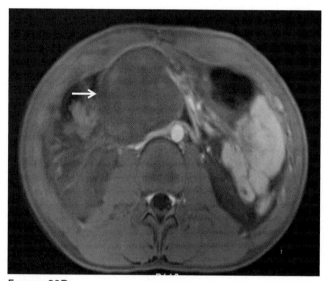

FIGURE 39D

FINDINGS Figure 39A: Axial noncontrast CT image of the upper abdomen demonstrates a large, heterogeneous intraluminal mass in the second and third portions of the duodenum, compatible with a hematoma (*arrow*). There are regions of internal hyperdensity, indicating acute hemorrhage. Figure 39B: Axial T1-weighted MRI image demonstrates a large, heterogeneous intraluminal mass in the second and third portions of the duodenum showing regions of T1 hyperintensity (*arrow*). Figure 39C: Axial T2-weighted MRI image demonstrates a large, heterogeneous duodenal mass with regions of T2 hyperintensity, indicating hematoma (*arrow*). Figure 39D: Axial

postcontrast T1 MRI image demonstrates no enhancement of the duodenal mass, indicating a hematoma (*arrow*).

DIFFERENTIAL DIAGNOSES Duodenal mass such as lymphoma or villous adenoma, duodenal hematoma, perforated duodenal ulcer, enteric duplication cyst.

DIAGNOSIS Duodenal hematoma.

DISCUSSION Duodenal hematoma usually results from trauma to the duodenum, such as blunt trauma or high-speed motor vehicle accidents. Iatrogenic injuries (from recent endoscopy), bleeding diathesis, and Henoch–Schonlein purpura (HSP) are also thought to be causes. The second or third portion of the duodenum is the most common area involved. Duodenal hematoma is the most common site of bowel injury in blunt abdominal trauma and is frequently associated with pancreatic injury in cases of blunt trauma. Duodenal hematomas are the fourth most common organ injury in children. They can be classically seen in children in the setting of bicycle handlebar, lap belt, or sports-related injuries as well as in child abuse. Common presenting signs and symptoms include abdominal pain/tenderness, nausea, and vomiting.

Duodenal injuries are graded on the basis of the American Association for the Surgery of Trauma grading scale:

- Grade 1—Hematoma or laceration involving single portion of duodenum.
- Grade 2—Hematoma or laceration involving one or more portions of duodenum; <50% disruption of circumference of duodenum.
- Grade 3—Laceration with 50% to 75% disruption of the circumference of the second portion of the duodenum; 50% to 100% disruption of the circumference of the first, third or fourth portion of the duodenum.
- Grade 4—Laceration with >75% disruption of the circumference of the second portion of the duodenum, or involvement of the ampulla or the distal common bile duct.
- Grade 5—Laceration or vascular injury with massive disruption of the duodenopancreatic complex or devascularization of the duodenum.

Computed tomography (CT) is the best imaging modality for duodenal injury. Imaging demonstrates the classic findings of high-density intramural hematoma and blood within the anterior pararenal space. Focal wall thickness greater than 4 mm is suspicious for duodenal hematoma in the setting of trauma. A large hematoma can also present with proximal distension of the stomach and proximal small bowel owing to obstruction. Intramural gas and pneumoperitoneum can be seen in duodenal perforation. A MRI or an upper gastrointestinal study is less commonly performed in the acute setting. An upper gastrointestinal study can demonstrate duodenal lumen narrowing and contrast extravasation into the peritoneum or retroperitoneum.

Clinical management is usually supportive therapy for isolated hematoma without perforation, which usually has a good prognosis. However, it is important to note that delayed perforation or stricture may occur. Surgery is usually performed if there is associated devascularization injury, duodenal perforation, or laceration injury to the pancreatic head, which has a higher mortality.

Question for Further Thought

1. What is the mechanism of injury for duodenal hematoma or laceration in the setting of blunt trauma?

Reporting Responsibilities

Duodenal hematoma should be emergently reported because it may lead to significant morbidity and mortality from hemorrhage, peritonitis, or sepsis. Additionally, other associated injuries may warrant emergent surgical repair.

What the Treating Physician Needs to Know

- Size and extent of the duodenal hematoma.
- Presence of partial or complete bowel obstruction.
- Signs of duodenal perforation or laceration injury to the pancreatic head.

Answer

1. Mechanism of injury for duodenal hematoma or laceration is thought to be blunt trauma causing compression of the duodenum against the vertebral bodies.

CLINICAL HISTORY *63-year-old female fell off the back of a pickup truck, landing on her left leg, now unable to bear weight.*

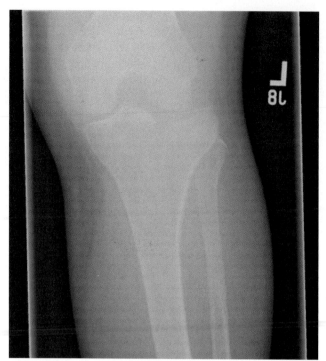

FIGURE 40A

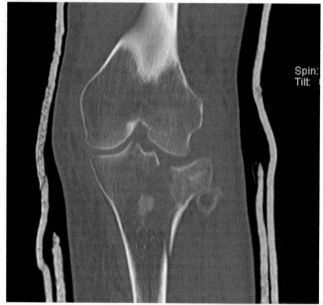

FIGURE 40B

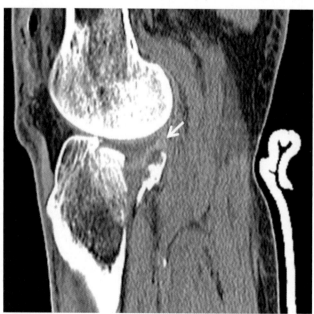

FIGURE 40C

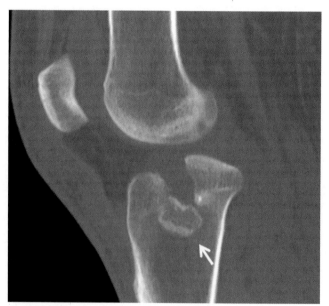

FIGURE 40D

FINDINGS Anteroposterior (AP) radiograph of the left knee (Fig. 40A) reveals a mildly comminuted lateral tibial plateau fracture with dominant sagittal plane split; a small amount of articular surface depression is likely present. Coronal CT image in bone window of the left knee (Fig. 40B) confirms the radiographic findings with additional involvement of the tibial spines also noted. Sagittal CT image in soft tissue window (Fig. 40C) demonstrates an avulsed lateral meniscus (*arrow*) displaced into a fracture cleft. A sagittal CT image through the knee of a different patient (Fig. 40D) demonstrates a nearly rectangular block of bone that has been depressed into the substance of the proximal tibia consistent with a "die-punch" fragment (*arrow*).

DIFFERENTIAL DIAGNOSIS Lateral tibial plateau fracture, lateral and medial tibial plateau fracture, medial tibial plateau fracture.

DIAGNOSIS Lateral tibial plateau fracture with extension to the tibial spines and avulsed lateral meniscus (Figs. 40A–C), lateral tibial plateau fracture with large associated die-punch fragment (Fig. 40D).

DISCUSSION Tibial plateau fractures account for between 1% and 2% of all fractures with the majority occurring in males ages 30 to 60.[1] They involve the articular portion of the proximal tibia and can result from a variety of forces including valgus stress, varus stress, axial loading, or a combination of forces. Injury to the tibial plateau can be sustained in a variety of settings including falls from a height, vehicle bumper-pedestrian collision, motor vehicle accidents, and sports-related injury. Tibial plateau fractures may be high-energy or low-energy. High-energy fractures tend to occur in younger patients with normal bone mineralization and result in splitting fractures. Low-energy fractures tend to occur in older patients with decreased bone mineralization and result in depression fractures. Although trauma to the tibial plateau can result in isolated osseous injury, the ligaments, menisci, and surrounding soft tissues are often involved.

The Schatzker classification is the most commonly used system for describing tibial plateau fractures.[2,3] The system is based on AP radiographs where sagittal and transverse plane fractures are best seen. The following list describes the classification along with data on relative frequency of associated soft tissue injury.

Type I—lateral plateau sagittal plane split fracture without depression (less than 4 mm); most associated with meniscal entrapment.

Type II—lateral plateau sagittal plane split with articular surface depression; high incidence of medial collateral ligament tears, low incidence of lateral collateral ligament tears; highest incidence of lateral meniscal tears.

Type III—lateral (A) or central (B) plateau articular surface depression without a split.

Type IV—medial plateau fracture; may be associated with knee dislocations with risk of neurovascular injury; highest relative incidence of medial meniscal and posterior cruciate ligament tears.

Type V—bicondylar (both medial and lateral plateau) fracture, usually sagittal plane splits.

Type VI—any plateau fracture with complete usually oblique transverse proximal (metadiaphyseal) tibia fracture; most severe form of plateau fracture; relatively high incidence of collateral ligament tears followed by cruciate ligament tears.

Types I through III are considered "low" energy, and Types IV through VI are considered "high" energy. An important variation of articular surface depression is the presence of a "die-punch" fragment, which are large tibial plateau ("die") articular surface fragments driven deep into the subchondral bone by the femoral condyle ("punch"). Wide variation in relative incidence of the various fracture types exists; for example, the incidence of Type II fractures varies from 25% to 60%, depending on the source. Type I fractures are the overall least common fracture type.

A high proportion of tibial plateau fractures have either a ligament or a meniscal injury. High-energy fractures are associated with overall greater incidence of soft tissue injury than low-energy fractures; among the high-energy patterns, Type IV has the highest overall incidence. Among low-energy fracture patterns, Type II has the highest overall incidence. Meniscal injury is very common, occurring from 40% to nearly 100%[4]; the majority of lateral meniscal tears are meniscocapsular separations. Cruciate ligament injuries are mostly caused by tibial footprint avulsions. Collateral ligament injuries are more likely in the high-energy fractures; lateral collateral ligament injury is least likely with Type II fractures. Associated neurovascular injury is uncommon, with injury to the peroneal nerve and popliteal artery occurring mostly in Type IV fractures.

AP and lateral radiographs are the initial imaging modality for evaluation of injury to the tibial plateau. Most tibial plateau fractures are readily identified on radiography; however, some may be radio-occult. A lipohemarthrosis on a lateral radiograph suggests an intra-articular fracture even if one is not otherwise seen. Although radiography provides a rapid assessment of the plateau, CT is far more accurate for determination of the fracture pattern as well as degree of articular surface depression and fracture gap. This information is essential for surgical planning. Evaluation of soft tissue structures, including ligaments and menisci, can also be performed with CT. If soft tissue kernel images are not separately generated, viewing the bone kernel images with soft tissue windows after smoothing improves the contrast resolution and decreases the noise needed for identification of soft tissue pathology. Menisci are bright/dense structures with an analogous triangular appearance to what is seen on MRI. Meniscal avulsion/meniscocapsular separation is more easily seen than intrasubstance tears; meniscal tissue between fracture fragments increases the risk of entrapment. Cruciate ligament avulsion fractures are common and can easily be seen on CT. Normal contours of ligaments exclude injury; abnormal contours suggest injury. MRI has the best contrast resolution for soft tissue assessment; most patients will undergo MRI either before fracture fixation or at a later time in a staged reconstruction procedure, although metal susceptibility artifact will degrade the soft tissue assessment after fracture fixation has occurred. In one study,

MRI was also shown to identify both radiographically and CT occult split fractures in a high proportion of patients classified as Type III, changing them to a Type II fracture.[4] CT angiography may be performed if there is suspected vascular injury.

Treatment of tibial plateau fractures aims to restore joint stability, correct alignment, and preserve full range of motion. Most tibial plateau fractures require surgical intervention; however, nondisplaced Type I to IV fractures with minimal depression may be amenable to conservative therapy. Nonoperative management includes skeletal traction, cast immobilization, and functional cast bracing. All Type V and VI fractures require surgical intervention. Internal fixation options for Type I to IV displaced fractures include lag screws alone or lag screws with plating. Depressed fractures and, in particular, "die-punch" fractures must be elevated, which requires the use of graft material. Type V and VI fractures are stabilized with lag screws and either one or two plates. External fixators may be used when extensive comminution prohibits internal fixation, but are contraindicated for Type VI fractures. Restoring the integrity of the menisci and ligaments is essential to stabilize the knee, but optimal timing for repair has not been established. Once fixation has been performed, rehabilitation involves early mobilization and early range of motion exercises.

Long-term complications associated with tibial plateau fractures include posttraumatic arthritis and knee instability. Infection is also a serious problem; the risk of infection increases with injury severity and use of open surgical approaches.[5]

Questions for Further Thought

1. Why are lateral tibial plateau fractures more common than medial tibial plateau fractures?
2. What are limitations of the Schatzker classification?

Reporting Responsibilities

Tibial plateau fractures are not emergencies; a timely report is required. One exception is the Type IV fracture, which may be associated with knee dislocations (and associated vascular injury); a phone call should be considered in this case.

What the Treating Physician Needs to Know

- CT is essential to properly characterize the fracture pattern.
- Displacement or depression of fracture fragments.
- Type IV injury is associated with knee dislocations.
- Evidence of meniscal or ligamentous injury.
- Evidence of vascular injury.

Answers

1. The preference for lateral tibial plateau fractures over medial tibial plateau fractures is multifactorial. The main reason likely centers on the valgus anatomic femorotibial angle in conjunction with the relatively more superior position of the lateral plateau articular surface (convex) versus the more inferior position of the medial plateau articular surface (concave). The medial tibial plateau also bears an asymmetrically increased load relative to the lateral plateau, which results in increased strength of the subchondral bone compared to the lateral tibial plateau, but the medial tibial plateau articular surface area is also larger than the lateral tibial plateau which serves to distribute the load over a wider area. A direct force applied to a convex surface (lateral plateau) is also more likely to result in compression with fragmentation than a concave surface (medial plateau).

2. The Schatzker classification system is based on injury patterns on AP radiographs and fails to evaluate injury patterns in the coronal plane. A coronal plane posteromedial fragment often occurs in higher-energy fractures; the presence of this fracture needs to be noted because fracture fixation may need to be altered to properly fix this fragment. The Schatzker classification system also does not include the severity of soft tissue injuries including the cruciate ligaments, menisci, and neurovascular structures.

CLINICAL HISTORY *20-year-old male with 6 days of worsening left-sided headaches, left eyelid swelling, and redness. The patient was seen previously at an outpatient urgent care and started on cefdinir and prednisone, but now reports worsening of his symptoms.*

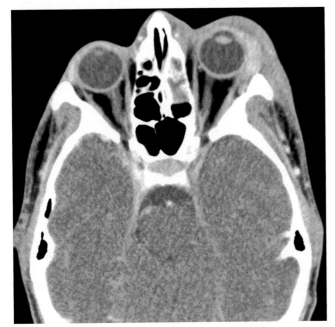

FIGURE 41A

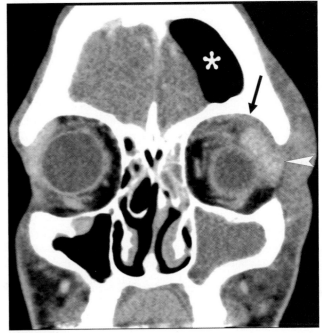

FIGURE 41B

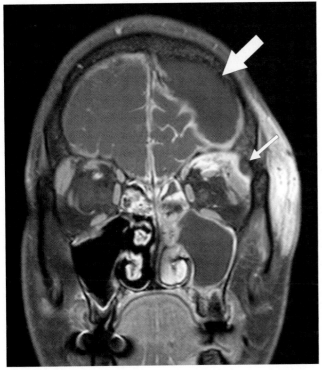

FIGURE 41C

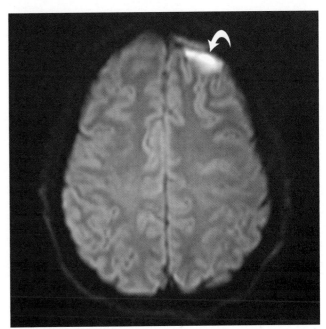

FIGURE 41D

FINDINGS Figure 41A: Axial contrast-enhanced CT at the level of the orbits. There is diffuse left-sided periorbital soft tissue stranding and edema as well as mild left proptosis. The lacrimal gland is prominently enlarged. The left anterior ethmoid air cells are opacified. Figure 41B: Coronal contrast-enhanced CT through the orbits. There is soft tissue stranding (*black arrow*) of the postseptal fat in the superior orbit that surrounds the superior rectus muscle and enlargement of the left lacrimal gland (*white arrowhead*). The left maxillary sinus and anterior ethmoid air cells are opacified, whereas there is only a minimal amount of mucosal disease in the right anterior ethmoid air cells and remaining paranasal sinuses. In addition, there is gas (*asterisk*) within the anterior cranial fossa. Figure 41C: Coronal gadolinium-enhanced fat-suppressed T1WI through the orbits, situated slightly posterior to Figure 41B. There is enhancing soft tissue in the extraconal fat in the superior orbit, displacing the superior rectus downward. There is a small fluid collection in the superolateral quadrant of the orbit abutting the frontal bone (*small white arrow*). There is an epidural fluid collection (*large white arrow*) in the anterior cranial fossa with enhancement of the adjacent dura. Note also abnormal thick leptomeningeal enhancement within the sulci of the frontal lobes. Figure 41D: Axial diffusion-weighted image through the brain demonstrates the epidural fluid collection (*curved arrow*) to have high signal intensity, suggesting restricted diffusion.

DIFFERENTIAL DIAGNOSIS The main differential to consider in this case is orbital cellulitis. Orbital cellulitis refers to an infection involving the soft tissues posterior to the orbital septum, whereas periorbital (or preseptal) cellulitis is limited to the soft tissues anterior to the orbital septum. In cases where there is both pre- and postseptal involvement, the infection should be referred to as an orbital cellulitis, given that more aggressive treatment is required when there is postseptal involvement. Orbital pseudotumor, sarcoidosis, lymphoma, or thyroid-associated orbitopathy are several other nontraumatic orbital pathologies that may involve the extraocular muscles and/or postseptal soft tissues. However, given the lack of medical history, prominent left pansinusitis, and obvious intracranial extension, these diagnoses would not apply in this case.

DIAGNOSIS Left orbital cellulitis complicated by left superior orbital subperiosteal abscess, epidural abscess, and meningitis.

DISCUSSION Orbital cellulitis is a postseptal orbital infection, with the vast majority of cases caused by underlying paranasal sinusitis. Less frequently, it may occur from direct spread of periorbital cellulitis, facial trauma resulting in direct inoculation of the postseptal soft tissues, or via hematogenous spread. The most common pathogens involved are streptococcal or staphylococcal species-hence the importance of gram-positive coverage in treatment - but these infections may be polymicrobial in children older than 9 years of age, the immunocompromised, or in cases of trauma.

Orbital cellulitis must be differentiated from a preseptal cellulitis. Clinically, there is some overlap of symptoms between the two processes, but the presence of proptosis and ophthalmoplegia should raise concern for postseptal involvement. Swelling and erythema of the eyelids are the most common symptoms with periorbital cellulitis, but are nonspecific because they may also be present in cases when both compartments are involved, as in this case. Chemosis is also a nonspecific finding that can be seen in both entities.

CT plays an important role in excluding orbital cellulitis in cases of obvious periorbital cellulitis. Careful inspection of the paranasal sinuses is mandatory on all orbital CTs because sinus disease should raise your suspicion of possible orbital cellulitis. The majority of cases of orbital cellulitis are unilateral, thus allowing for comparison of normal postseptal soft tissues. CT has the benefit of being extremely fast and may be the only imaging modality available in cases of retained periorbital metallic fragments (e.g. welders, prior trauma). CT may also demonstrate areas of bone dehiscence; however, intact bone does not exclude the possibility of intraorbital or intracranial involvement, because infection can spread through vascular channels in the bone.

If there is any concern for intracranial extension based either clinical suspicion or on CT imaging, a contrast-enhanced MRI should be performed for further evaluation. Orbital cellulitis can result in a multitude of possible intracranial complications including epidural abscess, subdural abscess, cerebral abscess, meningitis, cavernous sinus thrombosis, optic neuropathy that may progress to permanent vision loss, or superior ophthalmic or retinal vein occlusion. In the above case, the epidural abscess was identified on CT, but the full extent of intracranial involvement including meningitis could be appreciated only on MR. As was seen in this case, epidural abscesses appear as lentiform extraaxial fluid collections demonstrating enhancement on their dural side on T1W MR, and DWI may demonstrate restricted diffusivity of the purulent abscess fluid. Fortunately, this patient showed no evidence of cavernous sinus thrombosis, cerebral abscess, or optic nerve involvement. These complications may result in significant morbidity and even mortality if not treated aggressively and expeditiously. IV antibiotics are standard, and surgical drainage is usually required in cases of abscess. In cases of prominent underlying sinus disease, sinus surgery is often also warranted.

Question for Further Thought

1. Infections of which paranasal sinuses are most associated with developing orbital subperiosteal abscesses?

Reporting Responsibilities

Although it is important to report the findings of orbital cellulitis and visualized complications, it is equally critical to be clear on the limitations of CT if an intracranial complication is suspected on the basis of either the clinical or the CT findings. MRI is warranted for further evaluation in these cases.

What the Treating Physician Needs to Know

- Is there any evidence of orbital cellulitis?
- If orbital cellulitis is present, can the source of infection be identified? Is there obvious sinus disease or apparent traumatic injury?
- Is there an alternative differential diagnosis that needs to be taken into account if infection is not suspected clinically?

- Is there a drainable collection, which might require surgical evacuation?
- Are there any obvious complications associated with the orbital cellulitis?
- Is any further imaging recommended?

Answer

1. Ethmoid sinuses.

CLINICAL HISTORY *36-year-old male after a motor vehicle accident.*

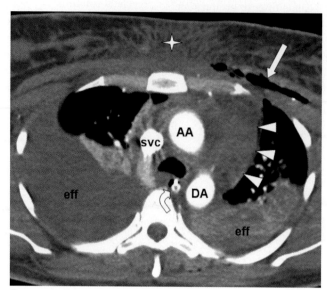

FIGURE 42A

FINDINGS Figure 42A: Axial contrast-enhanced CT image of the chest just below the aortic arch shows mediastinal hematoma (*arrowheads*). Ascending aorta (AA), descending aorta (DA), and superior vena cava (SVC) are intact. Large right pleural effusion is present, and higher density left effusion is likely hemothorax (*eff*). Note anterior chest wall contusion (*star*), subcutaneous air (*arrow*), and nasogastric tube (*curved arrow*).

DIFFERENTIAL DIAGNOSIS Mediastinal hematoma, thymoma, lipoma.

DIAGNOSIS Mediastinal hematoma.

DISCUSSION The source of mediastinal hematoma is usually from laceration of small veins within the mediastinum[1,2] caused by a blunt chest injury or high-speed deceleration injury. The hematoma is an indirect indicator of potential aortic injury, and does not alone constitute an aortic injury. The majority of patients with mediastinal hematoma do not have acute traumatic aortic injury, but the majority of patients with aortic injury have a mediastinal hematoma.[3,4]

Question for Further Thought

1. What large veins may be injured in blunt chest injury or high-speed deceleration injury?

Reporting Responsibility

In addition to the size and location of the mediastinal hematoma, reporting the presence or absence of acute traumatic aortic injury is paramount.

What the Treating Physician Needs to Know

- The treating clinician needs to know whether a mediastinal hematoma is present, and whether or not it is associated with an acute traumatic aortic injury, because acute traumatic aortic injury is treated surgically, whereas mediastinal hematoma alone may be managed conservatively.

Answer

1. SVC and azygous injuries are more rare, but can also cause mediastinal hematoma.

CLINICAL HISTORY *11-year-old female with history of acute onset of left pelvic pain.*

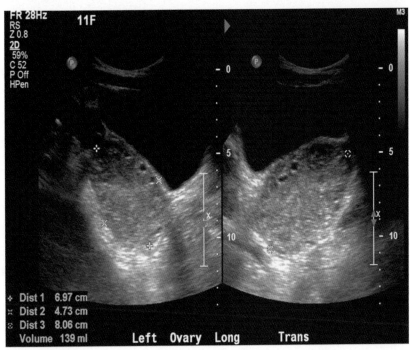

FIGURE 43A

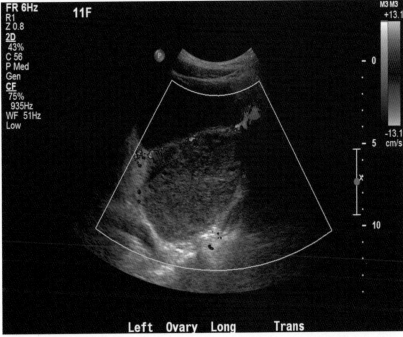

FIGURE 43B

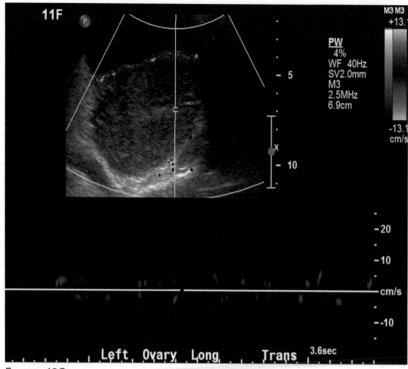

FIGURE 43C

FINDINGS Figure 43A: Longitudinal and transverse gray-scale US images show an enlarged left ovary (*between cursors*) with peripheral follicles. Figure 43B: Color Doppler sonogram of the left ovary shows absence of blood flow. Figure 43C: Spectral Doppler examination of the left ovary demonstrates no arterial or venous Doppler waveforms.

DIFFERENTIAL DIAGNOSIS Ovarian mass, hemorrhagic cyst, adnexal mass, pelvic inflammatory disease.

DIAGNOSIS Ovarian torsion.

DISCUSSION Ovarian torsion is caused by the rotation of the ovary and/or the fallopian tube about its vascular pedicle, compromising blood flow to the ovary. It has a bimodal distribution occurring mainly in young females (15 to 30 years of age) and in postmenopausal females. Signs and symptoms include acute onset of pelvic pain, nausea/vomiting, and leukocytosis. Unfortunately, these findings are nonspecific and can mimic a wide range of other pathologies including acute appendicitis, nephrolithiasis, pelvic inflammatory disease, tubo-ovarian abscess, ectopic pregnancy, endometriosis, and ruptured ovarian cyst. Factors that predispose to ovarian torsion include hypermobility of the vascular pedicle, ovarian or paraovarian masses, or an enlarged ovary such as in the setting of ovarian hyperstimulation syndrome. Interestingly, ovarian torsion does not commonly occur after pelvic inflammatory disease, endometriosis, or malignant neoplasms because of development of adhesions.

Pelvic ultrasound is the modality of choice for imaging ovarian torsion. The most sensitive imaging feature is an enlarged ovary compared with the contralateral, normal ovary with a volume frequently greater than 15 cc. The torsed ovary can demonstrate a variable grayscale appearance with a solid, heterogeneous, or cystic echotexture. Multiple peripherally located follicles are a secondary sign of ovarian torsion. Often, free fluid in the pelvis is present. The color Doppler examination may demonstrate decreased or absent blood flow, depending on the degree of vascular compromise. With spectral Doppler, a decrease or absence of the venous and/or arterial flow may also be seen. However, the presence of arterial flow or venous flow in the ovary does not exclude ovarian torsion. The whirlpool sign, indicating twisting of the vascular pedicle, is another secondary sign of ovarian torsion and appears as a swirling, round mass with concentric stripes or coiled vessels adjacent to the ovary. Ultrasound can also be used to assess for the presence of a lead point, such as an ovarian mass, that led to the torsion.

MRI can be used as an adjunct imaging modality in particularly challenging cases. However, MRI is not recommended as the initial imaging modality primarily because of the time it takes to acquire the images. As with ultrasound, the affected ovary will be enlarged, and the whirlpool sign of the twisted vascular pedicle is frequently seen. If contrast was given, the torsed ovary will be hypoenhancing relative to the normal ovary.

Management of ovarian torsion relies on emergent surgical exploration. As with testicular torsion, the more timely the diagnosis, the greater the likelihood that the ovary may be salvaged. In cases when the ovary is not salvageable, a salpingo-oophorectomy is frequently required. If the necrotic ovary is not removed, the ovary can become infected and lead to abscess formation. In the case of noninfarcted ovary, surgical untwisting is performed with or without oophoropexy.

Questions for Further Thought

1. Is hypermobility of the ovaries the most common cause of ovarian torsion, as is the case of testicular torsion?
2. Which ovary is more likely to undergo torsion?

Reporting Responsibilities

Ovarian torsion is a surgical emergency, and the referring physician should be notified immediately. Early recognition and restoration of blood flow is important in increasing the odds of salvaging the ovary.

What the Treating Physician Needs to Know

- Detection of an associated ovarian mass.
- The viability status of the contralateral ovary.

Answers

1. No, the most common cause of ovarian torsion is an ovarian mass as a lead point. Common adnexal masses causing ovarian torsion are dermoids or large ovarian cysts. The bell-clapper deformity, or inadequate fixation of the testis to the tunica vaginalis, results in increased mobility of the testis and thus increased risk of torsion.
2. There is a slight increased rate of torsion of the right ovary relative to the left. This is thought to be caused by the presence of the sigmoid colon helping to prevent torsion of the left ovary.

CLINICAL HISTORY *Foot pain after jumping off bunk bed.*

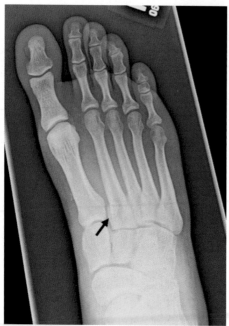

FIGURE 44A

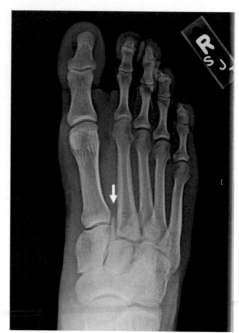

FIGURE 44B

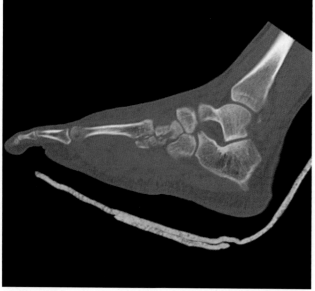

FIGURE 44C

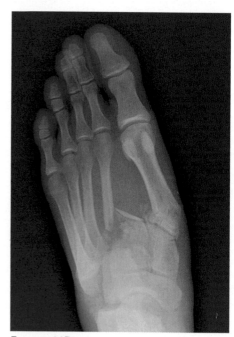

FIGURE 44D

FINDINGS Dorsal–plantar non–weight-bearing radiograph of the right foot (Fig. 44A) demonstrates a subtle incongruity along the medial aspect of the 2nd metatarsal base (*black arrow*). A weight-bearing dorsal–plantar radiograph was subsequently obtained (Fig. 44B), demonstrating an overt 2nd metatarsal base fracture (*white arrow*). Sagittal CT image through the second ray (Fig. 44C) demonstrates fractures of the 2nd metatarsal base and middle cuneiform as well as

inferior subluxation at the naviculocuneiform joint and dorsal subluxation at the tarsometatarsal (TMT) joint. Dorsal–plantar non–weight-bearing radiograph of the left foot in a different patient (Fig. 44D) demonstrates comminuted fractures of the 1st through 3rd metatarsal bases as well as all three cuneiforms. There is marked lateral displacement of the 2nd through 5th metatarsals and medial displacement of the distal 1st metatarsal fracture fragment. Lateral radiograph (not shown) revealed dorsal subluxation of the 2nd through 4th metatarsals and dorsal displacement of the 1st metatarsal distal fracture fragment.

DIFFERENTIAL DIAGNOSIS Homolateral Lisfranc fracture-dislocation, divergent Lisfranc fracture-dislocation, Lisfranc ligament avulsion, metatarsal fracture, tarsal bone fracture, Lisfranc ligament injury.

DIAGNOSIS First case: 2nd TMT joint fracture-dislocation. Second case: divergent Lisfranc fracture-dislocation.

DISCUSSION Lisfranc fracture-dislocations represent a spectrum of injuries from sprains of the Lisfranc ligament to overt fracture-dislocation of a part or all of the TMT joints. The Lisfranc fracture-dislocation accounts for only 0.2% of all fractures.[1] Despite its relative rarity, knowledge of this type of injury is essential to make a timely diagnosis; delayed diagnosis is associated with poor outcomes. A missed diagnosis rate of 20% has been estimated in the emergency department setting.[2] Chronic pain, dysfunction from ligamentous instability, arthritis, and deformity are all potential sequelae of delayed or inappropriate treatment.

The most common mechanism of injury at the TMT joint usually involves an indirect injury such as axial load and/or forced pronation/supination on a plantar flexed foot. A direct crush mechanism may also occur, but is not as common as an indirect injury. Examples of the indirect mechanism include a child jumping from a height to land on a plantar flexed foot or axial load of a foot on the floorboard during a motor vehicle crash. When this injury occurs during athletic activity, overpronation or supination in the plantar flexed foot is the likely mechanism.

The TMT or Lisfranc joint (after the surgeon in Napoleon's army who gained fame for an expeditious amputation through this joint in the field) is the articulation of the midfoot with the forefoot. The TMT ligaments connect the cuneiforms and cuboid with their respective metatarsal bases, and are present at each TMT joint. Intermetatarsal ligaments connect the bases of adjacent metatarsals. Both the TMT and the intermetatarsal ligaments have strong plantar components and relatively weaker dorsal bundles. There is no intermetatarsal ligament connecting the base of the 1st metatarsal to the 2nd metatarsal base, however, so the Lisfranc ligament connecting the medial cuneiform to the 2nd metatarsal base plays an important role in stabilizing the 2nd TMT joint.

Several classifications for Lisfranc fracture-dislocation injuries exist, but there is no strong evidence that any classification system accurately determines treatment and prognosis. One of the more widely used classifications is the system developed by Hardcastle et al., which described three broad categories of injury[3]: A, B, and C. In type A injury (total or homolateral), the entire TMT articulation is disrupted with lateral displacement. In type B injury (partial), either the 1st metatarsal is displaced medially, or there is lateral displacement of some or all of the 2nd through 5th TMTs, but with intact 1st TMT. In type C injuries (divergent), the 1st metatarsal is displaced medially, and some (partial) or all (total) of the remaining TMT joints are displaced laterally. Although the vast majority of the Lisfranc fracture-dislocations involve some portion of the 2nd through 5th TMT joints, an isolated fracture-dislocation of the 1st metatarsal is possible (type B injury). Fractures of the cuneiform and navicular bones are more likely with a divergent injury. Regardless, displaced/unstable injuries require surgery. Only stable, nondisplaced injuries do well with nonoperative management.

Radiographs of the foot are the first step in the evaluation of a suspected Lisfranc injury. Standard dorsal–plantar, internal oblique, and lateral radiographs will be sufficient to diagnose severe injuries to the TMT joints. More subtle injuries are likely to be missed, radiographs have sensitivity only in the range of 25% to 33% for midfoot fractures[4]; a systematic approach is therefore essential when analyzing radiographs for a Lisfranc injury. There are three key anatomic relationships to be scrutinized on the dorsal–plantar view. First, the medial margin of the 2nd metatarsal base should be aligned with the medial margin of the middle cuneiform. Second, the lateral margin of the 1st metatarsal base should be aligned with the lateral margin of the medial cuneiform. Third, the medial margin of the 4th metatarsal base should be aligned with the medial margin of the cuboid. The space between the 1st and the 2nd metatarsals should also be analyzed because it may be increased; comparison with the normal contralateral side may be helpful. This finding, however, is not as reliable as the relationships of the metatarsal bases with their respective tarsal bones. The 3rd and 5th metatarsals are usually difficult to analyze directly because of bony overlap. The lateral view is useful in detecting dorsal displacement at the TMT joint owing to rupture of the relatively weaker dorsal TMT ligaments. The base of the fifth metatarsal should be the inferior-most structure in this region, if it is not, then a midfoot dislocation is present. A tiny fragment of bone present between the 1st and the 2nd metatarsal bases on the dorsalplantar view, sometimes referred to as the "fleck" sign, indicates an avulsion injury. Non–weight-bearing radiographs have been shown to miss up to 50% of Lisfranc injuries.[1] If only a subtle injury is present, spontaneous reduction can occur. In cases with high suspicion and equivocal findings, weight-bearing radiographs may reveal the injury. Weight-bearing views can be painful for the patient; some form of analgesia should be considered in this setting. A contralateral comparison may also be helpful. Because of the ability of CT to provide an unobstructed view of all the bones and joints of the TMT joints, CT is much better able to detect small fractures and more subtle subluxations.[4] CT should be considered in the setting of negative radiographs with an appropriate clinical history.

Missed or inappropriately managed Lisfranc injuries may lead to deformity, instability, and/or arthritis. Stable, nondisplaced injuries may be treated nonsurgically with a non-weight-bearing cast for 6 weeks with possible extension to 10 or 16 weeks with a weight-bearing orthotic device as indicated. Patients with unstable or displaced injuries are treated surgically with anatomic reduction and internal fixation. Internal fixation may be with K-wires, screws, or dorsal plate, each of which has advantages and disadvantages. The role of primary arthrodesis is controversial, but there is some evidence that it may be useful in complex cases with cartilage damage and/or complete ligamentous disruption.

Question for Further Thought

1. How does TMT joint anatomy and residual instability relate to future functional impairment and arthritis?

Reporting Responsibilities

A Lisfranc fracture-dislocation is not an emergency; a timely report is required.

What the Treating Physician Needs to Know

- Presence of and general category of Lisfranc fracture-dislocation (homolateral vs. divergent, partial vs. total).
- Location of all fractures and direction of displacement.
- Obtain weight-bearing views and/or CT for cases with equivocal radiographic findings.
- Accurate description of alignment after reduction and treatment to ensure anatomic alignment and prevent long-term sequelae.

Answer

1. Myerson et al.[5] have proposed a functional model of the TMT joint composed of three columns. The medial column consists of the navicular, medial cuneiform, and 1st metatarsal. The middle column consists of the middle and lateral cuneiforms along with the 2nd and 3rd metatarsals. The lateral column is composed of the cuboid and 4th and 5th metatarsals. The lateral column is able to tolerate the most amount of normal motion, followed by the medial and then middle columns. This may explain why residual instability in the three different columns after treatment leads to varying degrees of functional impairment and/or osteoarthrosis, with the lateral column able to tolerate the most amount of instability.

CLINICAL HISTORY *23-year-old male with sudden onset of left arm weakness, left facial droop, and dysarthria.*

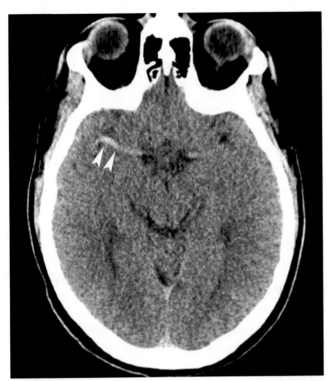

FIGURE 45A

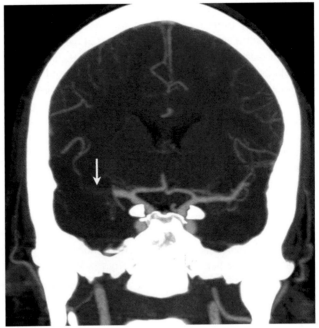

FIGURE 45B

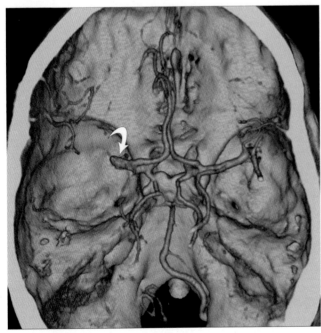

FIGURE 45C

FINDINGS Figure 45A: Axial noncontrast enhanced CT image reveals increased density (*arrowheads*) of the M1 segment of the right middle cerebral artery (MCA). No obvious parenchymal hypodensity or hemorrhage is present. Figure 45B: Coronal thick MIP image from a CT angiogram of the circle of Willis demonstrates an occlusive filling defect in the lateral half of the right M1 segment (*arrow*) extending into the proximal M2 branches. Figure 45C: 3D surface shaded reconstruction from the CTA again demonstrates occlusion of the right MCA. The *curved arrow* indicates the proximal stump of the right MCA.

DIFFERENTIAL DIAGNOSIS In this particular case, there is no real differential. The primary diagnostic consideration given the history and imaging findings is an acute stroke caused by thromboembolic occlusion of the right MCA. Entities that can produce hyperdensity of the MCA on unenhanced CT imaging include high hematocrit, usually from dehydration, high atherosclerotic burden, partial volume averaging, recent administration of intravenous contrast, and very rarely herpes simplex encephalitis. Recognizing these false positives can have great implications on patient management and outcome, especially in the recombinant-tissue plasminogen activator (t-PA) era. In this case, the CTA findings are diagnostic of MCA occlusion.

DIAGNOSIS Acute right MCA occlusion.

DISCUSSION The hyperdense MCA sign refers to the hyperattenuation of the MCA seen on non-enhanced CT scan images in an acute stroke setting caused by a thromboembolus (usually from a large vessel such as the common or internal carotid arteries) becoming lodged in the vessel. The sign is a marker of vascular occlusion rather than a marker of focal parenchymal infarct changes. Therefore, it is one of the earliest signs of an acute ischemic stroke on NECT imaging. There are few publications which have suggested an objective measurement for a true hyperdense arterial sign. Koo et al. suggest using an absolute density of greater than 43 HU and a MCA ratio (ratio of the density of the MCA to that of the contralateral MCA) of greater than 1.2 to define hyperdensity.

There is a companion sign to the hyperdense MCA sign, known as the MCA dot sign. This sign is depicted by a punctate focus of hyperattenuation usually located in Sylvian fissure. The MCA dot sign represents a thromboembolus within a more distal segment of MCA, usually the M2 or M3 segments. In these cases, a thrombus in one of these branches appears as a hyperdense dot rather than a linear focus of hyperattenuation because M2 and M3 segments do not course in the transverse imaging plane. A similar finding can be seen in the setting of basilar artery thrombosis, with a hyperdense dot being seen anterior to the pons.

Since the hyperdense MCA sign represents proximal occlusion of a major cerebral vessel, a larger territory is at risk for hypoperfusion in comparison to the more distal vessel occlusion represented by the MCA dot sign. Therefore, differentiating and reporting these two signs have important implications since the hyperdense MCA sign is associated with higher morbidity and mortality. In addition, more distal occlusions may be more difficult to treat using intra-arterial thrombectomy devices.

Questions for Further Thought

1. What is the major role of noncontrast enhanced CT scan in the setting of acute stroke?
2. What is the sensitivity and specificity of hyperdense artery sign on a noncontrast enhanced CT scan in an acute stroke setting?
3. What might possibly be the reason for the sensitivity and specificity of hyperdense arterial sign?

Reporting Responsibilities

In the acute stroke setting, the report of a non-enhanced CT scan should include any areas of acute hemorrhage, the location and extent of hypodensities, sulcal effacement with loss of gray–white matter differentiation, and the presence of hyperdense arterial vessels, which may suggest the location of occlusion. The presence of any of these findings in an acute stroke setting has significant implications on clinical management of the patient and need to be promptly communicated with the requesting physician. If an acute large vessel stroke is suspected and the possibility of endovascular therapy is being entertained, vascular imaging—typically with CTA—is warranted to determine the presence and location of an occlusion. Proximal lesions (M1 and M2) are generally amenable to attempts at mechanical thrombectomy. Significant areas of completed stroke (>1/3 the MCA territory) or the presence of hemorrhage are contraindications to both intravenous t-PA and intra-arterial thrombolysis or thrombectomy.

What the Treating Physician Needs to Know

- Is there acute hemorrhage?
- Are there areas of hypodensity, sulcal effacement, loss of gray–white matter differentiation? If there is evidence of parenchymal hypodensity, does it involve more than 1/3 of the MCA territory?
- Is there midline shift and/or brain herniation?
- Is there is a hyperdense vessel?

Answers

1. Approximately 87% of acute strokes result from an ischemic etiology. The most common cause of the ischemic etiology is thromboembolism of atherosclerotic plaques in a large vessel such as common carotid or internal carotid arteries. Noncontrast enhanced CT scan is done to rule out acute hemorrhage in the acute stroke setting so that the patient can be stratified as a potential t-PA candidate.
2. Noncontrast enhanced CT scan is not particularly sensitive in evaluating for acute infarction and is even less sensitive for findings such as the hyperdense MCA sign. The sensitivity and specificity of the hyperdense arterial sign are 30% and 90% to 100% respectively.
3. The reason for the low sensitivity of the hyperdense MCA sign is probably related to the ~5 mm slice thickness with which routine NECT are often reconstructed compared to the size of vessels in question, which are usually only about 2 to 3 mm in diameter. Despite the low sensitivities of this sign and other signs related to infarction, these findings when present are helpful for accurate and prompt management of patients with acute stroke symptoms.

CLINICAL HISTORY *62-year-old female with chest pain, who underwent CTA to assess for aortic dissection.*

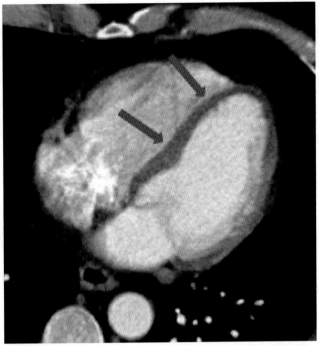

FIGURE 46A

FINDINGS Figure 46A: Axial contrast-enhanced arterial-phase computed tomography angiography (CTA) image of the heart shows decreased attenuation of interventricular septum (*arrows*) of the left ventricle, compared with the lateral wall, which shows normal enhancement.

DIFFERENTIAL DIAGNOSIS Myocardial ischemia, subendocardial infarct, artifact.

DIAGNOSIS Myocardial ischemia.

DISCUSSION Assessment of myocardial ischemia using CT is best assessed using a multiphase contrast-enhanced technique on a dual-source scanner with high temporal resolution, but areas of decreased perfusion and evidence of myocardial infarcts can be detected using routine contrast-enhanced CTA, although not reliably.[1] It is important to carefully review images of the heart to assess for myocardial perfusion abnormalities, evidence of old subendocardial or transmural infarcts, and coronary calcium. In this patient, the area of decreased attenuation was in the left anterior descending (LAD) coronary artery territory; confirmation with traditional coronary angiogram confirmed an LAD stenosis, which was treated with a stent. During the early contrast phase (arterial), myocardial segments with diminished perfusion have a reduced delivery of contrast material, resulting in a characteristic hypoattenuation.[1,2] Again, ischemia cannot reliably be detected on routine CTA, but when findings are present, the diagnosis should be suggested and discussed with the referring clinician.

Question for Further Thought

1. What are the next test(s) this patient should undergo?

Reporting Responsibilities

The referring clinician should be immediately notified so that he or she may administer appropriate medications or supportive care, and that the cardiac catheterization team may be activated if history, symptoms, and ECG findings are correlative.

What the Treating Physician Needs to Know

- Suggestion of myocardial ischemia.
- Coronary territory.
- Chronicity (if old studies are available for comparison).
- Presence of pulmonary edema.

Answer

1. If not already performed, cardiac markers, ECG, and echocardiogram.

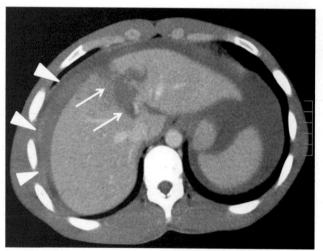

FIGURE 47A

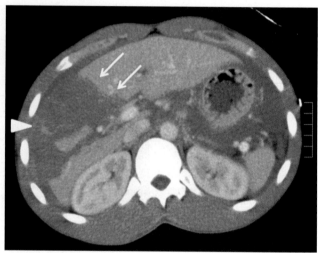

FIGURE 47B

FINDINGS Figure 47A: Axial contrast-enhanced CT of the liver at the level of the hepatic veins. Multiple linear and branching low-attenuation lacerations involving hepatic segments VIII and IVa extend to the vascular pedicle of the porta hepatis (*arrows*). Associated hemoperitoneum in the perihepatic region identified (*arrowheads*). Figure 47B: Contrast-enhanced CT at the level of the portal veins. Extension of the laceration into a large region of low attenuation involving most of hepatic segments V and VI (*arrows*). Amorphous high-density material within the large laceration/hematoma (arrowhead), representing active contrast extravasation..

DIFFERENTIAL DIAGNOSIS Hepatic laceration, fatty infiltration, cholangiocarcinoma.

DIAGNOSIS Grade V hepatic laceration.

DISCUSSION Liver lacerations can be seen in up to 25% of patients who receive a computed tomography (CT) exam at the time in blunt force injury. The liver is the most frequently injured organ in blunt force trauma.

Contrast-enhanced CT is the modality of choice to evaluate a trauma patient for hepatic lacerations. The injuries are usually identified on arterial and portal phase images. Hepatic lacerations appear as linear or branching areas of low attenuation and are graded according to the depth of hepatic parenchymal injury and damage to vascular structures. Lacerations that extend to the porta hepatis can be associated with bile duct leak and biloma. Ovoid or lobulated regions of low attention, which follow the contour of the hepatic capsule, represent subcapsular hematomas. Intraparenchymal hematomas are focal low-attenuation areas with poorly defined irregular margins within the liver. Acute contrast

extravasation appears as irregular linear or wispy high-attenuation material as opposed to a pseudoaneurysm that usually appears rounded. CT angiogram (CTA) images of the hepatic vessels should be carefully inspected to determine the presence of acute extravasation or pseudoaneurysm.

Liver injuries resulting from blunt force trauma are graded on the basis of the American Association for the Surgery of Trauma liver injury grading scale. To determine the final grade of the injury, the most severe characteristics of the injury are used.

Grade I: Subcapsular hematoma, <10% surface area
  Laceration: Capsular tear <1 cm parenchymal depth
Grade II: Subcapsular hematoma, 10% to 50% surface area or intraparenchymal hematoma <10 cm in diameter
  Laceration: 1 to 3 cm parenchymal depth, <10 cm length
Grade III: Subcapsular hematoma, >50% surface area or expanding or ruptured subcapsular or parenchymal hematoma with active bleeding
  Intraparenchymal hematoma >10 cm or expanding or ruptured
  Laceration: >3 cm parenchymal depth
Grade IV:
  Laceration: Parenchymal disruption involving 25% to 75% of a hepatic lobe or 1 to 3 Couinaud segments in a single lobe
Grade V: Laceration: parenchymal disruption involving >75% of hepatic lobe or >3 Couinaud segments within a single lobe
  Juxtahepatic venous injuries, that is, retrohepatic vena cava/central major hepatic veins
Grade VI: Hepatic avulsion

Management decisions for traumatic liver injuries depend on the hemodynamic stability of the patient, severity of the injury, presence of other injuries and medical comorbidities of the patient. Many of the less severe hepatic injuries and higher grade injuries in hemodynamically stable patients can usually be managed conservatively with supportive care. Treatment of grade III and higher injuries in hemodynamically unstable patients may require angiography and/or surgery.

Question for Further Thought

1. What treatment can interventional radiology offer in the setting of blunt force trauma to the liver?

Reporting Responsibilities

High-grade hepatic lacerations are severe injuries. The surgical team should be immediately notified of these findings.

What the Treating Physician Needs to Know

- The grade of the hepatic injury. Extension and size of the laceration and hematoma.
- Presence of vascular injury and pseudoaneurysm.
- Presence of acute contrast extravasation indicating active hemorrhage.

Answer

1. Interventional radiology can perform angiography in the setting of blunt force liver injuries when acute extravasation is seen on the initial CT. If the extravasation is present on the angiogram of the hepatic artery, embolization can be performed. Achieving hemostasis through embolization can stabilize the patient, possibly avoiding the need for surgical intervention. Also, posttraumatic complications of liver injury, including delayed hemorrhage, abscess, pseudoaneurysm, and biloma formation, can be successfully managed with interventional techniques.

CLINICAL HISTORY *Patient in high-force MVA trauma with neck pain, limited mobility, and upper extremity tingling and weakness.*

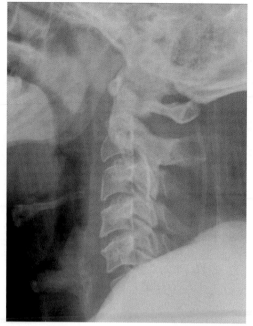

FIGURE 48A

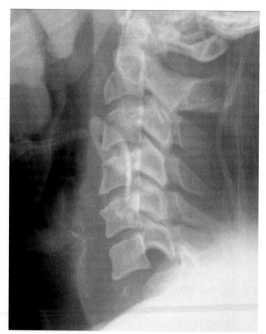

FIGURE 48B

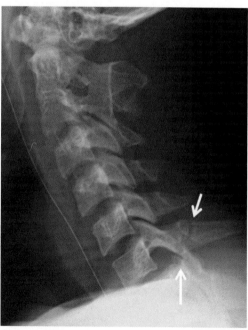

FIGURE 48C

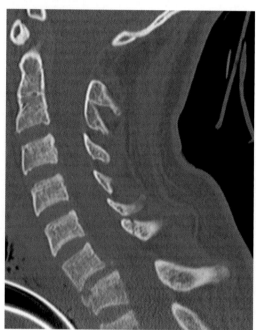

FIGURE 48D

FINDINGS Lateral radiograph of the cervical spine demonstrates incomplete visualization of the cervical spine, only to approximately the superior endplate of C6 (Fig. 48A). Lateral radiograph of the cervical spine with improved visualization to the superior endplate of C7 (Fig. 48B) demonstrates marked anterolisthesis of C6 on C7 as well as an anteriorly dislocated facet joint. Lateral radiographic view of the cervical spine in another patient with visualization only to the inferior endplate of C6 (Fig. 48C) reveals a perched facet at this level (*long arrow*) and C6 spinous process fracture (*short arrow*). Anterolisthesis of C6 on C7 as well as focal kyphosis is better appreciated on CT (Fig. 48D). Additional findings seen on CT are a C7 anterosuperior endplate fracture, narrowing of the C6/C7 disk space, and splaying of the C6 and C7 spinous processes.

DIFFERENTIAL DIAGNOSIS Hyperflexion translational injury, flexion–distraction injury, flexion–rotation injury, clay shoveler fracture, whiplash injury.

DIAGNOSIS Originally obscured cervicothoracic junction (CTJ) with cervical spine hyperflexion anterior translation with perched facet upon further imaging.

DISCUSSION Cervical spine injuries are reported in 5% to 10% of patients with blunt trauma. The majority of cervical spine injuries (75%) and fractures (65%) occur in the subaxial (C3 to C7) spine. Of subaxial spine injuries approximately 17% occur at the C7–T1 level.[1] Trauma patients are immobilized until the cervical spine is cleared of injury, and imaging plays a role in this process. Among the most severe consequences of missing a cervical spine injury on initial imaging is neurologic injury resulting from spinal cord or nerve root compression. Prolonged immobilization can also result in morbidity such as soft tissue ulcers, increased CSF pressure, pulmonary complications, and pain. Technically adequate imaging with clear visualization of the entire cervical spine and the CTJ is critical for these reasons. The most common reason that cervical spine injuries go unrecognized is that the region of injury is not adequately visualized, and decisions may be made on the basis of suboptimal visualization. This occurs most frequently at the upper and lower cervical spine, specifically the skull base to C2, and the CTJ at C7–T1. The most common type of injury missed at the CTJ is translation/subluxation or dislocation. Translational injury of the cervical spine occurs when one vertebral body displaces in the horizontal plane in relation to another, also known as listhesis. Any of these injuries may result in spinal canal narrowing and spinal cord impingement.

A cervical spine radiographic series often consists of an anteroposterior (AP), lateral, odontoid, and submental vertex views for initial evaluation. The CTJ level (C7/T1) is often difficult to visualize on trauma cervical spine radiographs, particularly on the lateral view, because of patient positioning and overlying osseous structures (particularly the shoulders). Severe, unstable injury may be missed at this level as a result, and careful inspection is needed to ensure proper visualization. If the CTJ is not clearly visualized, additional imaging should be acquired. In this case, a Swimmer's lateral view may be obtained that may provide improved visualization of the CTJ and the ability to exclude injury. However, Swimmer's views often remain nondiagnostic in this context due to underexposure and overlying bones (mainly the humerus and clavicle) that obscure the CTJ despite the attempt to move these structures out of the way.[2] Flexion/extension radiographic series have also proven inadequate, may potentially cause neurologic injury, and are not reliable at initial imaging for detecting ligamentous injury in part because of muscle spasm. Radiography has a low sensitivity compared with CT for cervical spine injuries (52% vs. 98%, respectively).[3] CT has also proven a faster evaluation than radiography and is complicated by fewer technical failures. In any patient who is not low risk for acute trauma involving the cervical spine, CT is recommended as first-line imaging, followed by MRI without contrast when there is concern for ligamentous, and/or spinal cord injury. If a CT is significantly compromised by motion, radiographs, specifically a single lateral radiograph, may be obtained to exclude a displaced fracture or dislocation. Because this remains a suboptimal evaluation, the patient should undergo a CT when otherwise stabilized.

Question for Further Thought

1. How do imaging recommendations differ in pediatric patients?

Reporting Responsibilities
If the CTJ is incompletely visualized, it is the radiologist's responsibility to report clearly that the study is technically inadequate and that additional imaging should be obtained; a phone call should be made to the referring clinician.

What the Treating Physician Needs to Know
- Whether initial imaging is technically inadequate and additional imaging is required.

Answer

1. Children under the age of 14 do not experience the same type of traumatic cervical spine injuries that adults do. They are more prone to injuries of the occiput, C1, or C2, which may lend itself to evaluation by radiography. Initial cervical spine evaluation in the child under 14 should consist of AP, lateral, and open mouth radiographs or cervical spine CT. If CT is necessary, radiation dose reductions should be made wherever possible. Children older than 14 have likely reached spinal maturity and should be treated as adults.

CLINICAL HISTORY *65-year-old female who became unresponsive after a fall at home. On arrival at the ED, the patient was noted to have nonreactive pupils with weak corneal reflexes and absent cough and gag reflexes.*

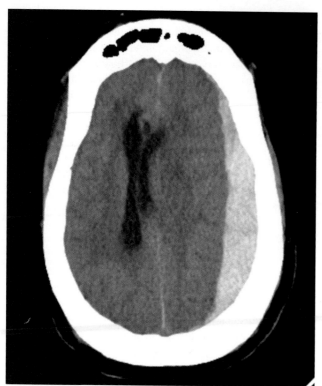

FIGURE 49A

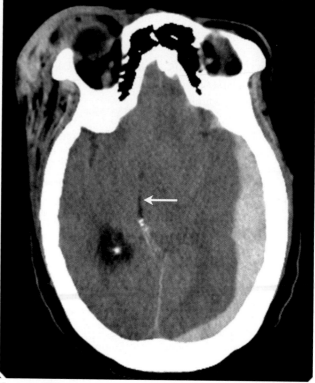

FIGURE 49B

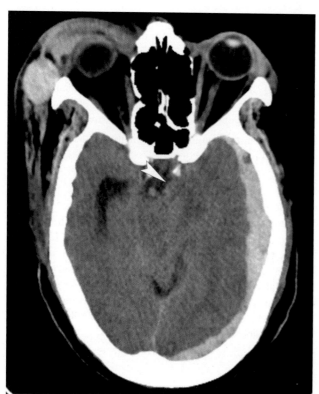

FIGURE 49C

FINDINGS Figures 49A to 49C: Axial noncontrast head CT images from superior to inferior demonstrate a hyperdense, crescentic extra-axial fluid collection extending along the left cerebral convexity. The collection crosses suture lines, but does not extend across the midline dural reflections. There is significant mass effect, evidenced by rightward shift of the lateral ventricles and third ventricle (*arrow* in Fig. 49B), indicating subfalcine herniation. In addition, in Figure 49C, the ambient and quadrigeminal cisterns are completely effaced, and the left uncus (*arrowhead*) appears to extend medially over the expected location of the left tentorial incisura, suggesting downward transtentorial herniation. Large right-sided periorbital hematomas are also evident on Figures 49B and 49C.

DIFFERENTIAL DIAGNOSIS The above findings are pathognomonic of an acute subdural hematoma (SDH) with associated subfalcine and uncal herniation. The differential diagnosis for a subdural collection is based mostly on the CT attenuation or MR intensity of the collection. Increased density of the collection relative to the adjacent brain parenchyma indicates hemorrhage. In the setting of trauma, an acute SDH needs to be distinguished from an *epidural hematoma*. The latter type of hemorrhage is typically biconvex in appearance, contained by the sutures, and often has an associated overlying calvarial fracture. Epidural hematomas can also cross dural reflections, whereas SDHs are limited by them.

When a subdural collection is hypodense relative to the adjacent brain, the differential includes *chronic SDH, subdural hygroma,* and *cerebral atrophy. Subdural hygromas* match the attenuation and signal intensity of the CSF in the ventricles. Although chronic SDHs may appear similar to CSF, they often demonstrate slightly higher density on CT and higher signal intensity on FLAIR compared with normal CSF. *Cerebral atrophy* is discerned from chronic SDH by noting the presence of cortical veins coursing through the extra-axial space and to the cortex. In infants, an entity known as *benign enlargement of the subarachnoid spaces* can also simulate chronic SDHs. Vessels are seen traversing the enlarged subarachnoid space in infants with former, and the findings typically resolve in 12 to 24 months without therapy. Acute on chronic SDHs in an infant should raise the possibility of nonaccidental trauma in children.

In the setting of signs of meningitis, a subdural fluid collection could represent a *subdural empyema.* These collections are typically hypodense compared with brain parenchyma and demonstrate peripheral enhancement on postcontrast imaging. On DWI, they show increased signal intensity centrally. Long-standing infections may lead to *subdural effusions* that lack the enhancement pattern and diffusion restriction associated with an empyema.

DIAGNOSIS Acute SDH with subfalcine and descending transtentorial herniation.

DISCUSSION *SDHs* usually develop as a result of trauma and occur between 10% and 20% of traumatic head injuries. They are believed to be caused by tears of the bridging veins as they cross the subdural space to drain into the dural sinuses. Blood accumulates between the inner layer of the dura and the arachnoid membrane, leading to a characteristic crescentic shape on imaging. Less common etiologies for subdural hemorrhage include blood that dissects from the subarachnoid space to the subdural space, as can be rarely seen in the setting of ruptured aneurysms or vascular malformations, although these primarily result in blood in the subarachnoid or intraparenchymal regions. Patients receiving anticoagulation or having intrinsic coagulopathies can also present with SDHs spontaneously or as a result of minor head trauma. In addition, subdural hemorrhages can be seen in the setting of vasculopathies including *Moyamoya* disease, and in patients with intracranial hypotension and aggressive shunting. In infants presenting with SDH, nonaccidental trauma should always be suspected.

SDHs occur across all ages; however, they are more common in the elderly secondary to cerebral atrophy and the higher likelihood that they may be on anticoagulation for various medical conditions. Most patients present after trauma, which may be relatively minor. The early clinical presentation is nonspecific, and many patients are asymptomatic. Classically, a lucid interval has been described in which patients are alert and oriented but then suddenly lose consciousness owing to the enlarging hematoma. Patients may also present with focal neurologic symptoms secondary to mass effect. Patients who are coagulopathic are at increased risk for extension of the hematoma and rebleeding with subsequent traumas.

The imaging findings in this case are typical for acute SDH. The collections may cross the sutures, but are contained by the dural reflections, giving the characteristic crescentic shape. The most common location is the supratentorial convexity. Attenuation and intensity may be affected by a superimposed arachnoid tear with CSF leaking into the subdural space, leading to a lower or mixed density collection. Inward displacement of the cortical veins can help distinguish chronic subdural from atrophic changes. Hyperacute blood may occasionally exhibit hypodensity (usually in the first 3–6 hours), but acute SDHs appear homogeneously hyperdense. In the absence of interval hemorrhage, the density of the collection should decrease by about 1.5 to 2 HU per day. Patients with blood dyscrasias and anemia may present with isodense SDHs. MRI may be obtained to determine the extent of the subdural findings and additional findings including infarction or associated traumatic brain injury. In the hyperacute setting, the hemorrhage demonstrates mild hyperintensity both on the T1WI and on the T2WI. MRI findings of acute SDH includes mildly hypointense signal on T1WI and hypointensity on T2WI.

Subfalcine herniation is the most common type of cerebral herniation and is easily recognized on cross-sectional imaging. The cingulate gyrus is displaced beneath the inferior free margin of the falx cerebri, resulting in midline shift. The degree of shift can be easily quantified by measuring the degree of displacement of the septum pellucidum. When midline shift is severe, obstruction of the foramina of Monro can occur, resulting in entrapment of the contralateral lateral ventricle. Transtentorial herniation occurs when brain tissue is displaced through the tentorial incisura, and can be subdivided into descending and ascending herniation. In descending transtentorial herniation, the uncus and/or parahippocampal gyrus are displaced inferomedially through the incisura. Transtentorial herniation is frequently preceded by subfalcine herniation. Early imaging findings of lateral descending transtentorial herniation include effacement of the ipsilateral suprasellar cistern, quadrigeminal plate, or ambient cisterns and widening of the ipsilateral cerebellopontine angle cistern (caused by displacement of the brain stem away from the herniating temporal lobe). As it is pushed away from its normal position by the herniated temporal lobe, the midbrain may become compressed against the opposite tentorial free edge, causing indentation along its lateral aspect opposite the side of the mass lesion, a finding referred to as the "Kernohan notch" sign. As herniation worsens, progressive obliteration of the basal cisterns will develop.

The treatment of a SDH is aimed at decreasing the mass effect and the intracranial pressure. Symptomatic SDHs require evacuation regardless of the size. Collections more than 1.0 cm in width or those causing more than 5 mm of midline shift are also potential indications for surgical management, depending upon the status of the patient. Smaller hematomas in asymptomatic patients can be observed and managed conservatively.

Question for Further Thought

1. What window settings on CT increase the sensitivity for subtle subdural hemorrhages?

Reporting Responsibilities

The official radiology report should include the location of the collection, the estimated age of the estimated blood products, and any associated mass effect. Evidence of mass effect warrants immediate communication with the clinical team. The possibility of nonaccidental trauma should be discussed with the referring physician in a child with SDH, especially if there is evidence of mixed age hemorrhage or there is no history of trauma.

What the Treating Physician Needs to Know

- Is there evidence of transtentorial herniation or midline shift?
- Is the mass effect explained by the hematoma?
- Is there evidence of other intracranial pathology such as parenchymal hemorrhage, subarachnoid hemorrhage, or infarction? Is there a skull fracture?
- What is the likely age of the subdural hemorrhage?
- In pediatric patients, are there additional findings to suggest the possibility of nonaccidental trauma? Is there evidence of hemorrhages of varying ages?

Answer

1. Use of relatively wide window settings increases the sensitivity for smaller subdural hemorrhages and isodense SDHs. Typical brain window settings use a window level of ~40 HU and a width of ~80 HU. Subdural window settings vary among institutions, but a window width of ~250 HU is typically used.

CLINICAL HISTORY *10-year-old female with chest pain and fever.*

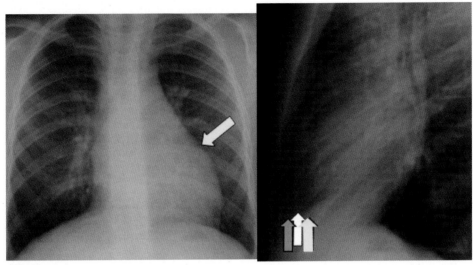

FIGURE 50A

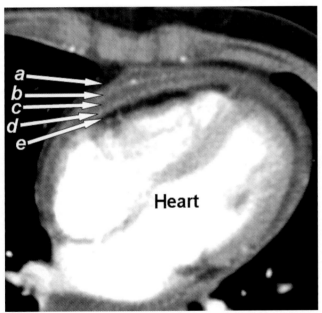

FIGURE 50B

FINDINGS Figure 50A: Posteroanterior (PA) chest film (*left*) shows some fullness of the left cardiac border (*yellow arrow*). Lateral chest film (*right*) shows subtle differences in density along the anterior heart border. Fluid in the pericardial space (*white arrow*) is more dense than pericardial fat (*orange arrow*) and more dense than epicardial fat (*yellow arrow*). These tissues together account for the layered appearance or "sandwich" sign of pericarditis and/or pericardial effusion. Figure 50B: Contrast-enhanced axial CT image of the heart. Pericardial fat (*a*) and epicardial fat (*e*) are on either side of thickened parietal (*b*) and visceral (*d*) pericardium with a small pericardial effusion (*c*). The pericardial layers are all the same density on plain film, composing the middle of the "sandwich."

DIFFERENTIAL DIAGNOSIS Pericarditis, pericardial effusion, cardiomyopathy, pneumopericardium.

DIAGNOSIS Pericarditis (viral).

DISCUSSION The "sandwich" sign seen on imaging is indicative of pericardial effusion (fluid between layers of epicardial and pericardial fat). There are numerous etiologies of pericardial effusions including viral infections, tuberculosis, uremia, myocardial infarction, cardiac surgery, Dressler's syndrome, and metastases. This case shows both pericardial thickening and a small pericardial effusion caused by Coxsackie virus infection. This thickening of the pericardium is consistent with inflammation as a result of infection. With larger pericardial effusions, it is possible to measure the attenuation in Hounsfield units (HU) to determine whether the fluid collection has attenuation close to water as with a simple effusion (HU < 10) or is proteinaceous or bloody (HU > 10, typically 20 to 30 HU) as with malignancy, hemopericardium, and so on.[1]

Question for Further Thought

1. What findings would provide clues to an effusion that is malignant in etiology?

Reporting Responsibilities

The interpreting radiologist should document acuity, size, attenuation, loculations, and presence of pericardial thickening or nodularity, as well as any other related findings (such as mediastinal lymphadenopathy). Depending on the clinical scenario and acuteness of the effusion, rapid intervention might be necessary, such as with cardiac tamponade.[2] Tamponade would demonstrate superior and inferior vena caval enlargement, hepatic and renal vein enlargement, and bowing of the interventricular septum.

What the Treating Physician Needs to Know

- Characterization of the pericardial fluid (simple or complex) based on attenuation.
- Severity/size of the effusion.

Answer

1. Irregular pericardial thickening, nodularity or masses, and pericardial enhancement along with mediastinal lymphadenopathy should provide suspicion for a malignant pericardial effusion.[3]

CLINICAL HISTORY *91-year-old female with pelvic pain after a fall.*

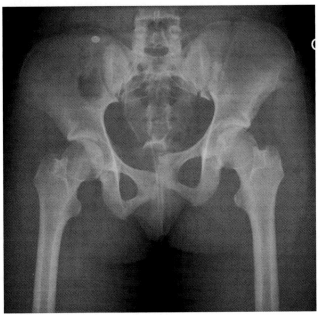

FIGURE 51A

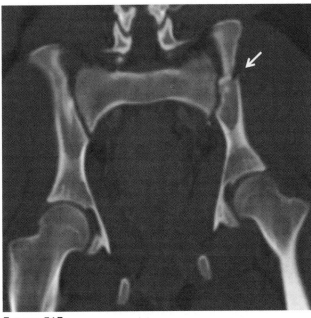

FIGURE 51B

FINDINGS Anteroposterior (AP) radiograph of the pelvis (Fig. 51A) demonstrates disruption of the pubic symphysis with marked superior displacement of the left pubis and mild widening of the left sacroiliac (SI) joint. A vertically oriented fracture through the left medial/posterior iliac wing adjacent to the SI joint is present; the lateral iliac wing fragment is superiorly displaced. Coronal CT image through the femoral heads (Fig. 51B) reveals a near sagittal plane fracture through the medial posterior ilium with superior displacement of the lateral iliac wing fragment (*arrow*). Involvement of the inferior left sacrum was also present, only indicated on this image by the small osseous fragment inferior and medial to the left SI joint. Note the relatively superior position of the left inferior pubic ramus compared with the right inferior pubic ramus.

DIFFERENTIAL DIAGNOSIS Vertical shear injury, AP compression fracture, isolated pubic ramus fracture.

DIAGNOSIS Vertical shear injury (Malgaigne fracture).

DISCUSSION Pelvic fractures can be classified by mechanism of injury on the basis of how they disrupt the anterior arch (pubic rami) and posterior arch (sacrum, SI joints, and posterior ileum) of the pelvis. The mechanism of injury may be a pure form, such as lateral compression, AP compression, or vertical shear, or have a combined mechanism. Vertical shear injury of the pelvis represents the most severe type of pelvic injury and may involve joint dislocations as well as fractures. A vertical shear injury occurs with disruption of both the anterior and the posterior arch, resulting in a disconnected hemipelvis. This is an unstable fracture, characterized by loss of both vertical and rotational stability of the pelvic ring; weight bearing on an unstable fracture will result in progressive displacement and may manifest as limb shortening on the affected side. Vertical shear injuries may be purely ligamentous, resulting in disruption of the pubic symphysis and one of the SI joints, or purely osseous, resulting in superior and inferior pubic ramus fractures along with either a posterior ilium or sacral ala fracture, or a combination of the two. When a fracture of the posterior ilium is involved, this form of injury has been referred to as a Malgaigne fracture. The mechanism of injury of a Malgaigne fracture is often high-energy axial loading, such as from falls or other high-energy trauma.

Initial clues to a vertical shear injury may be present on the standard supine AP radiograph of the pelvis obtained in the initial trauma evaluation. Fractures of the anterior ring are often immediately evident. Posterior ring fractures, although often evident on initial radiographs, can be more difficult to identify, and further imaging may be necessary. Inlet/outlet views of the pelvis could be obtained, by centering on the pelvis but with caudal and cranial angulation of the X-ray tube, respectively. Inlet views aid in evaluation for anterior/posterior displacement of pelvic structures as well as sacral arch or crush fractures. Outlet views aid in evaluation of hemipelvis elevation, SI joint widening, and for characterization of sacral fractures. Clues may also be present on initial imaging that can raise suspicion for a vertical shear injury. Vertical displacement at the inferior margin of the SI joint implies disruption of the posterior SI ligaments. Broadening of the ipsilateral iliac wing may be caused by external rotation of the hemipelvis. L5 transverse process fractures could indicate iliolumbar ligament injury. This ligament attaches the tip of the transverse process to the inner iliac crest, and its injury suggests high-energy forces acting on the pelvis.

The presence of a vertical shear injury is an indicator of high-energy trauma not just to the bony pelvis, but to the intrapelvic structures. Vascular injury is the most serious injury to be aware of; in patients with pelvic fractures and hemorrhagic shock, the mortality rate ranges from 36.4% to 54%.[1] Unstable patients may need to be sent immediately to angiography for transcatheter arterial embolization. If the patient undergoes CT imaging first, the presence of presacral hemorrhage should raise suspicion for a pelvic fracture, and the pelvis should be closely scrutinized if a fracture has not already been identified. In addition to detailed characterization of the pelvic fractures, CT will also provide information on the presence of active bleeders as well as signs of other intrapelvic organ injuries. There is a high incidence of trauma to adjacent structures, including the bladder and sacral plexus. There should be low threshold to suggest CT cystography at any sign of soft tissue injury near the bladder. Involvement of the sacral neural foramina should also be commented on, which may indicate a nerve injury.

Treatment initially involves external fixation with traction to stabilize mobilized pelvic fragments followed by more definitive treatment with internal fixation once the patient has stabilized.

Question for Further Thought

1. What is the relevant pelvic anatomy when approaching pelvic arterial hemorrhage?

Reporting Responsibilities

A pelvic ring vertical shear injury is an emergency; direct communication with the referring clinician is required.

What the Treating Physician Needs to Know

- Presence of a vertical shear pelvic ring injury.
- Specific components of the ring injury (joint disruptions and fractures).
- High association with life-threatening vascular injury as well as other injuries such as urinary tract and nerve injury.

Answer

1. Accurate reporting of the location of all pelvic hematomas and contrast extravasations, as well as the suspected corresponding arteries as seen on CT, will aid in future angiographic studies. Branches of the internal iliac artery have a close relationship with the pelvic ligaments and are at risk for injury in the setting of pelvic trauma. Most of these branches (as well as nerves) leave the pelvis through the greater sciatic foramen, bounded by the sacrum posteriorly, sacrospinous ligament inferiorly, ischium anteriorly, and ilium superiorly. The piriformis muscle also passes through the greater sciatic foramen and inserts onto the greater trochanter of the femur. The superior gluteal vessels course along the upper border of the piriformis muscles, and the inferior gluteal vessels course along the inferior border. The pudendal vessels leave the pelvis through the greater sciatic foramen more inferiorly. The obturator artery passes through the obturator foramen, the large rounded opening formed by the pubic rami. The somatic branches of the iliac artery (iliolumbar, lateral sacral) are usual the most proximal branches of the internal iliac artery and course anterior to the sacrum, SI joints, and iliacus muscles. The visceral branches (uterine/prostatic, vesicle, middle rectal) may be difficult to identify on portal venous phase contrast-enhanced CT, but course toward their respective organs low in the pelvis.

   The need for transcatheter arterial embolization is determined according to response to initial resuscitation, pelvic fracture pattern, volume and location of pelvic hematoma, and the visualization of contrast extravasation ("active bleeder"). The visualization of extravasations is highly predictive of the need for arterial embolization. In the unstable patient, urgent arteriography may be warranted; however, given the fast scanning time of modern multidetector helical CT, noninvasive imaging will often be obtained first.

CLINICAL HISTORY *5-year-old with refusal to bear weight.*

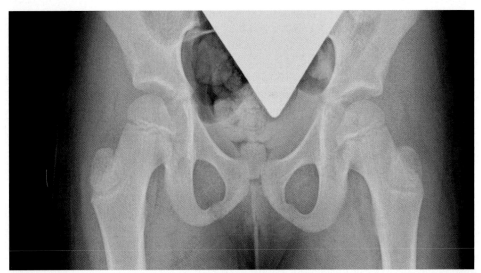

FIGURE 52A

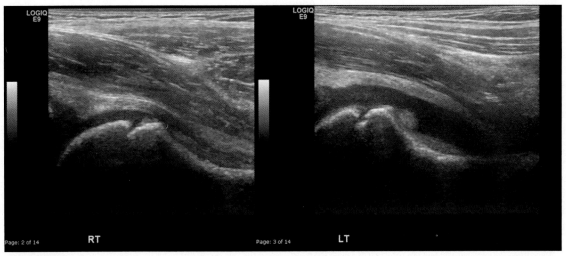

FIGURE 52B

FINDINGS Anteroposterior (AP) radiograph of the pelvis (Fig. 52A) is essentially normal. Sonographic images of the right and left hips obtained parallel to the long axis of the femoral neck (Fig. 52B) reveal a left hip effusion with mild thickening of the synovium; the right hip is normal.

DIFFERENTIAL DIAGNOSIS Transient (or toxic) synovitis, inflammatory arthropathy; osteomyelitis with reactive effusion; nondisplaced fracture with associated effusion.

DIAGNOSIS Septic arthritis.

DISCUSSION Children presenting with hip pain are a not-in-frequent sight in the emergency room. One of the most worrisome conditions to exclude is septic arthritis, a diagnosis requiring urgent treatment. In contradistinction, the diagnosis of transient synovitis is benign because it is a self-limiting phenomenon typically seen after a viral illness. Differentiating these two entities is challenging both clinically and on imaging. Laboratory data and history may be helpful in distinguishing these diagnoses with elevated inflammatory markers and WBC more suggestive of a septic process.

Septic arthritis most frequently occurs after a transient bacteremia, resulting in seeding of the synovium. Bacterial infections, frequently in the head and neck, may precede the development of septic arthritis. More rarely, septic arthritis may result from direct spread either from penetrating trauma or from osteomyelitis in the adjacent bone. In those instances, the history is typically more revealing, with a longer duration of more indolent symptoms in the setting of osteomyelitis, or a known trauma predisposing to the development of septic arthritis and/or osteomyelitis. The most frequent pathogen implicated in the development of osteomyelitis is *S. aureus*. Other causative organisms include *H. influenzae*, *N. meningitidis*, and *N. gonorrhoeae*. Through a yet undetermined pathway, these organisms cause the rapid destruction of articular cartilage. The cartilage may be greatly injured within 2 to 5 days of infection, explaining the urgency for diagnosis and therapy.

The workup for the affected child typically begins with a radiograph. Unfortunately, the radiographic manifestations may be subtle or nonexistent. For a radiograph of the hip, there are some nonspecific signs to suggest the presence of an effusion including asymmetric widening of the joint space and lateral displacement of the fat planes.

The next step in the workup is typically a hip ultrasound, using a high-frequency transducer. Images are obtained in the sagittal oblique plane, parallel to the femoral neck. The images are obtained at the junction of the capital femoral epiphysis and the proximal femoral metaphysis. A small amount of fluid noted in the concavity of the anterior femoral neck is normal. A common threshold for the diagnosis of an effusion is >5 mm of fluid measured from the anterior cortex of the femur to the joint capsule or greater than 2 mm of difference in fluid depth between the symptomatic hip and the contralateral hip. The effusion is normally anechoic, but may be of mixed echogenicity. Capsular thickening and hyperemia are secondary signs of an inflammatory process, but are somewhat subjective.

The presence and sonographic characteristics of the effusion are not helpful in distinguishing septic arthritis from transient synovitis. Analysis of the joint fluid is the best method for differentiating these two entities. Aspiration of the joint fluid is frequently performed in this setting via sonographic or fluoroscopic guidance owing to their relative ease and low risk of complication. If the joint fluid is suggestive of infection, the patient is typically taken to the operating room for a thorough lavage of the joint space.

MRI with contrast can be performed in equivocal cases, but, as with ultrasound, is not helpful in differentiating a septic from an aseptic effusion. Both forms of effusion may demonstrate marked synovial enhancement with varying degrees of synovial thickening. Enhancement of the femoral head may be diminished, presumably because of the pressure from the effusion diminishing blood flow.

The long-term sequelae of septic arthritis, particularly if left untreated, are many and include premature arthritis related to damage of the articular cartilage, osteonecrosis of the proximal femur, and increasing localized infection (osteomyelitis) or systemic infection (sepsis). Two of the most important factors implicated in long-term disability include delay in treatment and concomitant osteomyelitis.

Questions for Further Thought

1. What other joints are frequently affected by septic arthritis?
2. What potential hip pathologies may be missed if hip ultrasound alone is used to assess etiology of hip pain?

Reporting Responsibilities

A hip effusion, which may represent a septic joint, has the potential to be an emergency; direct communication with the referring physician is required.

What the Treating Physician Needs to Know

- Presence and/or signs of effusion.
- Secondary signs suggesting infection, although these are nonspecific.

Answers

1. The elbow, shoulder, and ankle are other frequent sites of septic arthritis. Sacroiliitis is also not uncommon, with *Mycobacterium tuberculosis* being a causative organism.
2. Slipped capital femoral epiphysis (SCFE) is an important diagnosis that could be missed with ultrasound. A hip fracture may also be easily missed with ultrasound. Both of these entities are better evaluated with radiographs of the hip.

CLINICAL HISTORY *60-year-old male with acute onset of left-sided weakness and facial droop. The patient had recently been complaining of new right-sided headaches.*

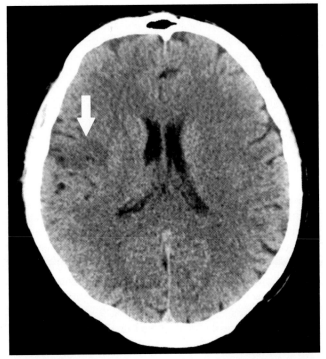

FIGURE 53A

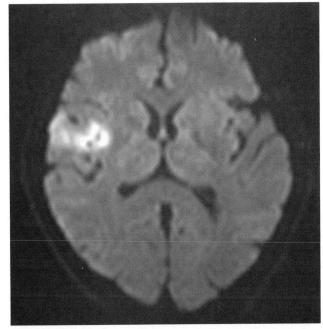

FIGURE 53B

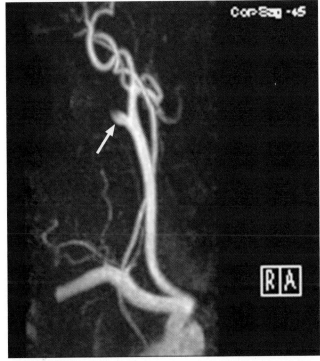

FIGURE 53C

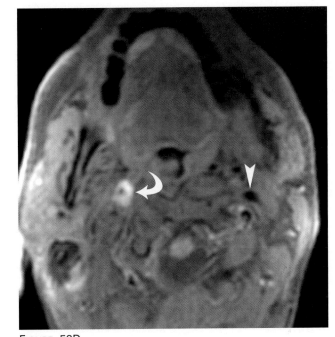

FIGURE 53D

FINDINGS Figure 53A: Axial unenhanced CT image demonstrates an area of hypodensity in the right frontal lobe (*large arrow*) involving the cortex and subcortical white matter, concerning for cerebral infarction. Figure 53B: Axial DWI image demonstrates high signal intensity in this region, confirming the diagnosis of infarction. Figure 53C: Right anterior oblique 3D MIP image from a contrast-enhanced MRA of the neck demonstrates occlusion of the right internal carotid artery (ICA; *small arrow*). The carotid bulb is relatively normal, and the vessel tapers proximal to the occlusion. Figure 53D: Axial fat-suppressed T1WI of the neck above the level of the carotid bifurcation demonstrates an eccentric crescent of high signal intensity encircling the lumen of the right ICA (*curved arrow*). Compare with the normal left ICA flow void (*arrowhead*).

DIFFERENTIAL DIAGNOSIS The primary differential in this case would be occlusion of the extracranial ICA secondary to atherosclerotic thrombosis or an arterial dissection. *Atherosclerosis* usually occurs in the elderly, affects multiple vessels, and commonly involves the vessel origin, carotid bifurcation, and carotid bulb. *Arterial dissections* usually spare the vessel origin, carotid bifurcation, and carotid bulb. Furthermore, dissections are usually solitary except in the setting of underlying vasculopathy or extensive trauma.

DIAGNOSIS Spontaneous internal carotid artery dissection with secondary thromboembolic stroke.

DISCUSSION An arterial dissection is caused by a tear in the vessel's intima or a rupture of the vasa vasorum, leading to the formation of an intramural hematoma that produces arterial stenosis or occlusion. Extracranial ICA dissections comprise 70% to 80% of all craniocervical artery dissections, and extracranial vertebral artery (VA) dissections account for about 15%. Approximately 60% of extracranial dissections are considered spontaneous, with the remainder being caused by blunt or penetrating injury.

Spontaneous dissections occur in the absence of significant trauma, but these dissections often follow a precipitating trivial event such as neck rotation, coughing, or vomiting. It is currently believed that spontaneous dissections may result from a combination of environmental and intrinsic factors, a theory supported by the observation that spontaneous dissections are associated with various connective tissue disorders, such as Ehlers–Danlos syndrome type IV, Marfan syndrome, cystic medial necrosis, polycystic kidney disease, osteogenesis imperfecta, and fibromuscular dysplasia (FMD), as well as with some infectious and inflammatory processes.

Traumatic dissections occur in approximately 1% to 2% of patients with direct or blunt trauma to the neck. Most result from motor vehicle accidents. Extracranial carotid artery injuries most often occur in the distal cervical ICA, particularly at the level of the C1–C3 vertebrae. In contrast, VA dissections usually occur in the V2 or in the V3 segment where the vessel travels through the transverse foramina or as it emerges from the transverse process of C2 and sweeps laterally to pass by the C1 vertebra before piercing the dural membrane. The majority of VA injuries are caused by subluxations and vertebral fractures that extend into the foramen transversarium.

The classic clinical presentation for carotid dissections consists of the triad of unilateral head, facial, or neck pain; Horner syndrome; and cerebral or retinal ischemia. Unfortunately, clinical diagnosis is often challenging because a minority of patients actually present with the complete triad. Furthermore, up to 5% of carotid artery dissections may be asymptomatic or have only minor symptoms. Headaches and neck pain are the most common clinical presentations, but patients can present with any of the above symptoms, as well as lower cranial nerve palsies and pulsatile tinnitus.

Typical findings of extracranial arterial dissection include eccentric narrowing of the vessel lumen that can range from mild stenosis to diffuse luminal narrowing (the "string" sign) or complete occlusion. Extracranial carotid artery dissections usually spare the carotid bifurcation and intracranial part of the ICA and are most commonly located 2 to 3 cm distal to the carotid bulb. Characteristic signs such as an intimal flap or double lumen are seen only in a minority of cases on cross-sectional imaging. Additional findings of EAD include a dissecting aneurysm and an intraluminal thrombus. Traumatic psuedoaneurysms develop in a minority of cases of traumatic cerebrovascular incidents, and usually occur in the middle or distal cervical vessels.

A common finding seen with carotid dissections on cross-sectional MRA imaging is an enlarged external diameter of the involved artery despite luminal narrowing. In the early and chronic stages, intramural hematomas are usually isointense to the surrounding structures. From 1 to 9 weeks, they tend to be hyperintense on T1-weighted images. Acute intramural hematoma can be easily missed on T1- and T2-weighted MR images because they tend to be hypointense and therefore difficult to delineate from an area of flow void. Subacute intramural hematoma appears as a crescentic hyperintensity surrounding an eccentrically located flow void on T1 fat-saturated sequences. Time-of-flight (TOF) MRA also allows for the visualization of a subacute intramural hematoma that can be easily overlooked on contrast-enhanced MRA. Contrast-enhanced MRA, on the other hand, is less time consuming, less susceptible to motion and flow artifacts, and better demonstrates luminal irregularities as well as stenoses. Contrast-enhanced MRA may also be superior at demonstrating dissecting aneurysms and vertebral artery dissections.

Distal ischemia is most commonly the result of emboli released from the injury site rather than hypoperfusion from focal stenosis or occlusion at the site of dissection. Intimal defects expose circulating blood to intrinsic clotting factors, leading to acute thrombosis, and thromboemboli from extracranial carotid dissections account for 5% to 22% of strokes in patients younger than 45 years. Therefore, treatment is typically aimed at preventing thromboembolic complications through the use of antithrombotic medication. Endovascular stenting is a treatment option in selected cases. Overall, neurologic outcome is good or excellent because the majority of stenoses and occlusions induced by dissections spontaneously resolve or recanalize on their own. The risk of recurrent dissection is reported to be 2% in the first year and 1% per year thereafter. Mortality rates associated with spontaneous extracranial cerebrovascular dissection range from 3% to 7%; however, they are higher for those induced by trauma. The higher mortality associated with trauma-induced dissections may relate to other coexisting injuries.

Question for Further Thought

1. Why do most extracranial carotid injuries associated with blunt trauma occur in the distal cervical ICA?

Reporting Responsibilities

Because of the risk of cerebral ischemia, findings of an acute cervical arterial dissection should be immediately communicated with the referring physician, so that appropriate antithrombotic therapy can be promptly initiated. If dissection is suspected but initial CTA imaging is equivocal, MRI imaging (including fat-suppressed T1-weighted images) should be recommended to rule out the presence of intramural thrombus.

What the Treating Physician Needs to Know

• Is there significant arterial stenosis, and is it more likely caused by atherosclerosis or a dissection?

• Is there evidence of cerebral infarction on concomitant brain imaging?

• Is there a pseudoaneurysm or arteriovenous fistula?

• In the setting of trauma, are there other traumatic injuries evident? Is there a foreign body or bone fragment penetrating the affected vessel?

• Are there findings to suggest an underlying vasculopathy (e.g., fibromuscular dysplasia)?

Answer

1. Carotid injuries associated with blunt trauma are believed to occur with combined hyperextension and contralateral rotation of the head. In these cases, the distal cervical ICA is the most commonly involved segment because it is especially susceptible to stretching over the lateral masses of the cervical vertebrae (particularly from C1 to C3) with rapid deceleration as well as to compression between the mandible and the cervical spine with hyperflexion.

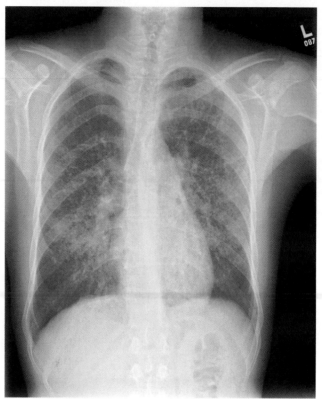

FIGURE 54A

FINDINGS Figure 54A: Posteroanterior (PA) plain film of the chest. The lungs are hyperinflated, and there are bilateral mostly central heterogeneous ground-glass opacities with some nodularity.

DIFFERENTIAL DIAGNOSIS *Pneumocystis jiroveci* pneumonia (PJP), viral pneumonia, aspergillus, pulmonary hemorrhage.

DIAGNOSIS *Pneumocystis jiroveci* pneumonia.

DISCUSSION PJP is thought of as an HIV-AIDS–defining illness that is usually found in patients with a CD4+ count <200 cells/mm³, although it can be seen in patients with higher cell counts. Cough and shortness of breath are common presenting symptoms. Radiographically, the principal finding is ground-glass opacities, with a slight predominance in the upper lung lobes. Reticular opacities or septal thickening can be present in more advanced disease. Pneumatoceles ("cysts") of varying size and wall thickness may occur in up to one-third of patients. It is notable that pleural effusions as

well as lymphadenopathy are rare in PCP. Some less common features include consolidation and granulomas, which may be cavitary.[2]

Question for Further Thought

1. What is an important complication that can be seen on imaging in patients with PJP?

Reporting Responsibilities
The interpreting radiologist should document the imaging findings as well as any associated findings such as pneumothorax or lymph node calcification.

What the Treating Physician Needs to Know
- Severity of disease.
- Differential diagnosis.

Answer

1. Pneumothorax. Rupture of cysts in the course of PJP can lead to spontaneous pneumothorax.

CLINICAL HISTORY *61-year-old man with severe abdominal trauma from a motor vehicle accident.*

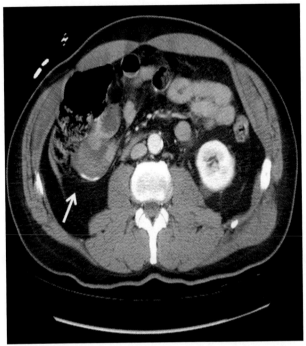

FIGURE 55A

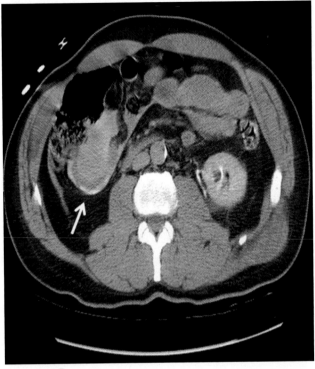

FIGURE 55B

FINDINGS Figure 55A: Axial contrast-enhanced CT image performed in the portal venous phase demonstrates active extravasation of contrast from an ileocolic arterial branch into the mesentery, showing similar attenuation with the contrast within the vessel lumen. Mesenteric hematoma with high attenuation is identified (*arrow*). Figure 55B: Delayed axial contrast-enhanced CT image at the same level demonstrates increased density and size of the mesenteric hematoma, indicating acute mesenteric injury and active bleeding (*arrow*).

DIFFERENTIAL DIAGNOSIS Mesenteric injury, bowel injury, renal or ureteral injury.

DIAGNOSIS Mesenteric injury.

DISCUSSION Mesenteric injury is a relatively uncommon event, constituting about 1% to 5% of all blunt abdominal injuries.[1] Active mesenteric bleeding, disruption of the mesentery, and mesenteric injury associated with bowel ischemia are considered significant mesenteric injuries. The mechanisms of injury include a crushing injury caused by direct force, a shearing injury caused by rapid deceleration, and a bursting injury caused by increase in intraluminal pressure.[2]

Computed tomography (CT) is the modality of choice for initial evaluation of blunt abdominal trauma. CT can help identify the location and extent of the injury. To facilitate imaging at an earlier time, some institutions will not give oral contrast. However, intravenous contrast is essential to evaluate for active extravasation.

CT findings for mesenteric injury include extravasation of contrast from a mesenteric vessel, mesenteric vascular beading, and abrupt termination of the mesenteric vessel. Extravasation of contrast material and presence of a mesenteric hematoma are pathognomonic of mesenteric injury, but not commonly seen. Mesenteric hematoma can indicate mesenteric injury, but as an isolated finding, it is nonspecific. Hematoma within the mesentery typically shows a geographic shape along the mesenteric folds with angular corners, often showing a triangular or polygonal morphology. Mesenteric vascular beading is irregularity of the mesenteric vessels resulting from changes in caliber related to vascular injury.

Intraperitoneal fluid and mesenteric stranding are also non-specific findings, but should be present in significant mesenteric injury. Hemoperitoneum in the absence of solid organ injury should raise the possibility of mesenteric or bowel injury. Bowel wall thickening and abnormal enhancement is a significant finding that may indicate bowel ischemia caused by mesenteric injury. A seat belt sign or subcutaneous fat stranding in the anterior abdominal wall can also be associated with mesenteric injury.

Mesenteric injury is associated with a high rate of mortality, especially if early intervention is not timely. Indications for surgery include presence of bowel ischemia or active mesenteric bleeding. Surgery may involve vessel ligation and/or resection of devitalized bowel.

Question for Further Thought

1. Should catheter angiogram be performed instead of CT mesenteric angiogram to evaluate mesenteric injury?

Reporting Responsibilities

Mesenteric injury is a surgical emergency and should be reported to the referring physician promptly.

What the Treating Physician Needs to Know

- Site and size of hematoma, and, if possible, site of the bleeding.
- Presence of extravasated IV contrast.

Answer

1. If there is strong suspicion of mesenteric injury with massive blood loss that requires urgent treatment, catheter angiogram or explorative laparotomy should be considered instead of CT mesenteric angiogram in the interest of timely management. This differs according to the availability of resources in individual hospitals. CT imaging is the preferred initial imaging study for blunt abdominal trauma in a hemodynamically stable patient.

CLINICAL HISTORY *27-year-old man who describes falling on an outstretched hand, now with pain and swelling of the elbow and proximal forearm.*

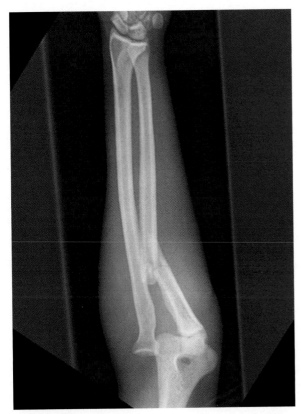

FIGURE 56A

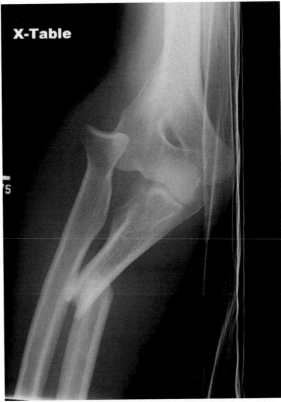

FIGURE 56B

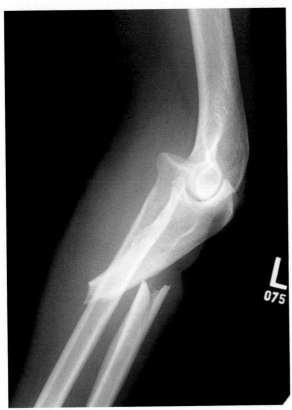

FIGURE 56C

FINDINGS Anteroposterior (AP) radiograph of the left forearm (Fig. 56A) and AP and lateral radiographs of the left elbow (Figs. 56B and 56C) demonstrate an ulnar diaphyseal fracture at the junction of the proximal and middle thirds with apex anterolateral angulation, posterior displacement of the distal fracture fragment, and overriding of the fracture fragments, resulting in foreshortening. The radial head is dislocated anterolaterally. Inspection of the coronoid process on the lateral view of the elbow reveals minimal irregularity, but no other evidence for coronoid process fracture. Apparent soft tissue defect over the posterior proximal ulna is caused by distortion from the displaced and overriding fracture rather than from a penetrating soft tissue injury.

DIFFERENTIAL DIAGNOSIS Anterior elbow dislocation, isolated radiocapitellar joint dislocation, isolated ulnar shaft fracture, ulna fracture with radiocapitellar joint dislocation.

DIAGNOSIS Ulna fracture with anterior radiocapitellar joint dislocation (Monteggia fracture-dislocation).

DISCUSSION The forearm functions as a ring composed of the radius and ulna as well as the proximal and distal radioulnar joints. A break in the ring is commonly associated with a fracture or dislocation in another part of the ring. When a forearm fracture is seen on radiographs, both the wrist and the elbow must be evaluated to exclude associated dislocations and additional fractures. Monteggia fracture-dislocations are unstable injuries composed of a proximal ulna fracture and dislocation of the radial head. Failure to recognize the associated radial head dislocation may lead to long-term complications, requiring more extensive surgery.

Monteggia fracture-dislocations are usually the result of a fall on an outstretched hand with forced pronation, fall with flexed elbow, or direct blow to the forearm. High-energy trauma, such as in a motor vehicle collision, can also result in this type of injury, but are often associated with additional injuries.

The most commonly used classification system for Monteggia fractures is the Bado classification.[1]

- Bado Type 1—The classic Monteggia fracture-dislocation. Most common in children. Anterior dislocation of the radial head and fracture of the proximal ulnar diaphysis, with apex anterior angulation.
- Bado Type 2—Most common in adults. Posterior or posterolateral dislocation of the radial head and fracture of ulna diaphysis with apex posterior angulation. Often associated with radial head fractures and lateral collateral ligament disruption. Associated with osteoporosis.
- Bado Type 3—Less common than Type 1 and also mostly seen in children. Lateral or anterolateral dislocation of the radial head and fracture of the ulna just distal to the coronoid process. Very similar to Type 1.
- Bado Type 4—Rare. Type 1 with fracture of the proximal radius shaft.

Additional variants to be aware of that are not captured by the Bado classification include very proximal ulna fractures with radiocapitellar joint dislocation, but relative preservation of the proximal radioulnar joint.

The diagnosis can usually be made with AP and lateral radiographs of the forearm. If there is any uncertainty about involvement of the elbow, dedicated elbow radiographs should be obtained. The ulna fracture is usually obvious; however, radial head dislocations can be subtle. A line drawn along the long axis of the radius should bisect the capitellum. One can also use the fact that the radial head often dislocates in the direction of the fracture apex. The radial head should also be scrutinized for fracture, which is common in posterior radial head dislocation. In complex cases, CT can be used to detect additional injuries, such as coronoid process fractures. MRI can be considered to evaluate for ligamentous injury.

The primary goal of treatment is restoration of normal ulnar alignment. If the interosseous membrane is intact, then the proximal radioulnar joint is generally stabilized. In adults, this necessitates open reduction with internal fixation. In children with buckle fractures, plastic deformation, or green stick fractures, closed reduction can be performed followed by cast immobilization. Successful treatment of

posterior Monteggia fracture-dislocations (Bado Type 2) requires evaluation and treatment of any associated fractures (radial head, coronoid process) and the likely torn lateral collateral ligament complex.[2] Delayed treatment may lead to further injury, requiring more extensive intervention.

The most common acute complication is posterior interosseous nerve (PIN) palsy, which may be caused by either direct contusion (usually in the setting of a Bado Type 2 injury) or stretch injury from radial head dislocation. The PIN is a deep motor branch of the radial nerve that wraps around the neck of the radius and supplies the wrist extensors except the extensor carpi radialis longus. Symptoms include weakness upon extension of the thumb or fingers and pain with supination and pronation. When associated with stretch injury, symptoms often resolve with radiocapitellar joint reduction. Common long-term complications include chronic proximal radioulnar and radiocapitellar joint instability, delayed union, malunion, nonunion, and proximal radioulnar synostosis.

Questions for Further Thought

1. How are Monteggia fracture-dislocations in children different from adults?
2. What is the terrible triad?

Reporting Responsibilities

Monteggia fracture-dislocations are not emergencies; a timely report is required. A phone call should be considered if the patient is referred from a setting other than an emergency department to ensure immediate orthopedic consultation.

What the Treating Physician Needs to Know

- Location and direction of the ulna fracture and the direction of the radial head dislocation.
- Associated injuries, such as radial head and coronoid process fractures.

Answers

1. In children, the predominant Monteggia-type injuries are Bado Types 1, 3, and 4. Adults more commonly have posterior Monteggia fracture-dislocations (Bado Type 2). Whereas open reduction and internal fixation is required in adults, closed reduction is often acceptable in children. In addition to simple plastic deformation, the ulnar fracture in children may present as a buckle or a greenstick fracture in addition to a complete fracture.
2. The "terrible triad" is an elbow dislocation with radial head and coronoid process fractures. These fracture-dislocations are difficult to treat and have overall poor outcomes; hence the name. Careful evaluation of the radial head and coronoid process should be undertaken; CT may be needed to evaluate the coronoid process if such a fracture is suspected.

CLINICAL HISTORY *5-month-old infant with a 2-week history of intermittent fevers, now presenting with left neck and chin swelling.*

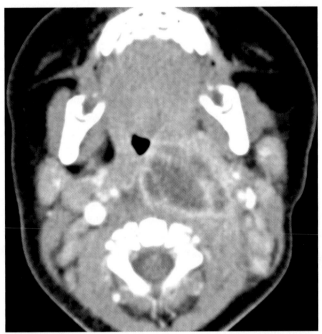

FIGURE 57A

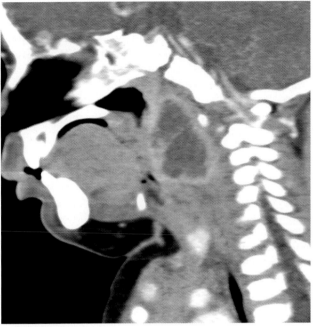

FIGURE 57B

FINDINGS Figures 57A and 57B: Axial (Fig. 57A) and sagittal (Fig. 57B) contrast-enhanced CT images reveal a large, ovoid fluid collection in the left lateral retropharyngeal space that demonstrates an irregular enhancing rim and internal septations. The fluid collection significantly displaces the oropharyngeal airway anteriorly and to the right. There is also enhancing cervical lymphadenopathy, which is slightly more pronounced on the left.

DIFFERENTIAL DIAGNOSIS The primary diagnostic consideration given the history and imaging findings is a *retropharyngeal abscess. Tonsillar and peritonsillar abscesses* are generally centered in the tonsils along the lateral pharyngeal wall and may extend laterally into the parapharyngeal space. *Suppurative retropharyngeal lymphadenitis* can also appear as a peripherally enhancing fluid collection in the lateral retropharyngeal space; however, these are typically smaller and less centrally located than abscesses. Sterile *retropharyngeal effusions/edema* also occur in the setting of upper respiratory tract infections and also appear as fluid collections in the retropharyngeal space; however, these effusions do not show peripheral enhancement, are typically midline, and demonstrate a more lentiform appearance on the sagittal images. *Lymphatic and mixed vascular malformations* can also appear as low-density masses and involve the retropharyngeal space; however, the pattern of enhancement in mixed vascular malformations is typically not isolated to the periphery of the lesions, and the clinical history in this case does not support the diagnosis.

DIAGNOSIS Retropharyngeal abscess.

DISCUSSION Retropharyngeal abscesses are usually the result of rupture of a suppurative retropharyngeal node into the retropharyngeal space. Less commonly, they develop from direct spread of infection from adjacent spaces in the head and neck. They are primarily a disease of childhood. When retropharyngeal abscesses develop in adults, they are more likely to be caused by regional trauma, foreign body ingestion, complications of medical procedures, or an immunocompromised state. Patients with retropharyngeal abscesses usually present with acute onset neck pain, fever, sore throat, decreased oral intake, or a neck mass. Neck stiffness and torticollis are also commonly observed. Complications can include airway compromise, sepsis, mediastinitis, and jugular vein thrombosis. An attempt to distinguish between a suppurative lymph node with an intact capsule and a true retropharyngeal abscess should therefore be made, as the former can usually be treated conservatively, whereas the majority of retropharyngeal abscesses require prompt surgical drainage owing to the potential for developing one of the above complications. Upper airway infections can give rise to effusions or edema of the retropharyngeal space. These collections are typically sterile and resolve with treatment of the underlying infection. Therefore, distinguishing between a simple effusion and a true abscess is also critical.

Lateral neck radiographs are still obtained in some instances when a retropharyngeal abnormality is suspected. On a true lateral radiograph, the width of the retropharyngeal

117

soft tissue stripe (measured at the inferior margin of C2) normally measures ≤7 mm in both adults and children, whereas the width of the retrotracheal soft tissue stripe (measured at the inferior aspect of C6) should be ≤14 mm in children and ≤22 mm in adults. Widening of either of these stripes should be viewed as suspicious for the presence of a retropharyngeal lesion, and merits further evaluation with either CT or MRI. The classic imaging finding of a retropharyngeal abscess on cross-sectional imaging, as demonstrated in this case, is that of a peripherally enhancing fluid collection in the retropharyngeal space. In some instances, the abscess may fill the entire space, whereas in other cases such as this one, it may primarily involve one side.

Question for Further Thought

1. Why are retropharyngeal abscesses more likely to occur in children than in adults?

Reporting Responsibilities

When imaging reveals a retropharyngeal abscess, the report should also reflect the presence or absence of findings that may indicate or herald development of significant complications, such as airway compression, mediastinal extension, or jugular vein thrombosis. The presence of any of these features should prompt an immediate call to the requesting physician.

What the Treating Physician Needs to Know

- Is the fluid collection more likely to represent a suppurative lymph node, or has the process extended beyond the nodal capsule and formed a true retropharyngeal abscess?
- Is the fluid collection more likely to be an abscess or a simple effusion?
- Is there evidence of significant airway compromise?
- Is there evidence of mediastinal extension of infection?
- Are the nearby vascular structures patent?

Answer

1. Retropharyngeal abscesses most commonly develop when infection from a suppurative lateral retropharyngeal lymph node breaks through the nodal capsule into the adjacent retropharyngeal space. These lateral retropharyngeal nodes are seen primarily in children, and over time begin to decrease in size, usually beginning at 4 years of age until the onset of puberty. As a result, suppurative retropharyngeal adenitis and, by extension, retropharyngeal abscesses are much less likely to develop in adults.

CLINICAL HISTORY *30-year-old male after motor vehicle crash.*

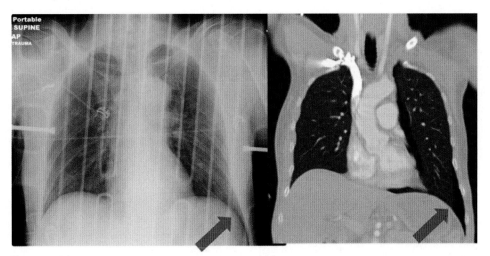

FIGURE 58A

FINDINGS Figure 58A: Anteroposterior (AP) supine chest film with patient on backboard shows abnormal lucency in the deep left costophrenic angle (*arrow*) with sharp demarcation of the left hemidiaphragm. No definite visceral pleural edge is appreciated. Coronal reformatted CT shows air in the pleural space in the left costophrenic angle (*arrow*), and also in the medial pleural space along the heart border.

DIFFERENTIAL DIAGNOSIS Pneumothorax with deep sulcus sign, emphysema, free intraperitoneal air.

DIAGNOSIS Pneumothorax with deep sulcus sign.

DISCUSSION On a supine chest film, pneumothoraces can be difficult to detect. With the patient in a supine position, the least dependent portion of the hemithorax is anterior and caudal, so air in the pleural space will collect in this region, often in the anterolateral diaphragmatic sulcus, creating what appears as a "deep" sulcus. Often, a definite visceral pleural edge cannot be appreciated in the supine position if the amount of air is small or small to medium. Depression of the ipsilateral hemidiaphragm and increased sharpness of the hemidiaphragm cardiac border may also be present, as seen in the figures above.[1]

Question for Further Thought

1. Can pneumothorax occur in the setting of trauma without a rib fracture?

Reporting Responsibilities

The referring clinician should be immediately notified, so (1) a CT can be obtained to verify and to assess for other thoracic injuries, or (2) the patient can be treated immediately with chest tube decompression if symptomatic.

What the Treating Physician Needs to Know

- Suspicion or presence of pneumothorax.
- Size of pneumothorax.
- Associated injuries.

Answer

1. Most often, pneumothoraces are associated with rib fractures, which cause direct injury to the visceral pleura, but high-speed deceleration injuries alone may cause a sheer injury of the visceral pleura, or a pulmonary laceration that involves the visceral pleura, causing a pneumothorax.

CLINICAL HISTORY *68-year-old female presenting with acute left lower quadrant abdominal pain, nausea, and vomiting. On physical exam, she has peritoneal signs and is diffusely tender to palpation.*

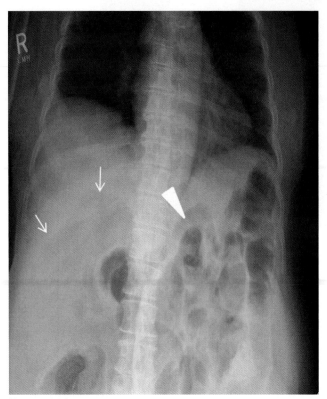

FIGURE 59A

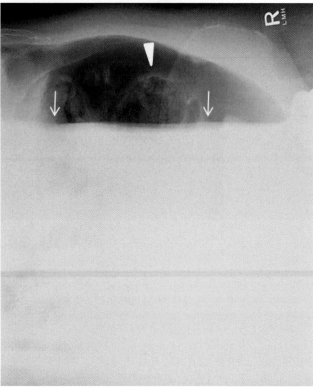

FIGURE 59B

FINDINGS Figure 59A: A supine abdominal radiograph demonstrates a large volume of free intraperitoneal air in the right hemiabdomen. The Rigler sign is identified with air present on both sides of the abdominal wall (*arrowhead*). The lucent liver sign is identified with increased lucency noted over the liver, which corresponds to free air anterior to the ventral surface of the liver (*arrows*). (Courtesy of Dr. Lauren Burke, Chapel Hill, NC, USA.) Figure 59B: A left lateral decubitus radiograph of the abdomen demonstrates a large volume of free intraperitoneal air in the nondependent abdomen between the abdominal wall and the liver, confirming pneumoperitoneum. The Rigler sign is again identified (*arrowhead*). There is an air–fluid level indicating fluid in the abdomen consistent with hydropneumoperitoneum (*arrows*). (Courtesy of Dr. Lauren Burke, Chapel Hill, NC, USA.)

DIFFERENTIAL DIAGNOSIS Chilaiditi syndrome (colonic interposition between liver and hemidiaphragm), biliary or portal venous gas, fat within the subdiaphragmatic space or ligamentum teres, abscess, pneumatosis, gas within skin folds, properitoneal fat stripe, pneumoperitoneum.

DIAGNOSIS Pneumoperitoneum.

DISCUSSION Pneumoperitoneum refers to the presence of free air within the peritoneal cavity. The most common cause is a perforation of an abdominal viscus. A number of other conditions, both benign and more worrisome, can cause pneumoperitoneum. These other conditions include penetrating trauma, postoperative free air, peritoneal dialysis, and air tracking inferiorly from the chest, such as in pneumothorax or pneumomediastinum.

Pneumoperitoneum is best visualized on an erect chest radiograph or a left lateral decubitus abdominal radiograph. However, many patients with acute abdomen are too sick or debilitated to stand or lie on their side, so the supine radiographs may be the only radiographic imaging that can be obtained. Pneumoperitoneum is able to be detected in the majority of patients on a supine abdominal image.

There are various signs of free intraperitoneal air that can be visualized on a supine radiograph, and a radiologist should be familiar with these signs. One of the more important signs is the Rigler sign or the "double wall sign." This is seen when air is visualized on both sides of the bowel wall. Frequently, air will collect between bowel loops forming lucent triangles known as the "triangle sign."

When the patient is supine, air will tend to collect anteriorly within the abdomen. This will frequently create lucency over the liver, known as the "lucent liver sign." When this lucent appearing liver is coupled with air outlining the falciform ligament, this is known as the "football sign" (the ribs crossing the falciform ligament, creating the laces on a football).

When pneumoperitoneum is suspected on a supine abdominal radiograph, an erect chest or lateral decubitus abdominal radiograph can be performed for confirmation. On erect chest radiograph, free air is typically seen under the hemidiaphragms. On a left lateral decubitus view, free air is typically seen between the liver and the right abdominal wall. Computed tomography can be obtained to confirm the suspicion of pneumoperitoneum and to evaluate the etiology of the pneumoperitoneum. In the case of a patient with acute abdomen and concomitant hemodynamic instability, exploratory laparotomy should be considered.

Questions for Further Thought

1. What views should you obtain to confirm your suspicion of free intraperitoneal air on supine plain radiographic imaging?
2. What imaging can be recommended in the case of suspected pneumoperitoneum in a pregnant patient?

Reporting Responsibilities

Diagnosis and prompt reporting of pneumoperitoneum is imperative in adequate management of the acute abdomen. Delay in diagnosis can cause a significant increase in morbidity and mortality for the patient with an acute abdomen. If the suspicion of pneumoperitoneum remains after lateral decubitus and erect chest radiographs, computed tomography should be recommended for a definitive diagnosis and to discern the etiology of pneumoperitoneum.

What the Treating Physician Needs to Know

- After the diagnosis of pneumoperitoneum, the cause of free intraperitoneal air needs to be determined. If the patient had recent surgical intervention or any instrumentation of the abdominal cavity, such as peritoneal dialysis catheter placement, pneumoperitoneum is likely a normal finding and does not require extensive workup. However, in the case of recent trauma, acute abdomen, suspected iatrogenic perforation, or in the case of gas-forming organism infection, further evaluation should be performed with computed tomography to discern the etiology. As noted above, in the case of a patient with acute abdomen and concomitant hemodynamic instability, urgent exploratory laparotomy should be considered.

Answers

1. Erect chest and left lateral decubitus abdominal radiographs. These two projections allow for air to rise in nondependent areas where it can be easily visualized. Left lateral decubitus allows air to be easily visualized on a liver background as compared with the right lateral decubitus projection, where the gastric air can conceal or make it difficult to appreciate free intraperitoneal air.

2. In a pregnant patient, erect lateral chest radiograph with appropriate shielding can be obtained to exclude the fetus from direct beam exposure. Ultrasound can also be performed, in which the free air will be identified as an echogenic peritoneal stripe accompanied by posterior reverberation/comet tail artifact. However, in the case of strong clinical suspicion of pneumoperitoneum, abdominal imaging, such as computed tomography, versus surgical exploration would have to be determined on an individual basis.

CLINICAL HISTORY *24-year-old male presents with pain in the upper neck and limited range of motion after cliff diving in shallower than expected water.*

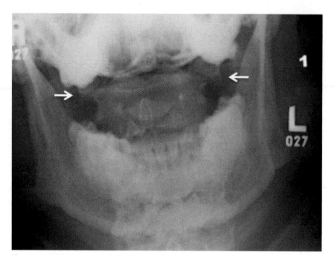

FIGURE 60A

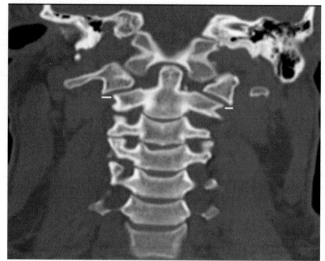

FIGURE 60B

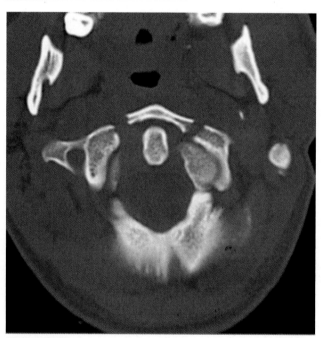

FIGURE 60C

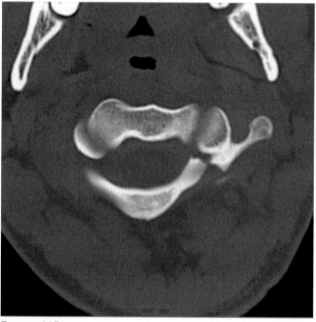

FIGURE 60D

FINDINGS Anteroposterior (AP) radiograph (Fig. 60A) demonstrates lateral offset of the lateral masses of C1 relative to the lateral margins of C2 (*arrows*). Coronal reconstruction from cervical spine CT (Fig. 60B) confirming lateralization of the lateral masses of C2 relative to the occipital condyles as well as the lateral margins of C2. *Short white lines* indicate the degree of lateralization of the lateral masses of C1; if the sum is greater than or equal to 7 mm, transverse ligament disruption is likely. Axial images from cervical spine CT confirm two anterior C1 ring fractures (Fig. 60C) and a displaced fracture of the left lateral C1 ring (Fig. 60D).

(Images courtesy of Jordan Renner, MD, University of North Carolina, Chapel Hill, NC, USA.)

DIFFERENTIAL DIAGNOSIS Congenital variant (cleft/malformation), C1 ring fracture (Jefferson).

DIAGNOSIS Three-part C1 ring fracture.

DISCUSSION Fractures of C1, although not as common as fractures of C2 or the subaxial cervical spine, still represent a significant portion of traumatic cervical injury, accounting for approximately 2% to 15% of acute cervical fractures.[1] Jefferson fractures result from axial loading force applied to the vertex of the head, such as from diving in shallow water. The applied force is transmitted through the occipital condyles onto the sloped C1 pillars. Sufficient applied force results in lateral displacement and eventual disruption of the C1 ring, which is a type of burst fracture. Isolated posterior arch fractures, alternatively, can also result from hyperextension, and resulting crush injury of the posterior ring. C1 fractures are not infrequently present with other cervical spine injuries, with approximately 50% associated with injury elsewhere in the cervical spine, and approximately one-third associated with concomitant C2 fracture.

Classification of C1 fractures can be described by the following:

- Type I: Isolated bilateral anterior arch or posterior arch fractures.
- Type II: Combined anterior and posterior arch fractures including the classic 4-part burst fracture, which was first described by neurosurgeon Dr. Geoffrey Jefferson. Stability determined by integrity of transverse ligament.
- Type III: Fracture involving unilateral C1 lateral mass. Stability determined by integrity of transverse ligament.

The gold standard for imaging evaluation of the cervical spine in the setting of suspected trauma, as designated by the American College of Radiology (ACR) appropriateness criteria, is CT of the cervical spine without contrast. CT is best able to delineate the fracture pattern (2, 3, 4 part fractures), and can visualize findings essential for establishing unstable injury, such as a transverse ligament avulsion fracture at its insertion on the inner C1 pillar. Coronal CT reconstructions are used to visualize and quantify lateral displacement of C1 lateral masses relative to lateral margins of C2. If the sum of C1 offset is greater than or equal to 7 mm, it is consistent with transverse ligament disruption, which is indicative of an unstable injury. Sagittal CT reconstructions can demonstrate widening of the atlantodental interval (ADI), which when greater than or equal to 4 mm but less than 7 mm is concerning for transverse ligament disruption. However, if the widening is greater than or equal to 7 mm, transverse ligament disruption is assumed, which is unstable. CT can also visualize other concerning soft tissue abnormalities, such as epidural hematoma.

Radiographs can also be used to visualize C1 fractures, which can demonstrate osseous disruption or associated paravertebral soft tissue swelling. The open mouth radiographic view can also be used to visualize lateral displacement of C1 lateral masses relative to lateral margins of C2, and lateral radiographs can be used to reveal widening of the ADI, as on sagittal CT projections. MRI can be performed as an adjunct, particularly when the patient has focal neurologic deficits or clinical examination for instability cannot be accurately performed; MRI is more sensitive for evaluation of ligamentous or spinal cord injury. If cervical spine fractures are present that extend to the vertebral foramina, or if there is clinical concern for vertebral artery dissection, CTA or MRA of the neck can be used to evaluate for vertebral artery injury.

There is a low rate of neurologic injury with isolated C1 fractures. The majority are stable fractures, thus requiring immobilization with hard cervical collar for 3 months. However, if the fracture is unstable, such as with transverse or alar ligamentous injury, surgical intervention is warranted with posterior C1–C2 or occipitocervical fusion.

Question for Further Thought

1. A sum of 2 mm of lateralization of the lateral masses of C1 is noted on the open mouth view of a 2-year-old patient who has no focal neurologic deficits or other clinical evidence of cervical spine injury. What is your level of suspicion of Jefferson fracture?

Reporting Responsibilities

Any trauma study of the cervical spine requires urgent assessment and reporting. Although Jefferson fractures are often stable, any evidence of instability (suggestion of transverse ligament disruption, concomitant unstable fracture at another level) requires immediate contact of the patient's care team.

What the Treating Physician Needs to Know

- If there is a history of significant cervical spine trauma, CT is the imaging modality of choice.
- Widening of the ADI $\geq$7 mm, combined offset of the C1 lateral masses $\geq$7 mm, or the presence of transverse ligament insertional avulsion fragment denotes unstable injuries and requires appropriate management.
- Concern for spinal cord injury (focal neurologic deficits, etc.) warrants further evaluation with MRI.

Answer

1. Jefferson fracture is less common in young children owing to the presence of forgiving synchondroses, and relative increased plasticity of children. Pseudospread of the atlas is seen in $\geq$90% of 2-year-olds evaluated for trauma, and is a result of disparity of growth rates of C1 and C2. However, although the flexibility seen leads to fewer fractures, children are more likely to suffer injury to the upper cervical spine with greater prevalence of neurologic injury.[2] Therefore, if there is clinical concern for neurologic injury, MRI should be performed.

CLINICAL HISTORY *56-year-old female presenting with acute onset of a severe headache.*

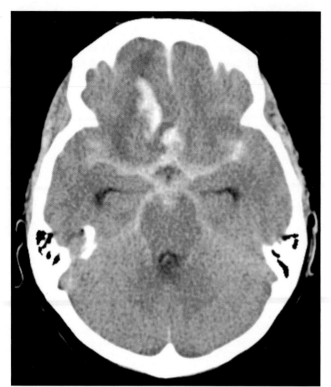

FIGURE 61A

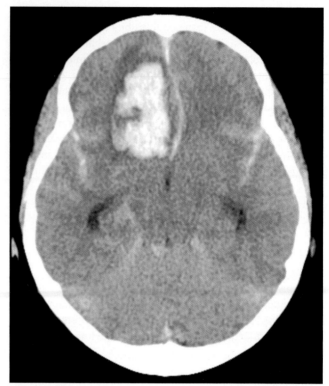

FIGURE 61B

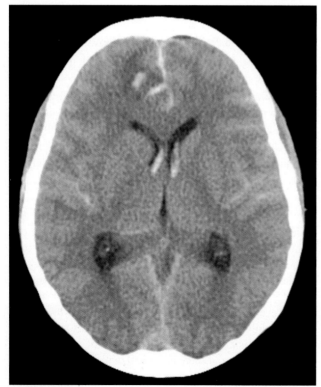

FIGURE 61C

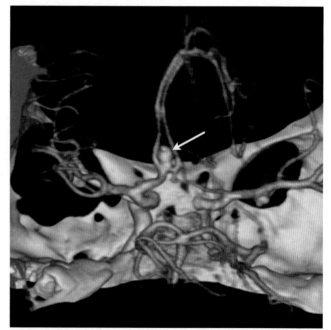

FIGURE 61D

FINDINGS Figures 61A–61C: Axial noncontrast head CT images from inferior to superior demonstrate diffuse subarachnoid hemorrhage in the suprasellar, interpeduncular, and ambient cisterns with extension laterally into the Sylvian fissures and superiorly along the interhemispheric fissure. There is also a parenchymal hematoma in the right frontal lobe (most apparent in Figs. 61A and 61B) as well as hemorrhage in both lateral ventricles (Fig. 61C). Figure 61D: 3D surface shaded reconstruction from a CTA of the circle of Willis demonstrates a superiorly oriented saccular aneurysm (*arrow*) arising from the anterior communicating artery.

DIFFERENTIAL DIAGNOSIS The above findings are pathognomonic of subarachnoid hemorrhage (SAH). When SAH is diagnosed, it is critical to distinguish *aneurysmal SAH* from nonaneurysmal causes, the latter of which include traumatic and perimesencephalic SAHs. *Traumatic SAH* is usually located along the cerebral convexities, and associated parenchymal contusions or other signs of traumatic brain injury may be present. The volume of SAH present in cases of trauma also tends to be less than what is seen in cases of aneurysmal SAH. Distribution of blood in the perimesencephalic cisterns and midbrain is usually suggestive of venous hemorrhages (*perimesencephalic SAH*). In cases of aneurysmal SAH, the distribution of blood can suggest the location of the ruptured aneurysm. Aneurysms distributed asymmetrically in a Sylvian fissure suggest rupture of a middle cerebral artery (MCA) aneurysm, whereas hemorrhages extending superiorly along the anterior interhemispheric fissure suggest an anterior communicating artery (AComA) aneurysm as the source of hemorrhage. Ruptured AComA aneurysms can also cause hemorrhage that dissects into the frontal lobes (as was the case in this patient); however, there will virtually always be a component of SAH as well. SAH secondary to rupture of aneurysms of the tip of the basilar or the posterior communicating artery can have a similar appearance and is located primarily in the perimesencephalic cisterns. Finally, *diffuse cerebral edema* can occasionally make the subarachnoid space and cisterns appear high in attenuation and mimic the appearance of SAH (pseudo-SAH).

DIAGNOSIS SAH and intraparenchymal hemorrhage secondary to a ruptured AComA aneurysm.

DISCUSSION *Aneurysmal SAH* is caused by the extravasation of blood into the sulci and cisterns due to the rupture of an intracranial aneurysm. Well-established risk factors for the formation of cerebral aneurysms and subsequent rupture include hypertension, use of alcohol, and sympathomimetic drugs. Genetic syndromes known to be associated include adult polycystic kidney disease and connective tissue disorders such as Ehlers–Danlos. Familial intracranial aneurysms are usually multiple and account for about 5% of ruptured

intracranial aneurysms. Vascular lesions such as aortic coarctation also tend to increase the risks of aneurysm formation and subsequent rupture.

Pathologically, aneurysmal SAH results from rupture of (1) saccular aneurysms, (2) fusiform aneurysms, or (3) blood blister aneurysms. Saccular aneurysms are the most common and are caused by the inherent weakness of the vessel walls at the branch points, which are inherently weak because of the absence of internal elastic lamina and tunica media. Fusiform aneurysms may result from previous trauma or high-flow arterial injuries. Blood blister aneurysms are the least common type and basically represent a rupture within a contained capsule. The most common location of intracranial aneurysm vessels is in the anterior circulation (90% compared with 10% in the posterior circulation), with the AComA, posterior communicating artery, and MCA bifurcation each accounting for roughly one-third of anterior circulation aneurysms.

Aneurysmal SAH is responsible for more than 80% of spontaneous SAH. The single most important risk factor for the rupture of an aneurysm is size. Aneurysm size >7 mm has a high risk of growth and subsequent rupture. The peak age distribution for aneurysmal SAH is between 40 and 60 years, and females are affected more frequently than males. The classic symptom of thunderclap headache or the worst headache of the patient's life is present in <50% of patients.

The Hunt and Hess grading system is commonly used for clinical assessment and prognosis, with patients being graded on a scale of 0 (unruptured aneurysm) to 5 (coma and decerebrate rigidity). The Fisher CT grading system is another commonly used grading tool in the management of aneurysmal SAH. Fisher Grade 1 represents no subarachnoid blood with an aneurysm present. Grade 2 correlates with diffuse SAH distributed in a thin layer (<1 mm). Localized clot or a thick layer of SAH (>1 mm) is Grade 3. Associated intraventricular hemorrhage from a ruptured aneurysm is Fisher Grade 4 and carries an ominous prognosis.

Initial diagnosis of SAH is made with a noncontrast CT showing blood in the subarachnoid regions. The sensitivity of a noncontrast head CT to detect SAH decreases with increasing time from the initial headache. A normal noncontrast CT of the brain but a high clinical suspicion for hemorrhage may prompt the clinician to perform a lumbar puncture to look for xanthochromia. MRI with FLAIR is highly sensitive but nonspecific for SAH. Hypointensity in the subarachnoid spaces may be seen on GRE and SWI sequences, depending on hemosiderin products. If atraumatic SAH is suspected, a CTA should be performed to identify an aneurysm and to determine its size, shape, orientation, and adjacent landmarks. CTA is usually sufficient to find the aneurysm. If the distribution of blood is suspicious for a ruptured aneurysm but no identifiable aneurysm is seen on noninvasive angiographic imaging, a four-vessel angiogram should be performed.

Aneurysms ≥2 to 3 mm can be treated with coils for occlusion. The morphology of the aneurysm, the width of the neck, and the relationship of the neck to the parent vessel are key features in determining whether endovascular treatment of the aneurysm is feasible. Open microsurgical treatment with clipping may be necessary in some cases, but is associated with a higher rate of mortality and morbidity than coiling.

The morbidity and mortality of SAH are usually caused by vasospasm that occurs because of irritation of the intracranial vessels. Vasospasm typically develops 3 to 4 days after rupture and peaks in incidence and severity at 7 to 10 days. It is best detected on catheter angiograms, but can also be seen in most cases on CTA as areas of focal stenoses of the intracranial vessels. Development of infarction is an indirect sign of vasospasm on CT. Maintenance of intracranial perfusion through high blood pressure, hypervolemia, and hemodilution (Triple H Therapy) is the mainstay of treatment for vasospasm. Treatment of vasospasm may also include calcium channel blockers or intra-arterial administration of vasodilators.

Question for Further Thought

1. What is the appropriate follow-up recommendation for incidental aneurysms <3 mm?

Reporting Responsibilities

The official radiology report should state the location of hemorrhage and amount of blood present. The CTA or MRA report should state the size, number, and morphology of any aneurysms present. Findings of hydrocephalus, infarction, or significant vasospasm should be communicated promptly to the referring physician.

What the Treating Physician Needs to Know

- Is the SAH distributed in an aneurysmal or nonaneurysmal pattern? Is there evidence of a focal clot or intraventricular hemorrhage?
- Is there an aneurysm present? If so, where is it and how large is it?
- What are the morphology and orientation of the aneurysm? If the aneurysm is saccular, does it have a wide or narrow neck?
- Are there direct or indirect signs of vasospasm (vessel narrowing or infarcts)?
- Is there hydrocephalus? If so, emergent shunting may be indicated.

Answer

1. MRA or CTA may be performed on an annual basis. There is no clear consensus on the type of study indicated, but the ability of an MRA to detect an aneurysm <3 mm is low.

CLINICAL HISTORY *36-year-old male after a motor vehicle accident.*

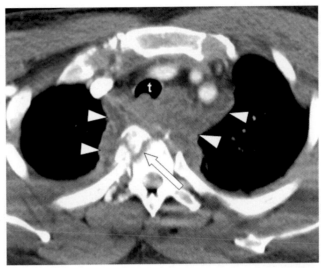

FIGURE 62A

FINDINGS FIGURE 62A: Axialcontrast-enhanced CT image of the chest just below thoracic inlet shows comminuted T4 vertebral body fracture (*arrow*) and abnormal high-density soft tissue (*arrowheads*) in the paraspinous region, posterior mediastinum, and extending into the middle mediastinum, displacing the trachea (*t*) and great vessels anteriorly.

DIFFERENTIAL DIAGNOSIS Posterior mediastinal hematoma, neurogenic tumor, osteomyelitis.

DIAGNOSIS Posterior mediastinal hematoma.

DISCUSSION Sources of posterior mediastinal hematomas are acute traumatic injury of the distal aortic arch or descending thoracic aorta, and vertebral fractures. Simple minimally displaced vertebral fractures may result in only a small paraspinal hematoma, but extensive or comminuted fractures often bleed extensively and extend into the mediastinum.[1,2] Paraspinal hematomas may also breach the parietal pleura into the pleural space. Concomitant aortic injury is not uncommon with comminuted thoracic vertebral body fractures.

Question for Further Thought

1. How is the hematoma treated?

Reporting Responsibility

In addition to the size and location of the mediastinal hematoma, reporting the presence or absence of acute traumatic aortic injury is paramount.

What the Treating Physician Needs to Know

• The treating clinician needs to know whether a mediastinal hematoma is present, and whether or not it is associated with an acute traumatic aortic injury, because acute traumatic aortic injury is treated surgically, whereas mediastinal hematoma alone may be managed conservatively. Posterior or middle column involvement[3] of vertebral fractures must be described carefully because of the potential for instability.

Answer

1. The hematoma will often resolve with conservative management. Large or rapidly increasing hematomas may have to be surgically evacuated to avoid compression of adjacent mediastinal structures.

CLINICAL HISTORY *35-year-old male with right lower-quadrant abdominal pain.*

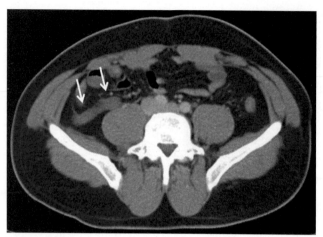

FIGURE 63A

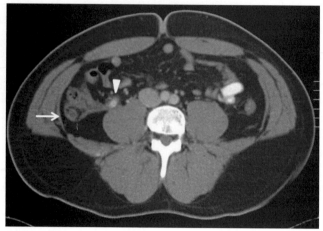

FIGURE 63B

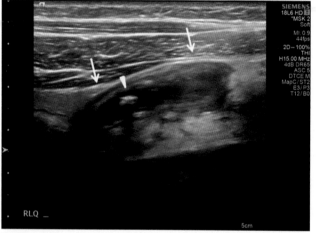

FIGURE 63C

FINDINGS Figure 63A: Axial contrast-enhanced CT scan of the appendix. The appendix is dilated and fluid-filled (*arrows*) with periappendiceal stranding. Figure 63B: Axial contrast-enhanced CT scan of the appendix of the same patient. The distal appendix is dilated and fluid-filled with appendiceal wall enhancement and periappendiceal stranding (*arrow*). An appendicolith is identified in the proximal appendix (*arrowhead*). Figure 63C: Grayscale ultrasound image of the right lower quadrant of a different patient shows a blind-ending, dilated tubular structure with thickened wall, consistent with a dilated, edematous appendix (*arrows*). Hypoechoic material fills the appendix. An echogenic round structure in the midappendix demonstrates posterior shadowing, compatible with an appendicolith (*arrowhead*). These findings are consistent with acute appendicitis.

DIFFERENTIAL DIAGNOSIS Appendicitis, active Crohn disease, appendiceal mucocele, cecal diverticulitis, omental infarction, epiploic appendagitis.

DIAGNOSIS Acute appendicitis.

DISCUSSION Acute appendicitis occurs most commonly in the second and third decades of life. The etiology of acute appendicitis is obstruction of the appendix, which may be caused by an appendicolith or lymphoid hyperplasia. The obstruction results in dilation of the blind-ending tube, which becomes fluid-filled, and thus thrombosis and obstruction of small vessels to the appendix. The resulting ischemia will progress to necrosis and rupture if not treated. Complications of appendicitis include perforation, abscess formation, phlegmon, peritonitis, bowel obstructions, and sepsis.

Although the imaging algorithm for the evaluation of appendicitis varies by institution, CT is typically the modality of choice in the nonpregnant adult patient. Pediatric patients can be initially evaluated with ultrasound (US) examination. There has been increased use of MRI in evaluating acute appendicitis in pediatric and pregnant patients.

Signs of appendicitis on CT include increased appendiceal transverse diameter (outer-to-outer wall) greater than 6 mm, fluid-filled appendix, appendicolith, wall thickening greater than 3 mm, and appendiceal wall hyperenhancement. CT findings of periappendiceal inflammation include mesenteric fat stranding surrounding the appendix, free fluid in the right lower quadrant, free intraperitoneal air, mesenteric lymph nodes in right lower quadrant, cecal wall thickening, and focal small bowel ileus. Enteric contrast or gas filling a normal caliber, thin-walled appendix excludes the diagnosis of acute appendicitis.

Signs of appendicitis on US examination include a dilated, blind-ended tubular structure that arises from the cecum with gut signature. The abnormal appendix is noncompressible and greater than 6 mm in diameter. Other supportive US findings include: an appendicolith—an echogenic, shadowing intraluminal structure; inflamed periappendiceal fat—echogenic material surrounding the appendix; and hyperemia-increased blood vascularity in the appendiceal wall on color Doppler examination. Signs of appendiceal perforation on US include periappendiceal fluid collections (phlegmon or abscess), and disruption of the submucosal layer. Graded compression helps to eliminate overlying bowel gas. Depending on the patient's body habitus and the skill of the sonographer, a normal appendix can be identified on US. The normal appendix should arise from the cecum, be blind-ending, and should be nonperistalsing. If these three criteria are met, one can confidently identify a normal appendix.

Treatment for acute appendicitis is classically an appendectomy, i.e., excision of the inflamed appendix. In the setting of abscess formation, treatment may include percutaneous drainage and IV antibiotics followed by delayed surgery.

Question for Further Thought

1. What are the MRI findings of appendicitis?

Reporting Responsibilities

Acute appendicitis is a surgical emergency, and the ordering physician should be notified immediately.

What the Treating Physician Needs to Know

- Signs of appendiceal perforation or abscess formation.
- Presence of a normal appearing appendix to exclude the diagnosis of acute appendicitis.
- Presence of atypical location of the appendix to help with surgical planning.

Answer

1. MRI imaging for acute appendicitis is becoming more frequently used in pediatric patients as well as pregnant patients. MRI features of appendicitis reflect the CT findings including appendiceal diameter greater than 6 mm, appendiceal wall thickness greater than 2 mm, high–signal-intensity luminal contents on T2-weighted images as a result of fluid or edema, and T2 hyperintense periappendiceal fat stranding and fluid. In nonpregnant patients, the administration of contrast to determine periappendiceal enhancement varies by institution.

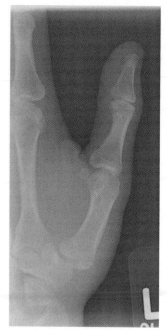

FIGURE 64A

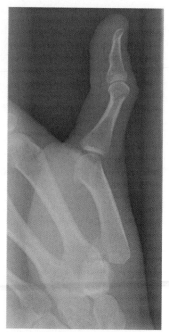

FIGURE 64B

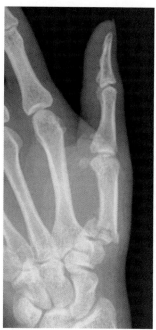

FIGURE 64C

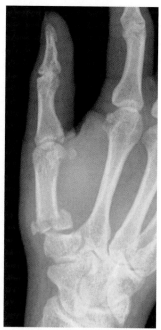

FIGURE 64D

FINDINGS Posteroanterior (PA) (Fig. 64A) and lateral (Fig. 64B) radiographs of the left thumb reveal an oblique intra-articular fracture at the volar medial aspect of the metacarpal base. PA (Fig. 64C) and oblique (Fig. 64D) views of the left hand coned on the thumb in another patient demonstrate an impacted comminuted intra-articular fracture of the thumb metacarpal base; the pattern of comminution can be described as either "T-shaped" or "Y-shaped."

DIFFERENTIAL DIAGNOSIS Bennett fracture, Rolando fracture, Epibasal fracture a.k.a. pseudo-Bennett fracture, first carpometacarpal (CMC) dislocation.

DIAGNOSIS Intra-articular first metacarpal fracture: Bennet fracture (Figs. 64A and B), Rolando fracture (Figs. 64B and C).

DISCUSSION The first CMC joint is a common site of degenerative disease and acute trauma. The majority of fractures involving the first metacarpal are seen at the metacarpal base. These fractures usually result from axial loading on a flexed thumb, as may occur in a fist fight. An oblique fracture involving the base of the thumb and the articular surface is called a Bennett fracture, of which the most common morphology is a triangular volar lip fragment. If the fracture is comminuted and intra-articular, it is termed a Rolando fracture; fracture lines may appear to form a Y-shape or T-shape. The Bennett fracture is more common than the Rolando fracture. A base of thumb metacarpal fracture that does not involve the joint surface has been called a pseudo-Bennett or epibasal fracture.

The strong thumb adductor muscles insert at the base of the thumb, making the metacarpal very prone to subluxation in the setting of a first metacarpal base fracture. The proximal medial fragment is likely to stay in articulation with the carpus because of the action of the volar oblique ligament, whereas the shaft is pulled dorsally and laterally by the actions of the extensor pollicis tendons and the abductor pollicis longus.

At first glance, these fractures may seem innocuous, but as discussed earlier, they can be very unstable because of the forces applied by the surrounding musculature. The majority of intra-articular base of thumb fractures will require surgery. Rolando fractures carry a worse prognosis than do Bennett fractures. Extra-articular, that is, epibasal or pseudo-Bennett, are much more likely to be stable and treated with more conservative measures. Posttraumatic osteoarthritis is a common complication of these injuries.

Orthogonal radiographs are usually sufficient for diagnosis. However, on routine views of the hand, the first CMC joint is always imaged in some degree of obliquity. A true lateral view of the first CMC joint, achieved by pronating the hand 15° to 35°, may be helpful. Occasionally, CT is used to search for occult fracture, and MRI to evaluate associated soft tissue injury.

Questions for Further Thought

1. A woman presents with hand pain after a skiing accident in which her hand was jammed into the base of her skiing pole. Radiographs show an avulsion fracture at the ulnar aspect of the first proximal phalanx. What is the name of this fracture?
2. A first metacarpal base fracture may be associated with fracture of what adjacent carpal bone?

Reporting Responsibilities

Bennett and Rolando fractures are not surgical emergencies; a timely report is required.

What the Treating Physician Needs to Know

- Degree of comminution, angulation, and involvement of joint surfaces is most important.
- Both Bennett and Rolando fractures are unstable and usually require internal fixation.

Answers

1. Gamekeeper's thumb or Skier's thumb. The ulnar aspect of the first metacarpophalangeal joint is the insertion site of the ulnar collateral ligament.
2. The trapezium. Trapezium fractures are rare, but when present, are often seen in association with a first metacarpal base fracture or dislocation. They most commonly result from direct or indirect axial loading.

CLINICAL HISTORY *57-year-old male presenting with an enlarging right neck mass and progressive dysphagia.*

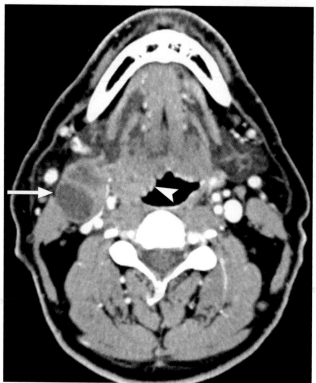

FIGURE 65A

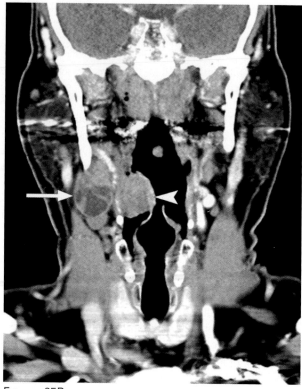

FIGURE 65B

FINDINGS Figures 65A and 65B: Axial (Fig. 65A) and coronal (Fig. 65B) contrast-enhanced CT images of the neck demonstrate an ovoid mixed solid and cystic density mass in the right neck (*arrow*) situated just inferior to the mandibular angle and anteromedial to the sternocleidomastoid muscle. In addition, there is increased and asymmetric soft tissue situated along the right tongue base and lateral pharyngeal wall (*arrowhead*).

DIFFERENTIAL DIAGNOSIS When faced with a new neck mass in a patient over the age of 40 years, malignancy should be considered the primary diagnosis until proven otherwise, and in this case, *metastatic lymphadenopathy* from an oropharyngeal cancer should be the main concern. Other neoplastic causes of cervical lymphadenopathy include metastases from cancers of the skin, parotid gland, and thyroid, as well as *lymphoma*. In children and adults under the age of 40, the majority of posterior and lateral neck masses represent *inflammatory lymphadenopathy* (although the likelihood of neoplasm goes up with increasing age). Infectious causes of lymph node enlargement include *suppurative bacterial adenitis, mycobacterial (tuberculous and nontuberculous) lymphadenitis, cat scratch disease,* and *actinomycosis.* These entities can all present with cystic or necrotic lymphadenopathy. A *second branchial cleft cyst* can also present as a cystic mass in this location; however, these usually present

in childhood and should not demonstrate significant soft tissue elements or enhancement, although they may show peripheral enhancement if infected.

DIAGNOSIS Squamous cell carcinoma (SCC) of the oropharynx with metastatic jugulodigastric (level II) lymphadenopathy.

DISCUSSION The differential diagnosis for neck masses is broad, but it is important to remember that in adult patients over the age of 40, most represent malignancy. In fact, roughly 80% of neck masses in this demographic are neoplastic, and of those, 80% are malignant. Among head and neck malignancies, SCC is far and away the most common, accounting for more than 90% of cases. Head and neck SCC affects men twice as often as women, and is strongly associated with tobacco and alcohol use. Although the overall incidence of head and neck SCC has declined over the past two decades because of a decline in smoking, there has been an increase in the incidence of oropharyngeal SCCs associated with high-risk human papillomavirus (HPV) infection, particularly HPV-16. As a result, the proportion of head and neck SCC caused by HPV has increased. Fortunately, HPV-associated tumors appear to have a better prognosis than HPV-negative tumors for both surgical and nonsurgical therapies.

Patients with SCC of the head and neck can present with symptoms related to the primary tumor that vary by site, but those with cancers of the pharynx and supraglottic larynx can also present with a painless neck mass because of metastatic lymphadenopathy, as was the case here. Depending upon the primary tumor site, anywhere from 30% to 90% of patients with head and neck SCC have evidence of regional nodal metastases at the time of presentation. The imaging features that should raise the most concern for lymph node metastases on imaging are the presence of central necrosis/lucency or extracapsular tumor extension (indicated by shaggy, irregular, or poorly defined nodal margins and surrounding fat stranding). Interestingly, lymph node metastases from HPV-positive cancers are more likely to appear cystic, and in some instances may appear completely cystic, mimicking the appearance of a developmental cyst. Increased nodal size is also a useful, though less specific, feature of metastatic disease. If one uses long-axis measurements, lymph nodes in the neck should be considered pathologic if they exceed 15 mm in maximal longitudinal diameter at the submandibular (level Ib) or jugulodigastric (level IIa) stations, and 10 mm elsewhere in the neck (excluding retropharyngeal nodes). If short axis diameter is used, nodes should be considered abnormal if they exceed 11 mm in minimal diameter at level IIa and 10 mm elsewhere. Regardless of the size criteria used, however, one can expect an overall error rate of roughly 15% to 20% for both false positives and false negatives when size alone is used. Lymph node morphology can be helpful in improving diagnostic specificity. Nodes that are rounded, have lost their normal fatty hilum, or are clustered in groups should be viewed with a higher degree of suspicion, particularly when they are borderline in size.

If metastatic lymphadenopathy is suspected, as it should be in this case, a careful survey of the aerodigestive tract should be undertaken to try to identify the primary site of malignancy. Primary sites that tend to metastasize initially to the jugulodigastric nodal group include the pharynx, supraglottic larynx, and posterior oral cavity, with the most common primary sites for isolated nodal metastasis being the oropharynx and nasopharynx. It is also particularly important to assess the number and laterality of lymph node metastases (relative to the primary site) and for the findings of extracapsular spread, as all of these factors can influence treatment decisions and overall prognosis.

Question for Further Thought

1. Why are cancers of the glottis less likely to present with metastatic cervical lymphadenopathy than cancers of the supraglottic larynx?

Reporting Responsibilities

It is critical in situations such as this one for the radiologist to clearly communicate the high likelihood malignancy based on the imaging findings, even if the clinical suspicion for cancer is low. Although it may be reasonable to treat patients conservatively in the emergency setting, particularly in situations in which an infectious or inflammatory etiology is suspected clinically and an aerodigestive tract lesion is not evident, these lesions should all be followed up to resolution. For lesions that fail to resolve with conservative treatment, fine needle aspiration for tissue sampling should be suggested.

What the Treating Physician Needs to Know

- What is the most likely etiology of the neck mass?
- If neoplastic lymphadenopathy is suspected, is it likely to be primary (i.e., lymphoma) or metastatic? If the latter, what is the most likely site for the primary tumor?
- For cases of metastatic lymphadenopathy, is the nodal disease solitary or multiple? In addition, is nodal involvement unilateral or bilateral?
- Is there evidence of extracapsular spread or involvement of nearby structures (e.g., the carotid artery)?

Answer

1. Cancers of the glottis (true vocal cord) are more likely to present at an early stage because they typically cause significant and persistent symptoms of hoarseness even when very small. On the other hand, cancers of the supraglottic larynx can present more insidiously with nonspecific symptoms and are frequently quite advanced at the time of diagnosis. In addition, compared to the supraglottic larynx, which has a rich lymphatic drainage system, the glottis has a paucity of lymphatics draining it. For these reasons, supraglottic tumors are much more likely to present with metastatic lymphadenopathy than those arising in the glottis. Nodal metastases from glottic cancers typically develop in advanced cases in which the tumor has extended into the supraglottic or subglottic larynx and acquired their lymphatic drainage.

CLINICAL HISTORY *57-year-old male with failure to thrive and cough.*

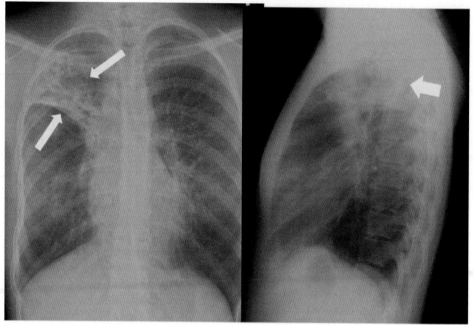

FIGURE 66A

FINDINGS Figure 66A: Posteroanterior (PA) and lateral chest films show a heterogeneous opacity with bronchiectasis and cavities/cysts in the right upper lobe (*yellow arrows*), as well as elevation of minor fissure and superior retraction of right hilum.

DIFFERENTIAL DIAGNOSIS Postprimary tuberculosis, lung cancer, sarcoid.

DIAGNOSIS Postprimary tuberculosis (TB).

DISCUSSION Parenchymal involvement in postprimary TB most commonly manifests as heterogeneous opacities in the apical and posterior segments of the upper lobes, and in the superior segment of the lower lobes, along with bronchiectasis, architectural distortion, calcifications, and residual cavities.[1,2] Predilection of postprimary TB to involve the upper lobes is likely caused by the relatively higher oxygen tension and less robust lymphatic drainage. Because architectural distortion and calcifications may be present in both nonactive and active disease, determination of active TB infection based on radiographs alone is not possible, and must be confirmed by sputum culture,[3] as was done in this patient.

Question for Further Thought

1. If this patient were to present with hemoptysis, what rare complication of TB should be considered?

Reporting Responsibilities

The referring clinician should be immediately notified, so that he or she may place the patient in isolation, then gather accurate history regarding prior TB infections or TB treatment, assess for symptoms of active TB, and collect sputum if necessary.

What the Treating Physician Needs to Know

- Possibility of active TB.
- Chronicity (if old studies are available for comparison).
- Presence or absence of effusions.

Answer

1. Rasmussen aneurysm, which is a pseudoaneurysm of a pulmonary artery caused by inflammation by an adjacent tuberculous cavity.[3]

CLINICAL HISTORY *24-year-old female restrained passenger in a high-speed motor vehicle collision.*

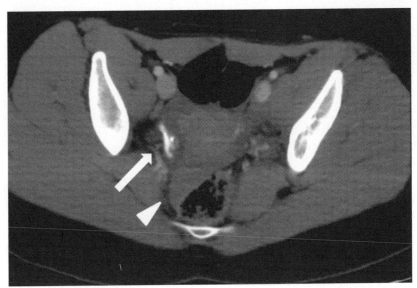

FIGURE 67A

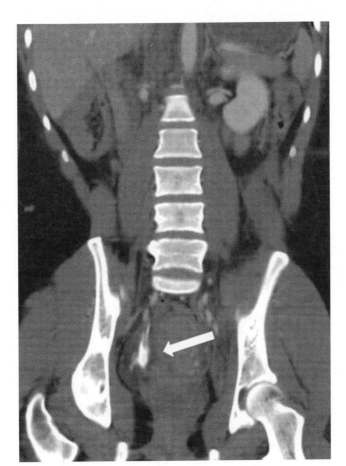

FIGURE 67B

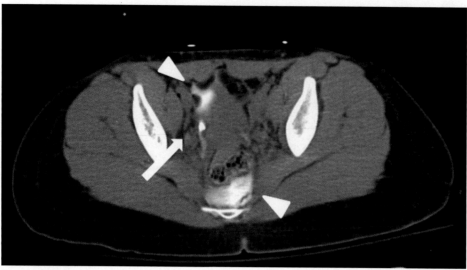

Figure 67C

FINDINGS Figures 67A and 67B: Axial and coronal contrast-enhanced CT images of the pelvis demonstrate a collection of high-density material surrounding the right distal ureter just above the level of the acetabula (*arrows*). The density is greater than that of the arteries. There is low- and high-density fluid in the pelvis (*arrowhead*), likely consisting of urine and hemorrhage. Figure 67C: Axial delayed CT image of the pelvis demonstrates increased amount of extravasated contrasted urine from the right distal ureter (*arrow*) in the anterior and posterior pelvis (*arrowhead*).

DIFFERENTIAL DIAGNOSIS Ureteral injury, active arterial hemorrhage.

DIAGNOSIS Right ureteral injury from blunt trauma.

DISCUSSION Most (80% to 90%) ureteral injuries are iatrogenic, seen after gynecologic surgery (most common), colorectal surgery, vascular surgery, ureteroscopy, or endourologic intervention.[1] Ureteral injury can occur from direct injury or ischemic injury from damage to ureteric vessels. The most common site of injury is the distal third of the ureter.

Traumatic ureteral injury is rare. Traumatic injury is usually from penetrating trauma causing direct ureteral injury, whereas injury from blunt trauma is extremely rare and usually affects the ureteropelvic junction. Delays in diagnosis are common and can occur in up to 50% of patients, usually secondary to the lack of suspicion for ureteral injury, particularly in the setting of significant multiorgan trauma.[1]

Signs and symptoms are nonspecific and may include gross hematuria, abdominal pain/tenderness, elevated blood urea nitrogen and creatinine levels, vaginal urinary leakage, and fever.

Contrast-enhanced computed tomography (CT) is the primary imaging technique used to evaluate the upper and lower urinary tract for trauma. Findings on CT include perinephric stranding, perinephric or periureter hematoma, and low-density fluid around the kidney and ureters. If these findings are detected on initial CT scan, delayed excretory phase imaging of the kidneys and ureters or CT urogram should be performed. On delayed images, contrast extravasation from the genitourinary (GU) tract or partial or complete ureteral obstruction can be seen in patients with ureteral injury. Also, urinary ascites and urinoma can be detected on CT.

If a CT cystogram is to be performed, a noncontrast scan should be performed prior to filling the bladder because contrast may track down the ureter around the bladder, which could mimic a bladder rupture. Cystoscopy with retrograde pyelography is the best procedure for detecting ureteral injuries in the stable patient, and also allows for ureteral stent placement in the same session, if needed.

Treatment includes nephroureteral stenting or surgical repair. Delayed diagnosis can lead to stricture and hydronephrosis with resultant kidney injury and sepsis.

Questions for Further Thought

1. Do ureteral injuries occur more often with laparoscopic or open surgery?
2. Does the ureteral injury have to occur at the time of surgery?
3. Should delayed images be performed routinely in trauma patients?

Reporting Responsibilities

Traumatic ureteral injuries are urgent findings requiring prompt reporting. However, other surgeries or interventions may take priority. Delayed excretory CT images or CT urogram should be recommended if subtle findings are found on the initial CT or if there is high clinical suspicion for ureteral injury.

What the Treating Physician Needs to Know

- The level of the ureteral injury.
- Complications of ureteral injury including urinoma, abscess formation, ureteral strictures, and fistula formation.

Answers

1. Ureter injury is believed to be more common with laparoscopic surgery than open surgery.
2. Thermal injury to a ureter during surgery can lead to delayed necrosis of the ureter, which usually presents 10 to 14 days after surgery. The initial cystoscopy or CT urogram may be normal with the ureteral injury presenting weeks later.
3. Routine delayed CT images of the kidney and ureters are not recommended unless subtle findings such as perinephric stranding, or perinephric or periureter hematoma or fluid are identified.

CLINICAL HISTORY *42-year-old female with lateral left foot pain following forced inversion injury while ballroom dancing.*

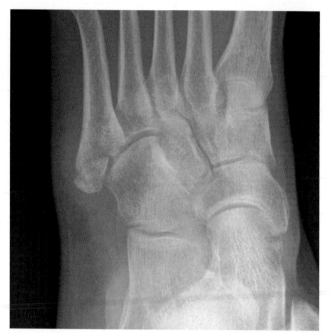

FIGURE 68A

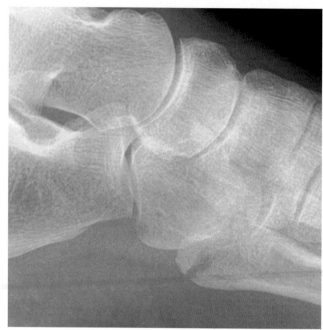

FIGURE 68B

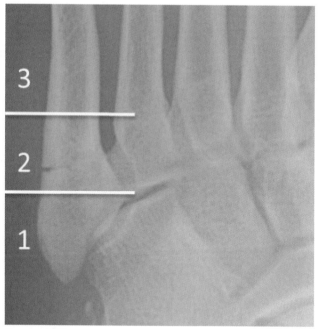

FIGURE 68C

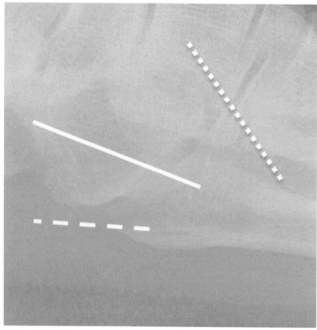

FIGURE 68D

FINDINGS Oblique and lateral views of the left foot (Figs. 68A and 68B) reveal a transverse fracture of the fifth metatarsal base approximately 1.0 cm from the proximal tuberosity with mild posterior displacement of the proximal fragment. The fracture extends into the tarsometatarsal joint. Annotations on an oblique radiograph of the foot in another patient (Fig. 68C) demonstrate the zones of fracture in the fifth metatarsal base. Zone 1 = avulsion fractures. Zone 2 = Jones fractures. Zone 3 = stress fractures. A transverse fracture of the fifth metatarsal base extends into the intermetatarsal articulation and lies within Zone 2. The zoomed-in portion of a lateral foot radiograph in another patient (Fig. 68D) demonstrates the important soft tissue attachment sites on the base of the fifth metatarsal: the *solid white line* represents the approximate course and attachment of the peroneus brevis tendon, the *dashed white line* represents the approximate course and attachment of the lateral bundle of the plantar fascia/aponeurosis, and the *dotted white line* represents the approximate course and attachment of the peroneus tertius tendon.

DIFFERENTIAL DIAGNOSIS Jones fracture, avulsion fracture (a.k.a. pseudo-Jones or dancer's fracture), unfused apophysis, os peroneum.

DIAGNOSIS Case 1: Fifth metatarsal base avulsion fracture extending into the tarsometatarsal joint (pseudo-Jones fracture). Case 2: Fifth metatarsal base avulsion fracture extending into the intermetatarsal joint (Jones fracture).

DISCUSSION The proximal fifth metatarsal is a common site of fracture in the foot. The term Jones fracture has been used to refer to any fracture of the proximal fifth metatarsal. However, differentiation between a true Jones fracture and an avulsion fracture of the proximal metatarsal tuberosity is important. Both fractures typically occur following forceful inversion and adduction of the foot while in plantarflexion. Although both fractures are caused by an avulsive force, the actual location of the fracture in relation to the surrounding tendon attachment sites (discussed in detail later) has consequences for prognosis and treatment course. The Jones fracture is a transverse fracture at the metaphyseal–diaphyseal junction 1.5 to 3 cm from the proximal metatarsal tuberosity that extends into the intermetatarsal articulation. The majority of avulsion fractures, also transverse in orientation, of the proximal tuberosity are either entirely proximal to the tarsometatarsal joint or may extend into the tarsometatarsal joint. Potential mimics of a base of fifth metatarsal fracture include an unfused apophysis, which is oriented longitudinally along the metatarsal, or os peroneum, which is a very common accessory ossicle within the peroneus longus tendon typically found proximal to the metatarsal base adjacent to the cuboid bone.

There are three primary tendinous attachments to the fifth metatarsal base.[1] The lateral component of the plantar aponeurosis (LPA) attaches to the most proximal, inferior surface. The peroneus brevis tendon (PBT) attaches distal to the LPA on the dorsolateral surface with a broad-based attachment site. The peroneus tertius tendon (PTT) attaches distal to the PBT on the dorsolateral surface. The attachment sites loosely correspond to the portions of the metatarsal associated with the tarsometatarsal and intermetatarsal joints, respectively. The primary avulsive mechanics in avulsion fractures of the proximal tuberosity are applied predominantly by the LPA.[2] These fractures may be treated conservatively with weight-bearing immobilization because

there is limited potential motion of the fracture fragment. In general, avulsion fractures of the proximal tuberosity have a low risk of nonunion. The avulsive mechanics in Jones fractures are applied predominantly by the PBT. The fracture occurs between the attachment sites of the PBT and PTT with proximal and superior tension placed on the proximal fracture fragment while the metatarsal shaft is held in a relatively stable position. Jones fractures have a higher rate of displacement and nonunion than do avulsion fractures of the tuberosity not just because of the forces exerted on it by the PBT, but also because of the relatively poor vascular supply as the metaphyseal–diaphyseal junction is a watershed perfusion zone. Therefore, Jones fractures are better treated with strict immobilization and non–weight-bearing status. If there is nonunion or displacement of more than 3 to 4 mm following conservative treatment, internal fixation with or without bone grafting may become necessary.

Imaging evaluation of traumatic lateral foot pain starts with dorsal–plantar, oblique, and lateral radiographs of the involved foot. Identification of the location of the fracture in relation to the proximal tuberosity is important to differentiate a Jones fracture from an avulsion fracture of the proximal tuberosity. It is also important to evaluate for extension into the tarsometatarsal joint or intermetatarsal articulation, a marker for the fracture's relative position in relation to the PBT and PTT. If the radiographs are unrevealing and there is continued clinical suspicion for a fracture, then appropriate management with repeat radiographs at least 14 days from the date of injury would be recommended. If a more immediate diagnosis is needed or if there is concern for tendon or ligament injury, then MRI can be considered.

Questions for Further Thought

1. How do the dynamic forces placed by the tendinous attachments on the fifth metatarsal affect the healing process of the fracture?
2. Where do fifth metatarsal stress fractures occur?

Reporting Responsibilities

Base of fifth metatarsal fractures are not emergencies; a timely report is required.

What the Treating Physician Needs to Know

- Simple versus comminuted.
- Fracture location in relation to the metatarsal proximal tuberosity (Jones fracture vs. avulsion fracture of the tuberosity).
- Extension into the tarsometatarsal or intermetatarsal joints.
- Presence of foreign body or soft tissue gas.
- Displacement of the fracture.

Answers

1. The dynamic forces of the tendons attached to the fracture fragments result in continued strain across the fracture site that can cause delayed healing, increased displacement, or nonunion. This is especially true of the PBT, where the pulley effect as it wraps around the lateral malleolus results in particularly high distractive force on the base of the fifth metatarsal.

2. Stress fractures of the proximal fifth metatarsal are the least common fracture type in this area. They occur distal to the typical site of Jones fracture, approximately 1.5 cm distal to the metaphyseal–diaphyseal junction (Zone 3 in Fig. 68C).

CLINICAL HISTORY *27-year-old man involved in a high-speed motorcycle-versus-car collision with a poor neurologic examination.*

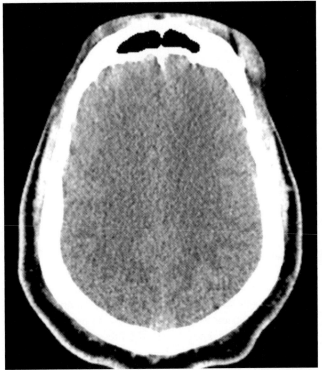

FIGURE 69A

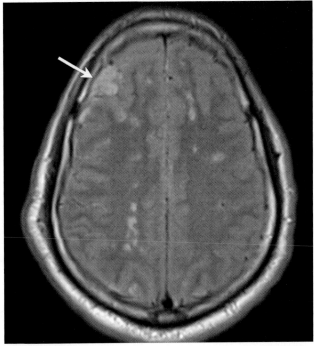

FIGURE 69B

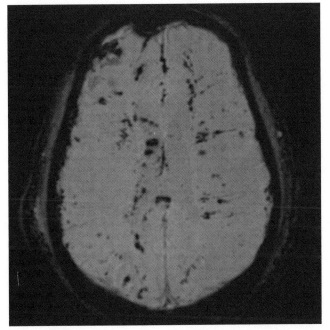

FIGURE 69C

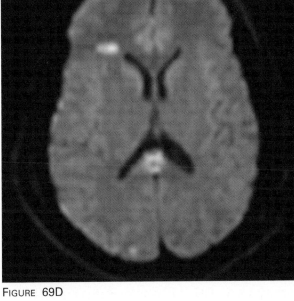

FIGURE 69D

FINDINGS Figure 69A: Noncontrast head CT image demonstrates effacement of the cortical sulci, suggesting edema, but preservation of gray–white differentiation. There was also evidence of subarachnoid and intraventricular hemorrhage (not shown), but no definite intraparenchymal hemorrhage is seen. Figures 69B to 69D are images from a subsequent MRI performed 3 days later because of continued poor neurologic examination and clinical suspicion for traumatic brain injury (TBI). Figure 69B: FLAIR image at a roughly comparable level to Figure 69A shows multiple punctate hyperintensities in the white matter of the centrum semiovale. There is also a more confluent area of cortical hyperintensity in the right frontal lobe, compatible with a cortical contusion. Figure 69C: Susceptibility-weighted imaging (SWI) demonstrates multiple punctate and linear foci of dark signal, most prominently at the gray–white matter junction throughout the cerebrum and corpus callosum. Figure 69D: Diffusion-weighted image (DWI) demonstrates areas of increased signal within the brain and splenium of the corpus callosum that were restricted on the ADC map (not shown). Postcontrast imaging is not shown, but these lesions did not demonstrate contrast enhancement.

DIFFERENTIAL DIAGNOSIS The history limits the differential to diffuse axonal injury (DAI) and related hemorrhages. Absent the history of trauma, the differential for multifocal nonhemorrhagic lesions include embolic infarcts, leukoaraiosis, and demyelinating disease. Multifocal hemorrhagic lesions could be due to cerebral amyloid angiopathy in the elderly, chronic hypertensive hemorrhages, multiple cavernous malformations, and hemorrhagic metastases. The distribution and signal characteristics of these lesions would not be characteristic these entities, however.

DIAGNOSIS Traumatic brain injury with DAI and cerebral hemorrhages.

DISCUSSION In cases of DAI, the neurologic examination typically does not improve over the days following the trauma and is often disproportionately worse than the findings on the initial trauma CT would lead one to suspect. This history should raise concern for TBI and DAI, and MRI is the next step in management. The underlying mechanism of DAI is shear injury caused by a sudden deceleration of the head and change in angular momentum. The predilection for hemorrhage and injury at the gray–white matter junction is caused by the cortex rotating at a different speed in relation to white matter. Despite multiple findings on MRI, the majority of lesions on autopsy are usually still occult on imaging secondary to factors at the cellular level.

The dark signal of the these lesions on SWI results from the high susceptibility effects of hemosiderin iron deposition following hemorrhage. Dark (black) signal on MR is typically one of three things: dense calcification, gas/air, or old hemosiderin/blood. FLAIR and T2 abnormalities represent edema, while foci of restricted diffusion represent decreased motion of water molecules indicative of focal neuronal injury and cell death.

SWI is an important sequence to include when TBI has occurred because of the sensitivity for hemorrhage and blood products. The FLAIR sequence is generally the most sensitive for nonhemorrhagic lesions.

The Adams–Gennarelli staging categorizes mild, moderate, and severe DAI and provides some basis for prognosis in regard to expected recovery and morbidity/mortality:

Stage 1: Frontal and temporal lobe gray–white matter interface lesions (mild traumatic brain injury [TBI])

Stage 2: Lesions in lobar white matter and corpus callosum (moderate TBI)

Stage 3: Lesions of dorsolateral midbrain and upper pons (severe TBI)

Because the development of DAI is usually caused by high-speed injuries, it is often seen in association with other intracranial abnormalities, including parenchymal contusions, subarachnoid hemorrhage, and subdural and epidural hematomas.

Question for Further Thought

1. What is the prognosis for patients with diffuse axonal injury?

Reporting Responsibilities

Communicating the extent of the injury is important to provide prognostic information to clinicians, patients, and family members. In the acute setting, it is important to let the treating physicians know about the presence of associated hemorrhages or mass effect that could cause imminent death or disability. The findings of DAI are ultimately only of prognostic value because there is currently no proven treatment for DAI.

What the Treating Physician Needs to Know

- Is there evidence of DAI? If so, how extensive is the lesion burden, and where are the lesions located?
- Are there other associated intracranial abnormalities?
- Is there significant mass effect or evidence to suggest impending brain herniation?

Answer

1. Mild TBI and DAI may cause persistent clinical symptoms for months or longer, with symptoms including headaches, memory loss, mild cognitive impairment, personality changes, and postconcussive syndromes. Severe DAI rarely directly causes death, but more than 90% of patients with severe shearing injuries will remain in a persistent vegetative state. Up to 10%, however, may return to almost normal function within 1 year. Neurocognitive deficits persist in approximately 100% of severe, 67% of moderate, and 10% of mild cases of DAI. A greater number of lesions correlate with a poorer outcome.

CLINICAL HISTORY *58-year-old male with shortness of breath.*

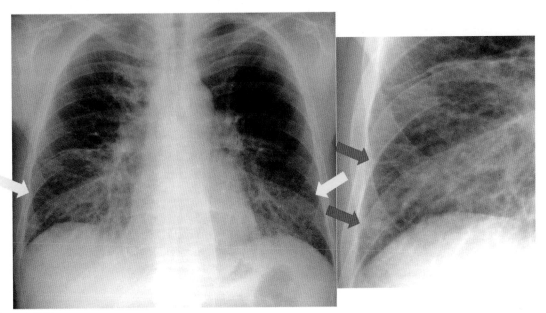

FIGURE 70A

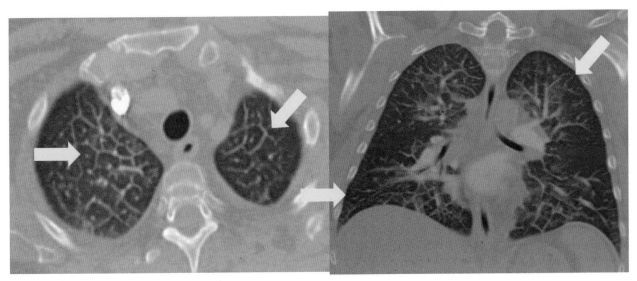

FIGURE 70B

FINDINGS Figure 70A: Posteroanterior (PA) plain film of the chest and coned-down view of the same image. Kerley B lines, or thickened interlobular septa (*yellow arrows*). Coned-down view shows Kerley B lines extending to the pleura (*red arrows*). The hila are indistinct and assume a "fluffy" appearance. Figure 70B: Axial and coronal CT image of the chest. Both images show interlobular septal thickening (*yellow arrows*), outlining the secondary pulmonary lobule.

DIFFERENTIAL DIAGNOSIS Pulmonary edema (interstitial), pulmonary fibrosis, lymphangitic carinomatosis, sarcoidosis.

DIAGNOSIS Pulmonary edema (interstitial).

DISCUSSION Pulmonary edema occurs owing to pulmonary venous hypertension and distension of the lymphatics within the lungs. The etiologies can be grouped into four general categories: (1) Increased hydrostatic pressure edema caused by left heart failure, fluid overload, acute mitral insufficiency, COPD, acute asthma, upper airway obstruction, pulmonary embolism, veno-occlusive disease, and near drowning, (2) Permeability edema caused by primary or secondary insult to the alveoli results in leaky vascular endothelium, common

143

in septicemia, (3) Permeability edema without direct alveolar insult may be caused by high altitude, cytokine administration, and opiate overdose, (4) Mixed edema, which occurs postpneumonectomy, postlung transplantation, after reexpansion of a collapsed lung, or after reperfusion. In addition to Kerley lines, indistinct hila, and peribronchial cuffing, azygos vein distension and enlargement of the cardiac silhouette can occur. If fluid begins to accumulate in the alveolar spaces, perihilar opacities and ground-glass opacities will be present. Pleural effusions occur when increased hydrostatic pressures in the pleural lymphatics cause leak into pleural space.[1]

Question for Further Thought

1. What is the most common cause of *asymmetric* pulmonary edema?

Reporting Responsibilities

The interpreting radiologist should consider clinical history and any previous chest imaging for comparison. The patient's history as well as disease chronology is critical for determining urgency and course of action. For instance, if the edema has worsened significantly in a short time or is related to acute respiratory distress syndrome (ARDS), this represents a clinical emergency requiring urgent diuresis or mechanical ventilation, respectively.

What the Treating Physician Needs to Know

- Extent and severity of the edema.
- Timing when compared with a previous imaging study (if available).
- Any associated findings that might provide a clue to the etiology if unknown.

Answer

1. Emphysema causes parenchymal destruction, which often results in patchy or asymmetric edema because areas of destroyed lung are less perfused (V/Q matching) and, therefore, are typically less prone to edema. Other causes of asymmetric edema include: dependent edema (patient position), acute radiation, pulmonary vein stenosis, and acute mitral valve disease.[2]

CLINICAL HISTORY *54-year-old man with recurrent suprapubic pain and diarrhea.*

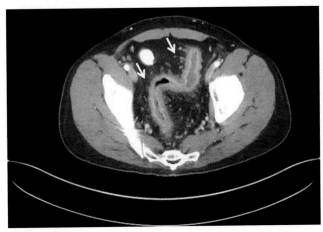

FIGURE 71A

FINDINGS Figure 71A: Axial contrast-enhanced CT scan of the pelvis demonstrates wall thickening and stratification of the rectum, sigmoid colon, and descending colon, with increased enhancement of the mucosa, prominent vasa recta, and stranding in the adjacent fat (*arrows*). The remaining bowel is normal.

DIFFERENTIAL DIAGNOSIS Inflammatory bowel disease—Crohn disease or ulcerative colitis, infectious proctocolitis, diverticulitis.

DIAGNOSIS Ulcerative proctocolitis.

DISCUSSION Proctocolitis refers to the inflammation of the rectum and colon. The causes of inflammation are myriad and often difficult to diagnose clinically or by imaging. Ulcerative colitis is a chronic idiopathic inflammatory bowel disease that involves the rectum and extends from the rectum to more proximal areas of the colon in a continuous fashion. Eventually, the entire colon may be involved. Typically, patients with ulcerative proctocolitis present with rectal bleeding and abdominal pain. The main role of imaging is to exclude other causes of abdominal pain at initial presentation and to exclude major complications, such as bowel perforation. Definitive diagnosis of ulcerative proctocolitis requires corroboration with clinical history, endoscopy, and histology.

In the acute to subacute phase of ulcerative colitis, erosion of the bowel mucosa may leave a residual island of regenerative tissue or pseudopolyp, which has been mistaken for a villous adenoma or polypoid carcinoma. Colonic polyposis syndrome may mimic multiple pseudopolyps related to ulcerative colitis. A constricting infiltrative or ulcerative mass indicates malignant transformation. Ulcerative colitis may also present with chronic strictures related to local sequelae of severe inflammation. Advanced cases may demonstrate diffuse loss of mucosal folds and decreased haustration, leading to a lead-pipe configuration. This may subsequently lead to recurrent pancolitis and toxic megacolon in about 5% of the patients with markedly dilated colon to at least 6 cm and associated symptoms. Backwash ileitis may also occur if the disease progresses from the cecum into the terminal ileum.

On computed tomography (CT), inflammation in ulcerative proctocolitis involves a continuous segment of the rectum and a variable amount of colon. There is concentric mural wall thickening and luminal dilatation of the involved bowel segment and increased prominence of the adjacent vessels. Increased enhancement of the colonic mucosa and the muscularis propria leads to stratification or a target sign when visualized en face. This may be identified in the acute phase, but ulcers are often difficult to appreciate. In more severe inflammation, pneumatosis may occur. Stranding in the pericolic fat and ascites are nonspecific signs that can be present.

Mild disease confined to the rectum may be treated with topical anti-inflammatory drugs. Combined oral and topical therapy, systemic steroids, immunosuppressants, monoclonal antibodies, and supportive treatment are considered for those with more advanced or severe disease. Fulminant disease or toxic megacolon refractory to medical management, uncontrolled bleeding, and bowel perforation with abscesses and peritonitis are indications for surgery.

Questions for Further Thought

1. Should barium enema be done after CT to confirm proctocolitis?
2. What are some major differences between ulcerative colitis and Crohn disease?

Reporting Responsibilities

Findings of acute ulcerative colitis and associated complications, including bowel perforation and peritonitis, should be emergently reported to the referring clinician.

What the Treating Physician Needs to Know

- Definitive diagnosis of ulcerative colitis requires endoscopy and histology. Imaging is more of a preliminary tool to exclude other sites of inflammation.
- Extent and location of disease, extraluminal findings, and complications.
- Signs of bowel perforation or malignancy, because the risks of lymphoma and carcinoma are increased.
- Etiologies of isolated proctocolitis without involvement of other viscera cannot be differentiated from each other.

Answers

1. Barium enema can demonstrate early superficial mucosal disease, with typical findings of stippled mucosa, punctate barium collections in flask-shaped collar-button-like ulcers, and inflammatory pseudopolyps. Depiction of the ulcerated mucosal pattern is superior on barium enema, although that requires trained expertise and is not favored for acute presentations. Consequently, because endoscopic evaluation with histology is essential, proceeding with barium enema after a CT study to evaluate the mucosa is often not necessary, unless the patient declines to undergo endoscopy. If the patient is too sick to undergo endoscopy, barium enema is also not advisable.

2. There are major differences between ulcerative colitis and Crohn disease. Ulcerative colitis is a continuous process from the rectum to the colon with predominantly distal and left-sided involvement, and superficial mucosal erosions, whereas in Crohn disease, there is transmural inflammation, deep fissuring, and fistulation with skip areas of bowel involvement.

CLINICAL HISTORY *10-month-old boy with left lower extremity erythema and tenderness.*

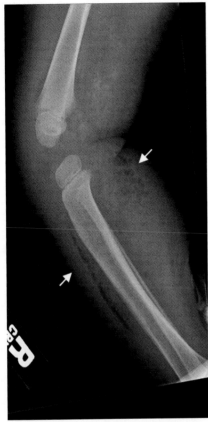

FIGURE 72A

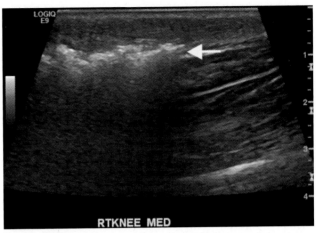

FIGURE 72B

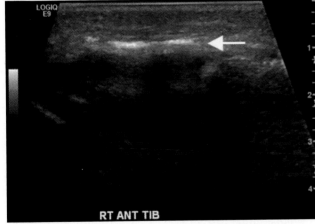

FIGURE 72C

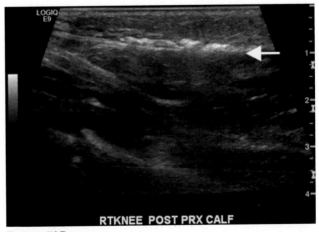

FIGURE 72D

FINDINGS Lateral radiograph of the right leg (Fig. 72A) demonstrates subcutaneous gas along the anterior and posterior lower leg (*arrows*); the anterior soft tissue gas is oriented in a linear fashion along the interface between the subcutaneous tissues and the underlying muscular compartment, which is invested by the deep fascia. Figures 72B to 72D demonstrate different sonographic appearances of soft tissue gas (*arrow*), from very echogenic reflectors with extensive posterior streak artifact resulting in complete obscuration of the tissues deep to the gas (Fig. 72B) to much more subtle foci of hyperintensity

147

along the superficial fascia with relatively preserved appearance of the soft tissues deep to the gas (Fig. 72D).

DIFFERENTIAL DIAGNOSIS Postsurgical changes, recent instrumentation or laparoscopic insufflation, infection with a gas-forming organism (necrotizing fasciitis).

DIAGNOSIS Necrotizing fasciitis.

DISCUSSION Necrotizing fasciitis is a rare form of a severe soft tissue infection with a high morbidity and mortality. The infection spreads from the subcutaneous tissues to the deep fascial layers that surround the musculature. Infection usually rapidly spreads along the fascia to involve large regions of the soft tissues.

Infections causing necrotizing soft tissue infections can be broadly divided into two categories. Type 1 consists of a polymicrobial infection, whereas type 2 infections are caused by group A *Streptococcus* and *Staphylococcus* species. In the pediatric population, type 1 infections have been described to be more prevalent in infants less than 1 year of age. In addition, there appears to be a predilection for younger children, in general, to develop the disease, with the annual incidence quoted as substantially higher in children younger than 5 years old (5.9 vs. 1.8 per million).[1] General risk factors for development of this condition in this population include a history of chronic illness, surgery, trauma, as well as recent infection with varicella.

Necrotizing infections can be very difficult to distinguish from their nonnecrotizing forms based on initial presentation. Physical examination usually reveals erythema, swelling, and pain for both. Although the diagnosis of necrotizing fasciitis does not rely on imaging, the absence or presence of gas within the soft tissues has been found to be highly associated with a necrotizing infection. One study found that of all the possible imaging findings on CT evaluation, subcutaneous gas was noted to be the most reliable finding that could help discern between necrotizing and nonnecrotizing infections (Odds Ratio 23).[2] Although described on CT, this distinguishing factor is likely to be generally applicable to gas identified on other modalities as well.

Radiography is a reasonable modality to begin with because soft tissue gas can be readily identified in an expeditious manner. Ultrasonography has also become a larger part of the initial Emergency Department evaluation. The lack of ionizing radiation and increasing availability of bedside sonography units makes this modality a reasonable first advanced imaging modality for the identification of soft tissue gas if radiographs are normal. Gas bubbles appear as small, highly echogenic foci; in the setting of necrotizing fasciitis, the gas bubbles are arrayed along a fascial plane and may move when observed in real time. Distal to the gas bubbles, there is often an echogenic streak caused by ring-down artifact that obscures the deeper tissues, a potential limitation if more information is needed about the status of the deep soft

tissues. The diagnostic image quality of ultrasonography diminishes with increasing thickness of adipose tissue because the intensity of sound waves returned to the transducer diminishes with increasing depth. Therefore, ultrasonography currently is felt to be of most utility in the pediatric population[2] or adult patients with lower body mass index.

Contrast-enhanced MRI can also be of use. However, the decreased sensitivity of the modality to the identification of gas, the otherwise largely overlapping findings between necrotizing and nonnecrotizing infections, and long acquisition times make it less desirable as an initial diagnostic tool. Therefore, MRI is more useful in delineating soft tissue extent once the diagnosis of necrotizing infection has been ruled in or out.

Initial therapy consists of appropriate antibiotic therapy and supportive therapy with IV fluids and pain control. Definitive therapy in both pediatric and adult populations remains surgical debridement, with the time to intervention being the most important factor in patient outcomes. Mortality has been quoted to be as high as 59% in the neonatal cohort, but as low as 9.4% in the pediatric population in general.[1] As a result, it is of critical importance that the surgeon be aware of any findings that would support the diagnosis of necrotizing fasciitis.

Questions for Further Thought

1. By definition, what is the Hounsfield unit value of air?
2. What does air look like on MRI? Which sequences would be the most sensitive to the absence/presence of soft tissue gas?
3. How fast can soft tissue destruction occur in the setting of necrotizing infection?

Reporting Responsibilities

Necrotizing fasciitis is a surgical emergency; direct communication with the referring clinician is required.

What the Treating Physician Needs to Know

- Presence or absence of soft tissue gas.
- Extent of involvement to direct the area of debridement.
- Any underlying osseous or joint involvement.

Answers

1. By definition, the Hounsfield unit (HU) of air is set as −1,000. Pure water, as a reference, is set as 0 HU, and fat tends to range from −100 to −50 HU.
2. Unlike in the case of CT, gas is very difficult to detect on MR images. Of the various sequences, the gradient echo sequences are the most sensitive to gas. In those sequences, gas is represented by an area of signal void that demonstrates "blooming" owing to susceptibility artifact.
3. Although estimates may vary, necrosis can occur up to a rate of approximately 1 inch per hour.[1]

CLINICAL HISTORY *26-year-old male involved in a rollover motor vehicle collision, now with right-sided hearing loss and facial paralysis.*

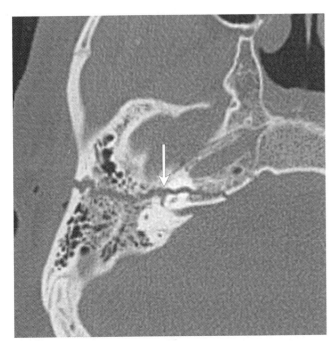

FIGURE 73A

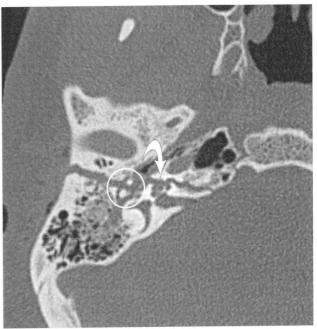

FIGURE 73B

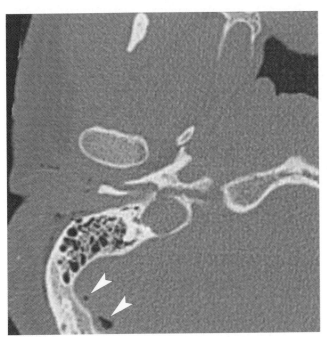

FIGURE 73C

FINDINGS Figures 73A to 73C: Axial unenhanced CT through the right temporal bone demonstrate an obliquely oriented fracture coursing from the lateral mastoid cortex through the petrous apex. The fracture line extends through the fossa for the geniculate ganglion of the facial nerve (*arrow* in Fig. 73A) and through the cochlea (*curved arrow* in

Fig. 73B). There is widening of the malleoincudal joint indicating joint dislocation (*circled area* in Fig. 73B). In Figure 73C, the fracture can be seen to extend through the anterior wall of the external auditory canal and between the carotid canal and jugular foramen. There is also pneumocephalus in the posterior fossa (*arrowheads*), indicating the presence of a CSF fistula.

DIFFERENTIAL DIAGNOSIS There is no differential diagnosis for this case. Occasionally, normal anatomic structures including sutures and fissures as well as neurovascular canals, such as the subarcuate canal and singular canal, may mimic a nondisplaced temporal bone fracture. Recognition of these normal structures can prevent one from misinterpreting them as fractures in the trauma setting.

DIAGNOSIS Oblique temporal bone fracture with involvement of the otic capsule and facial nerve and associated malleoincudal dislocation.

DISCUSSION Among patients presenting to trauma centers with closed head injuries, roughly 10% to 20% have temporal bone fractures evident clinically or by CT. Historically, temporal bone fractures have been classified based on their course relative to the long axis of the petrous pyramid as either longitudinal or transverse fractures. Longitudinal fractures, which account for approximately 80% of temporal bone fractures, classically result from a blow to the temporoparietal region and are directed parallel to the long axis of the petrous pyramid, typically involving squamosal portion of the temporal bone and the posterosuperior wall of the external auditory canal (EAC), with extension through the tegmen mastoideum and tegmen tympani. These fractures often course through the region of the malleoincudal joint and the anterior genu of the facial nerve and, as a result, are often associated with ossicular fractures/dislocations and facial nerve injury. The facial nerve is injured in roughly 25% of patients with longitudinal fractures. Transverse fractures usually occur as a result of severe trauma to the frontal or occipital regions often resulting in loss of consciousness and are oriented perpendicular to the long axis of the petrous pyramid. These fractures may extend through the internal auditory canal (IAC) or across the cochlea and vestibule, so transverse fractures often cause sensorineural hearing loss and vertigo. In addition, approximately 50% of patients with transverse fractures suffer facial nerve injury.

In reality, as is demonstrated in the case here, most temporal bone fractures are obliquely oriented in relationship to the axis of the petrous bone or demonstrate mixed features. Because of this, it has been suggested that it may be more useful to classify these fractures based on whether they involve or spare the otic capsule, as otic capsule disrupting fractures almost always result in sensorineural hearing loss and are also associated with a much higher incidence of facial nerve paralysis.

Dedicated temporal bone CT imaging should be performed for suspected temporal bone fractures and provides information regarding the course of the fracture and the structures involved, including the IAC, otic capsule, facial nerve canal, and ossicular chain. In all cases, the status of the tegmen tympani and tegmen mastoideum should also be determined, because fracture extension through these areas places patients at higher risk for CSF leak and recurrent meningitis. The majority of temporal bone fractures are associated with ipsilateral opacification of the mastoid air cells, and patients who present with signs of a basilar skull fracture and an opacified mastoid without an obvious fracture by CT should be assumed to have an occult temporal bone fracture. Most patients with temporal bone fractures will demonstrate some degree of conductive hearing loss owing to hemotympanum or tympanic membrane perforation; however, persistent conductive hearing loss after these acute findings are resolved (usually by 3 weeks) suggests ossicular chain disruption.

Question for Further Thought

1. What is the most common site of traumatic ossicular chain disruption? What is the second most common?

Reporting Responsibilities

In addition to describing the course of the fracture and structures involved, the report should include a comment on any potentially reversible causes of facial nerve palsy such as hematomas or bone fragments impinging on the facial nerve, as emergent decompressive surgery or intravenous steroid administration may be warranted in certain instances in order to preserve facial nerve function. In addition, extension of the fracture through the petrous carotid canal should be sought for and described as this finding is associated with carotid artery injury in 18% of cases, therefore warranting further imaging with either CTA or MRA.

What the Treating Physician Needs to Know

- What is the course and orientation of the fracture?
- Does the fracture involve the otic capsule?
- Is there evidence of ossicular chain injury?
- Does the fracture involve the course of the facial nerve? If so, is there evidence of correctable causes of facial paralysis (e.g., displaced bone fragments impinging on the nerve)?
- Does the fracture involve the petrous carotid canal?
- Is there evidence of a perilymphatic or CSF fistula? If so, where is the site of communication?

Answer

1. Traumatic ossicular chain disruption most commonly occurs at the incudostapedial joint. The next most common traumatic ossicular abnormality is a fracture of the stapedial arch.

CLINICAL HISTORY *52-year-old male with cough and shortness of breath.*

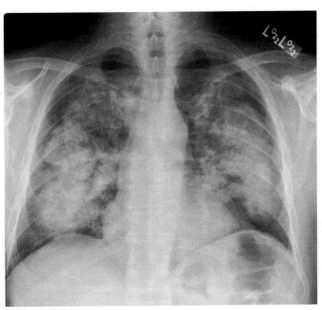

FIGURE 74A

FINDINGS Figure 74A: PA chest film shows bilateral symmetric mostly central parenchymal opacities without pleural effusion.

DIFFERENTIAL DIAGNOSIS Multifocal pneumonia, multifocal well-differentiated adenocarcinoma, sarcoidosis, pulmonary hemorrhage caused by granulomatosis with polyangiitis.

DIAGNOSIS Pulmonary hemorrhage due to granulomatosis with polyangiitis.

DISCUSSION Granulomatosis with polyangiitis (GPA), formerly known as Wegener's granulomatosis, is a cause of pulmonary hemorrhage or diffuse alveolar hemorrhage (DAH). DAH caused by GPA results in diffuse intra-alveolar bleeding from small vessels towing to damage of the alveolocapillary membrane of the lungs.[1] Large alveolar or ground glass opacities are the radiographic manifestation of DAH, and is the second most common radiographic finding after nodules in GPA.[2] The symmetry suggests the process may be systemic, favored over pneumonia or adenocarcinoma.

Question for Further Thought

1. Does hemoptysis have to be present in patients with DAH?

Reporting Responsibilities

DAH should be considered a medical emergency because of the significant morbidity and mortality associated with delayed treatment and should be reported immediately. Correlation with hemoglobin level is paramount.

What the Treating Physician Needs to Know

- Extent of opacities.
- Presence of other manifestations of GPA including nodules, cavitary lesions, and bronchiectasis.

Answer

1. One-third of patients with DAH will not have hemoptysis.[3]

CLINICAL HISTORY *41-year-old female with right upper-quadrant pain, fever, and vomiting.*

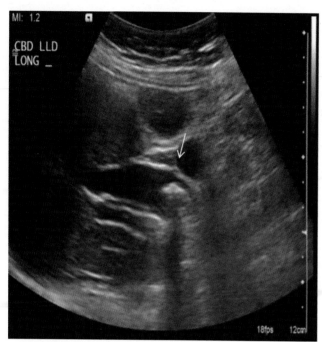

FIGURE 75A

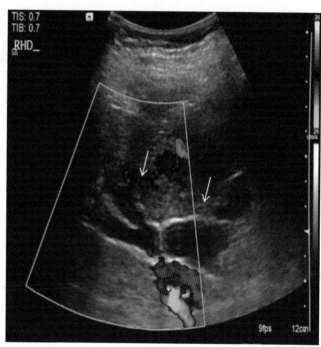

FIGURE 75B

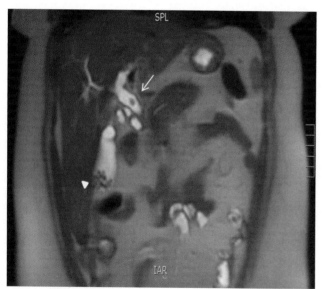

FIGURE 75C

FINDINGS Figure 75A: Longitudinal US image of the common bile duct demonstrates an echogenic focus with posterior shadowing in the distal common bile duct (*arrow*), compatible with choledocholithiasis. The common bile duct is dilated. Figure 75B: Longitudinal color Doppler image of the proximal common bile duct demonstrates dilation of the intra and extrahepatic bile ducts (*arrows*) proximal to the common bile duct stone. Figure 75C: Coronal T2-weighted

MRI image of the abdomen demonstrates a hypointense gallstone in the common bile duct surrounded by hyperintense bile (*arrow*). Common bile duct dilation is identified. In addition, multiple small hypointense gallstones are identified in the gallbladder (*arrowhead*).

DIFFERENTIAL DIAGNOSES Pancreatic or ampullary cancer, cholangiocarcinoma, choledocholithiasis, chronic pancreatitis, blood clot—hemobilia.

DIAGNOSIS Choledocholithiasis.

DISCUSSION Ultrasound imaging is the screening modality of choice for evaluating the biliary tree for choledocholithiasis and biliary obstruction. On ultrasound, a common bile duct stone appears as a round or curvilinear echogenic focus with posterior acoustic shadowing in the common bile duct. There is usually dilation of the bile ducts proximal to the stone depending on the size of the stone. Many common bile duct stones are found in the distal common bile duct near the ampulla of Vater. However, this area is commonly obscured by bowel gas, and an echogenic focus is usually not seen. In these cases, dilation of the common bile duct is usually the characteristic finding that suggests the possibility of an obstructing stone, which then leads to obtaining a magnetic retrograde cholangiopancreatography (MRCP) or endoscopic retrograde cholangiopancreatography (ERCP). Of note, 10% of stones do not produce posterior acoustic shadowing owing to their small size, or soft and porous composition.[1]

MRCP is increasingly used in patients with suspected common bile duct stones because of high sensitivity and specificity. On T2-weighted images, choledocholithiasis appears as characteristic low signal filling defects in the common bile duct. There is typically common bile duct dilation. MRCP can identify other biliary abnormalities and biliary anatomic variations that may potentially lead to complications in surgery.

Choledocholithiasis is defined as stones in the bile ducts and classified into two types based on etiology: primary or secondary. Approximately 5% of bile duct stones are primary, whereas 95% are secondary bile duct stones. Primary duct stones form within the bile ducts and are largely composed of pigment, typically calcium bilirubinate. These bile duct stones typically form in conditions of stasis and/or infected bile. Primary duct stones can be associated with congenital anomalies of bile ducts, such as Caroli's disease, sclerosing cholangitis, cirrhosis, chronic hemolytic disease, low fat/protein diet, biliary surgery, and parasites. Secondary duct stones are gallstones that travel from the gallbladder into the common bile duct.

Choledocholithiasis leads to obstruction and bile stasis that can lead to infection and cause ascending cholangitis and pancreatitis. Stones less than 3 mm usually pass spontaneously and no treatment is necessary. An ERCP with sphincterotomy and stone retrieval is usually performed if a stone is between 3 and 10 mm. For stones larger than 10 mm, lithotripsy is usually required.

Questions for Further Thought

1. In Asian countries, where primary duct stones are more common than the US, what is the etiology?
2. What are some mimics of filling defects on MRCP?

Reporting Responsibilities

Choledocholithiasis should be promptly reported to the referring clinician, so the patient can receive appropriate treatment. If there is suspicion for choledocholithiasis based on the ultrasound, an MRCP or ERCP should be recommended in order to further dictate care.

What the Treating Physician Needs to Know

- Presence of biliary dilatation.
- Size and level of biliary obstruction.
- Presence of other biliary abnormalities and biliary anatomic variations.

Answers

1. Brown pigment stones are more common in Asian populations. Parasites, such as *Ascaris lumbricoides* and *Clonorchis sinensis*, are one of the major causes of pigment common bile duct stones.
2. Artifacts that have the appearance of filling defects on MRCP include gas, blood clot, surgical clip susceptibility artifact, motion/reconstruction artifact, and vascular compression or arterial pulsation artifact.

CLINICAL HISTORY *47-year-old male with a history of shoulder pain secondary to a motor vehicle collision.*

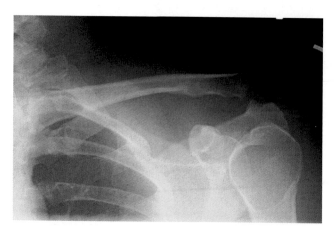

FIGURE 76A

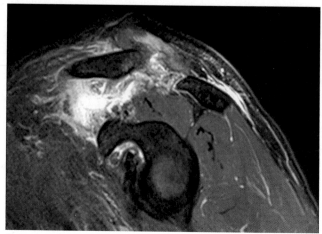

FIGURE 76B

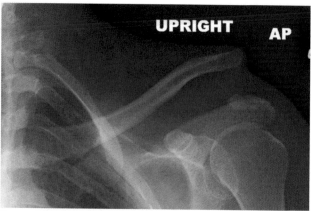

FIGURE 76C

FINDINGS AP view of the left shoulder (Fig. 76A) demonstrates inferior subluxation of the acromion at the acromioclavicular joint of one full clavicular shaft width. The coracoacromial distance is increased. Sagittal T2-weighted fat-suppressed MR image (Fig. 76B) demonstrates a discontinuous coracoclavicular ligament complex with a large amount of intervening fluid. AP view of the left shoulder in another patient (Fig. 76C) demonstrates marked relative inferior dislocation of the acromioclavicular joint associated with marked superior displacement of the distal clavicle, resulting in focal convexity of the subcutaneous tissues.

DIFFERENTIAL DIAGNOSIS Acromioclavicular joint separation with or without coracoclavicular ligament disruption, distal clavicle fracture.

DIAGNOSIS Case 1: Type III acromioclavicular (AC) Joint Separation. Case 2: Type V AC Joint Separation.

DISCUSSION AC joint injuries are involved in 9% to 12% of all shoulder dislocations and account for nearly half of all shoulder injuries among athletes involved in contact sports.[1,2] AC joint injury is usually the result of direct or, less commonly, indirect forces. The most common cause is direct trauma to the acromion, which occurs frequently during contact sports. Falling onto an outstretched arm or elbow can also indirectly lead to an AC joint separation via a superior or lateral force directed through the shoulder, although this is less common.

AC joint separations represent a spectrum of injuries involving the AC joint capsule/ligament, the coracoclavicular (CC) ligament, and the surrounding muscular and fascial structures. The Rockwood classification defines six subtypes of AC joint separation, which are listed here with associated soft tissue pathology and usual radiographic findings:[3]

- Type I: AC joint capsular sprain with intact CC ligament. Normal radiographs.

- Type II: AC joint capsular tear with CC ligament sprain. Widened AC joint with minimal, if any, superior subluxation of the clavicle.

- Type III: Complete disruption of the AC and CC ligaments. Superior subluxation/dislocation of the distal clavicle (no more than one full clavicular shaft width) with associated widening of the CC interval.

- Type IV: Type III plus distal clavicle displaced posteriorly into or through the trapezius muscle.

- Type V: Type III with disruption of the muscular and fascial attachments of the distal clavicle. Marked superior displacement of the distal clavicle; skin tenting may be present.

- Type VI: Type III with inferior displacement of the clavicle disrupting the muscular supporting structures.

Radiographic evaluation of the AC joint is usually sufficient for the diagnosis of an AC joint separation. Routine shoulder radiographs, which include an AP view, should be obtained. Obtaining an AP internal rotation view has been suggested in lieu of a weight-bearing view to separate type I and II separations from type III separations; in the internally rotated position, the scapula (and acromion) is rotated medially forcing the untethered distal clavicle superiorly.[4] An axillary view to establish the AP direction of the distal clavicle is needed for diagnosis of a type IV separation. Evaluation of the AC joint and CC interval should be performed. If findings are subtle or indeterminate, a 10° cephalad view (Zanca view) and/or comparison to the contralateral side can be made. Measurements can also be used: the AC joint width should be no more than 7 mm and the CC distance in an adult should be no greater that 13 mm. It is also important to identify associated injuries such as coracoid fractures, clavicle fractures, or glenohumeral injuries that could be concomitant with an AC joint injury. If there is concern for additional soft tissue injury (e.g., concern for a type V injury, but radiographs are most consistent with a type III injury; concern for a type IV injury with inconclusive axillary radiograph), MRI can be obtained; the coronal plane should be obliqued into the plane of the AC joint.

Type IV to VI AC joint separations always undergo surgical fixation, and type I and II AC joint separations are managed conservatively. Type III AC joint separations may be treated either way depending on the circumstances. A high-performance athlete will likely get a surgical repair, whereas a sedentary individual will more likely be treated conservatively. Conservative treatment consists of rest, ice, pain management, and protection with a sling.

Type V and VI separations may be accompanied by neurologic symptoms related to brachial plexus injury in the acute setting. Long-term complications of an AC joint injury include: pain and weakness, development of AC joint osteoarthrosis, clavicular instability, and posttraumatic osteolysis of the distal clavicle.

Question for Further Thought

1. Is it possible to have a high-grade AC joint separation with an intact CC ligament? If so, how?

Reporting Responsibilities

Acromioclavicular joint separations are in general not emergencies; a timely report is required.

What the Treating Physician Needs to Know

- High-grade separations (types IV to VI) require surgery.
- If there is uncertainty about the presence of concomitant adjacent soft tissue injury or the status of the CC ligament, MRI should be considered.

Answer

1. Yes. A type VI AC joint separation, for example, owing to inferior displacement of the clavicle, reduces tension on the CC ligament initially. Depending on the degree of forces involved, the CC ligament may be ruptured or remain intact. In general, the AC joint capsuloligamentous structures stabilize the AC joint in the AP direction and the CC ligament stabilizes the clavicle against superior motion.

CLINICAL HISTORY *11-year-old female presenting with the worst headache of her life, which began abruptly after jumping up and cheering at a basketball game. She quickly developed left-sided weakness and numbness.*

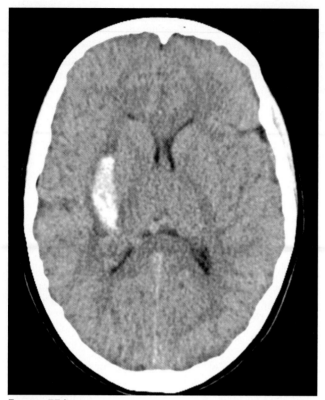

FIGURE 77A

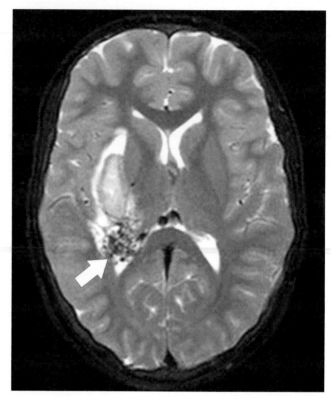

FIGURE 77B

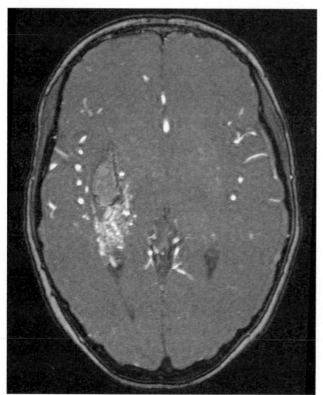

FIGURE 77C

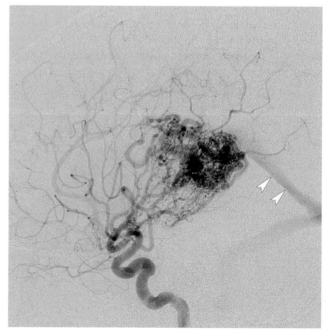

FIGURE 77D

FINDINGS Figure 77A: Noncontrast head CT demonstrates acute hemorrhage centered in the posterolateral putamen and external capsule. Note also the subtle area of subtle hyperdensity just posterior to the hemorrhage. Figure 77B: Axial T2WI demonstrates a cluster of hypointense flow voids in this area (*arrow*) posterior to the hematoma. Figure 77C: Axial source image from a 3D-TOF MRA demonstrates punctate and serpiginous flow-related enhancement in the area posterior to the hematoma, suggesting arterial flow. Figure 77D: Lateral projection from cerebral angiography with injection of the right internal carotid artery demonstrates a tangle of abnormal vessels supplied by perforators from the right middle cerebral artery and anterior choroidal artery, as well as early filling of the straight sinus (*arrowheads*).

DIFFERENTIAL DIAGNOSIS The constellation of findings presented previously are pathognomonic for a ruptured arteriovenous malformation (AVM). Atraumatic intraparenchymal hemorrhages can also be a result of *hypertension, tumors,* and *amyloid angiopathy*; however, the clinical history, age of the patient, and MR findings rule these entities out. Other intracranial vascular malformations include *cavernous malformation, developmental venous anomaly, capillary telangiectasia,* and *dural arteriovenous fistula*; however, none of these entities would be mistaken for the AVM in this case.

DIAGNOSIS Hemorrhage secondary to a ruptured AVM.

DISCUSSION Cerebral AVMs are developmental vascular malformations that consist of at least one feeding artery and draining vein, with an intervening tangle of abnormal blood vessels (nidus) that shunt blood from artery to vein. The estimated annual incidence of cerebral AVMs is less than 0.1%, but the risk of hemorrhage from an AVM is approximately 3% to 4% per year. Vascular malformations account for approximately 1% to 2% of strokes and 20% of all spontaneous intracerebral hemorrhages (ICHs), and they are the most common cause of nontraumatic ICH in children and young adults. Therefore, a spontaneous intracranial hemorrhage occurring in a young patient should immediately prompt a search for an underlying vascular malformation. In addition, a high index of suspicion for an underlying vascular anomaly should be entertained if there are no obvious risk factors for hemorrhage, such as trauma, hypertension, or anticoagulation, or if the location or appearance of the bleed is atypical. Noninvasive imaging can be performed with either CTA or MRA. Although generally less accurate than DSA, both CTA and MRA are still sensitive (up to 90%) for detecting underlying secondary causes of ICH, making them excellent first-line screening tools if a vascular lesion is suspected. DSA remains the gold standard for diagnosis of AVMs, however, and is generally indicated for treatment planning in order to identify the feeding arteries and draining veins. Intranidal aneurysms may also be present, which carry a greater risk for hemorrhage. In addition, aneurysms may be seen arising from the feeding arteries.

A primary goal of AVM treatment is to lower the risk of AVM bleeding and complications relative to the natural history of an untreated AVM. The mainstay of treatment has been through surgical removal. The classification system described by Spetzler and Martin provides a relative risk of open surgery-related morbidity for treatment of cerebral AVMs based on certain criteria: deep venous drainage (1 point) versus superficial drainage only (0 point); eloquent (1 point) versus noneloquent cortex (0 point); and size of nidus <3 cm (1 point), 3 to 6 cm (2 points), or >6 cm (3 points). This allows for a grading of AVM from a 1- to 5-point scale. An inoperable AVM is classified as a grade 6. Removal of AVM from eloquent areas carries greater risk of disabling neurologic morbidity. In the Spetzler–Martin classification, eloquent cortex is defined as: sensorimotor, language, and visual cortices; hypothalamus and thalamus; internal capsule; brainstem; cerebellar peduncles and deep cerebellar nuclei. Noneloquent cortex (i.e., incidental damage may not result in a permanent disabling deficit) is defined as: anterior portion of the frontal and temporal lobes, and cerebellar cortex.

Treatment options for AVM include microsurgery, endovascular embolization, and radiosurgery techniques. Often a combination of methodologies is employed, depending on specific characteristics of a particular lesion and patient factors. Microsurgery has been shown in several studies to be an optimal treatment for many AVMs. Embolization can be employed as an exclusion method, as an adjunct to surgical or radiation therapy, as a targeted treatment of a bleeding site, or as a palliative measure. Embolization as a lone treatment of AVM may be unfavorable in the setting of multiple feeding arteries or multiple draining veins.

Radiosurgery has been employed as an alternative for patients who are unable to undergo surgical removal, with relatively low morbidity and mortality rates, especially for smaller AVMs. Although the Spetzler–Martin classification was developed for surgical treatment of AVMs, it has been shown in some studies to accurately predict outcome in patients undergoing radiosurgery. Newer and more comprehensive grading scales have been developed specifically for radiosurgery, and are of additional benefit in pretreatment algorithms. Higher-grade AVMs are often currently treated with gamma-knife radiosurgery. However, treatment of larger lesions often requires a larger dose. Delayed effects of radiation treatment may manifest several years after treatment, including edema, hemorrhage, radiation necrosis, or cyst formation. Follow-up MRI of the brain is often performed for several years post treatment, even in the setting of initial complete obliteration.

Question for Further Thought

1. What is the most common cause of subarachnoid hemorrhage in a pediatric patient and in an adult patient?

Reporting Responsibilities

In patients with an AVM, the most critical finding to communicate is the presence of acute intracranial hemorrhage or mass effect. If a hemorrhage is suspected to be a result of a vascular malformation, CTA or MRI should be recommended to search for the lesion. If these studies are negative and the suspicion for an AVM remains, catheter angiography should be suggested.

What the Treating Physician Needs to Know

- If an AVM is suspected, where is it located and is there involvement of eloquent cortex? What is the size of the nidus?

- What is the predominant arterial supply? What is the venous drainage?
- Is there an associated aneurysm?
- Has there been prior therapy or embolization?
- If there is hemorrhage, is there evidence of significant mass effect or hydrocephalus?

Answer

1. The overall most common cause of intracranial hemorrhage, young or old, is trauma. The most common cause of spontaneous subarachnoid hemorrhage in pediatric patients is AVM. In an adult patient, it is a ruptured aneurysm.

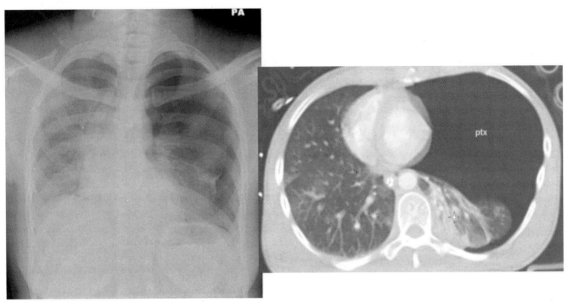

FIGURE 78A

FINDINGS Figure 78A: Upright PA chest X-ray: Abnormal lucency in the left hemithorax, with partially collapsed left lung. Note visceral pleural edge (*arrow*) of left upper lobe, and mediastinal shift toward the right, and increased space between the left ribs compared to right. Axial contrast-enhanced chest CT: There is a large left pneumothorax (*ptx*), and the heart and mediastinum are shifted across midline. The left lower lobe is collapsed (*star*), and air fills remainder of hemithorax.

DIFFERENTIAL DIAGNOSIS Pneumothorax, tension pneumothorax, collapsed right lung, pneumomediastinum, Poland syndrome.

DIAGNOSIS Tension pneumothorax.

DISCUSSION Clinical signs of a tension pneumothorax include tachypnea, hypotension, pleuritic chest pain, tracheal deviation, jugular vein distention, and unilateral absence of breath sounds. They occur when a perforation of the visceral pleura occurs with continuous air leak, but without chest wall injury. This causes accumulation of air in one hemithorax with subsequent increased pressure, compressing the lung and mediastinal structures to the contralateral side. Tension pneumothoraces often occur after trauma. Other risk factors include recent procedure such as central line placement, bronchoscopy, mechanical ventilation, and underlying lung disease. If a tension pneumothorax is strongly suspected, radiologic evidence is not necessary and the clinician should proceed with a needle thoracostomy at the second or third

intercostal space at the midclavicular line to decompress the thorax followed by chest tube placement once the patient is stabilized. For patients in whom the diagnosis is less certain, chest radiograph is the initial study of choice. Findings suggesting a tension pneumothorax include hyperlucency in one hemithorax with increased intercostal space compared to the contralateral hemithorax, and tracheal, esophageal, and mediastinal deviation away from the pneumothorax.

Questions for Further Thought

1. How common are iatrogenic pneumothoraces?
2. What is the effect on patient outcome?

Reporting Responsibilities

Given the acuity and life-threatening nature of the condition, immediate reporting is essential so that the treating physician can proceed with treatment and stabilization of the patient. Associated trauma or findings should also be reported.

What the Treating Physician Needs to Know

- Side of mediastinal deviation, location of pneumothorax.

Answers

1. Pneumothorax is estimated to occur in 4% to 15% of ICU patients and is a potentially life-threatening complication. In a critically ill or unconscious patient, the diagnosis can be more difficult to make, as the locations are often atypical or complicated by other disease processes. High index of suspicion is required as pneumothorax progresses

to tension pneumothorax in an estimated 30% to 97% of iatrogenic pneumothoraces and can rapidly progress if left untreated. Presenting features of a tension pneumothorax in this setting are nonspecific (acute drop in blood pressure, fall in O_2 sat).

2. Prompt diagnosis and treatment with chest tube drainage is key. Mortality ranges from 46% to 77% in patients in whom pneumothorax is a complication of mechanical ventilation.[3]

CLINICAL HISTORY *35-year-old female with acute onset abdominal pain. Initially, the abdominal pain significantly improved with pain medications and she was sent home. At home, the patient attempted to eat, but the abdominal pain returned.*

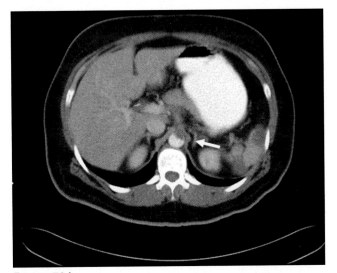

FIGURE 79A

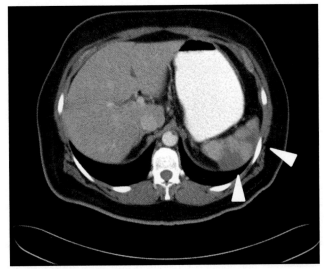

FIGURE 79B

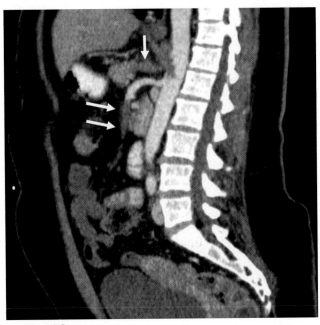

FIGURE 79C

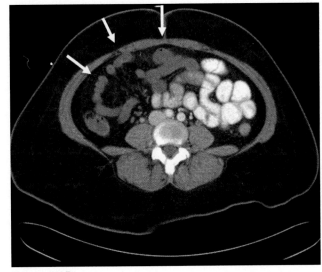

FIGURE 79D

FINDINGS Figure 79A: Axial contrast-enhanced CT image of the upper abdomen demonstrates thrombus within the anterior abdominal aorta (*arrow*). Figure 79B: Axial contrast-enhanced CT image of the upper abdomen demonstrates multiple peripheral wedge-shaped regions of hypodensity in the spleen (*arrowheads*), compatible with splenic infarcts. Figure 79C: Sagittal contrast-enhanced CT image of the abdominal aorta demonstrates filling defects in the enlarged proximal celiac artery and mid and distal superior mesenteric artery, consistent with acute thromboemboli (*arrows*).

Figure 79D: Axial contrast-enhanced CT image of the abdomen demonstrates absent mural enhancement of the small bowel (*arrows*). The bowel was nonviable during surgery.

DIFFERENTIAL DIAGNOSIS Superior mesenteric artery (SMA) and celiac artery thrombosis, aortic dissection, atherosclerotic disease.

DIAGNOSIS Thromboemboli causing splenic infarcts and acute arterial mesenteric ischemia.

DISCUSSION Acute mesenteric ischemia is caused by decreased blood flow in the mesenteric vessels, resulting in ischemia of the bowel wall. Subsequently, bowel infarction, perforation, peritonitis, and sepsis will follow unless reperfusion occurs. Acute mesenteric ischemia is the one of the most worrisome abdominal CT findings with high morbidity and mortality. The findings can be subtle early on or quite obvious in the later stages and vary depending on the cause, acuity, duration, site, and amount of collateral circulation. Mesenteric ischemia can be caused by mesenteric arterial occlusion, mesenteric venous occlusion, strangulating/closed loop obstruction, or nonocclusive vascular disease.

Acute mesenteric arterial ischemia is the most common cause of mesenteric ischemia and can result from embolic or thrombotic arterial occlusion of the mesenteric vessels. Acute mesenteric arterial occlusion caused by thromboembolism is associated with cardiovascular abnormalities, such as arrhythmias, myocardial infarction, valve disease, or endocarditis. Emboli are typically located at the branching points near the middle colic artery and typically collateral vessels are not present. Of note, bowel wall thickening is usually not seen or is a very late sign of arterial ischemia.

Arterial thrombosis of the mesenteric vessels is a late complication of atherosclerotic disease and typically occurs at or near the origin of the mesenteric arteries in an acute on chronic mesenteric ischemia. When there is slow flow to the stenotic mesenteric vessels, thrombus will form, further decreasing the flow to the bowel. Typically, collateral vessels are present.

Acute mesenteric venous ischemia can be secondary to portal hypertension, infection, pancreatitis, recent surgery, or hypercoagulable states. Mesenteric venous thrombus will lead to poor venous drainage, resulting in increased hydrostatic pressure, causing bowel wall thickening, mesenteric edema/stranding, and free fluid. If the pressure increases high enough, arterial inflow can be compromised and cause bowel wall ischemia. Bowel infarction is relatively infrequent.

Strangulated bowel obstruction or closed loop obstruction are mechanical small bowel obstructions (SBO) that can lead to mesenteric ischemia. This usually occurs secondary to an adhesion, or internal or external hernias. There is initial impairment of the venous outflow followed by arterial ischemia.

Nonocclusive mesenteric ischemia is seen in 20% to 30% of acute mesenteric ischemic cases.[1] Mesenteric arterial vasoconstriction occurs when there is hypoperfusion without vascular occlusion. This can occur as a reflex to a hypotensive episode or vasospasm.

Computed tomography (CT) and CT angiography (CTA) are the modality of choice for diagnosing mesenteric ischemia and identifying emboli and thrombi in the mesenteric arteries and veins. MR angiography is a good noninvasive screening technique; however, CTA has higher spatial resolution and faster acquisition times. Catheter angiogram is the gold standard and can be used for confirmation and interventional treatment, but is invasive with increased radiation exposure.

CT findings of bowel ischemia include bowel wall thickening, nonenhancement of the bowel wall, dilatation of the bowel lumen, mesenteric fat stranding, and ascites. Pneumatosis, venous gas, and free intraperitoneal air are indicators of bowel infarction and perforation.

Treatment options for acute thrombosis include surgical intervention; percutaneous transluminal angioplasty with stenting; and thrombolytic therapy if within 8 hours of presentation and the patient does not have signs of bowel necrosis or peritonitis. Treatment may involve watchful waiting in nonocclusive mesenteric ischemia; anticoagulation with mesenteric vein thrombosis; and emergent surgical exploration for strangulated/closed loop obstruction.

Questions for Further Thought

1. Where do most emboli lodge within the SMA and the celiac artery?

2. When would ischemic bowel demonstrate high-density wall thickening?

Reporting Responsibilities

Acute mesenteric ischemia is an emergency and should be reported to the referring physician immediately.

What the Treating Physician Needs to Know

- Cause of the mesenteric ischemia.

- Patency of the mesenteric arteries and veins.

- Presence of pneumatosis, venous gas, free fluid, and free air indicating bowel infarction and perforation.

Answers

1. Most emboli in the SMA lodge near the middle colic artery branch. Because of its small takeoff angle from the aorta and higher flow, the SMA is the visceral vessel most susceptible to emboli; the IMA is less commonly affected. Most emboli from the celiac artery lodge at the segmental splenic arteries, causing segmental splenic infarctions.

2. Ischemic bowel would demonstrate hyperdense bowel wall thickening from intramural hemorrhage (which can be seen in anticoagulation, trauma to the duodenum, or Henoch Schonlein Purpura) or from hyperenhancement if the ischemic bowel becomes reperfused.

CLINICAL HISTORY *76-year-old woman fell on her left side while walking at the supermarket and now complains of hip pain. Radiographs are negative for fracture.*

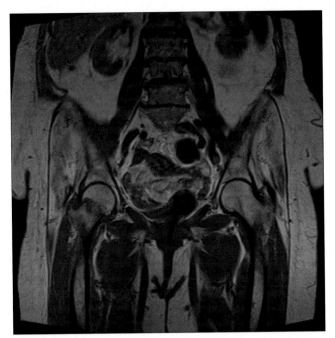

FIGURE 80A

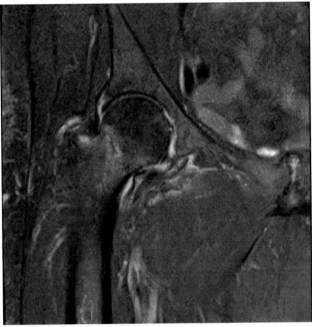

FIGURE 80B

FINDINGS Coronal T1-weighted MR image (Fig. 80A) through the entire pelvis reveals a curvilinear hypointensity within the lateral right subcapital femoral neck that extends approximately half the width of the femoral neck with adjacent, more ill-defined hypointensity consistent with edema. Coronal T2-weighted fat-suppressed image (Fig. 80B) of only the right hip demonstrates a curvilinear hypointensity that matches the course of the hypointensity on the T1-weighted image with a thin rim of marked adjacent hyperintensity. More ill-defined hyperintensity of the adjacent bone marrow is also noted. Radiographs immediately preceding the MRI were normal.

DIFFERENTIAL DIAGNOSIS Osteoarthrosis, intertrochanteric bursitis, radio-occult hip fracture, soft tissue tumor or metastases.

DIAGNOSIS Radio-occult right subcapital femoral neck fracture.

DISCUSSION Hip fractures in the elderly are associated with high morbidity and 1-year mortality, which may be as high as 30%.[1] A nondisplaced hip fracture, particularly in the elderly patient with osteopenia, is at times difficult to visualize. With our population increasingly outliving historical average age estimates, hip fractures are expected to double in the next 20 years. The typical mechanism in the elderly is minor

trauma, usually a fall from a standing position, to a bone that is already weakened by osteoporosis.

Radiographs are the first diagnostic test when a hip fracture is clinically suspected, although they only have about 55% to 60% sensitivity for a hip fracture.[2] Radiographs may be limited by osteopenia, patient positioning, and large body habitus. If the radiograph is negative and clinical suspicion remains, other imaging modalities should be pursued. MRI is the diagnostic study of choice after a negative radiograph, because changes are seen within 4 hours of the injury. A recent 10-year retrospective study showed fractures in 83 of 98 patients with negative radiographs suggesting radiographs alone cannot exclude a fracture in older patients.[3] T1-weighted images will show a low-signal fracture line with effusion and edema better visualized on fluid-sensitive sequences. CT scanning can miss impacted fractures or nondisplaced fractures that are parallel to the axial plane, but might be considered in the acute setting when MRI is unavailable or contraindicated. A radionuclide bone scan is an alternative choice; 24 to 72 hours must pass from the time of injury to show a fracture and is also reserved for patients who are unable to have an MRI.

A delay in the diagnosis of occult fractures can lead to subsequent displacement and osteonecrosis of the femoral head. As the prognosis worsens with displacement, MRI following negative radiographs is recommended in patients older than age 50.[1] Treatment is usually surgical, ranging from screw fixation to total hip arthroplasty. Displaced fractures require more aggressive intervention.

Questions for Further Thought

1. Stress fractures (fatigue fractures) and insufficiency fractures are more likely to be radio-occult than traumatic fractures. How do these present and how are they managed?

2. What are some mimics of radio-occult proximal femur fractures that may also be radio-occult?

Reporting Responsibilities

Nondisplaced hip fractures are not emergencies; a timely report is required. In the outpatient setting, a phone call might be considered to emphasize the need for MRI in the setting of negative radiographs.

What the Treating Physician Needs to Know

- The sensitivity of radiographs for hip fracture is less than perfect, especially in the setting of osteoporosis. If there was sufficient suspicion for a hip fracture in an elderly patient to prompt imaging in the first place, then an MRI should be obtained.

Answers

1. Stress fractures result from abnormal repetitive stress on normal bone and insufficiency fractures result from normal stress on abnormal bone. Stress fractures are more common in young adults such as athletes, whereas insufficiency fractures tend to occur in elderly patients with underlying primary or secondary osteoporosis. Radiographs identify 28% of acute stress fractures; so it is important to obtain an MR or bone scan if clinical suspicion persists. Radiographs usually show linear sclerosis and possibly periosteal reaction, and MR shows a low-signal fracture line with marrow edema. Treatment usually involves conservative management including protection from weight-bearing or even immobilization. The majority of stress fractures heal. However, if no protection is instituted the fracture may progress and require surgical management. Of note, our patient from the aforementioned case suffered a low energy fall (near normal stress) (fall) on abnormal bone (osteoporosis) most consistent with an insufficiency fracture.

2. Patients suspected of having a hip fracture with negative radiographs can later be found to have fractures other than proximal femoral fractures on MRI. The most common include acetabular fractures and fractures of the obturator ring. Sacral insufficiency fractures are also not uncommon following a fall. Soft tissue injury may also occur. The most common muscle that is injured is the obturator externus. Usually, surgery is not required for obturator ring fractures and muscle injury.

CLINICAL HISTORY *42-year-old patient with a history of IV drug abuse presenting with low back pain, which has progressively worsened over several weeks.*

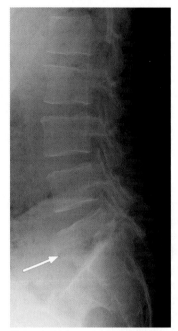

FIGURE 81A

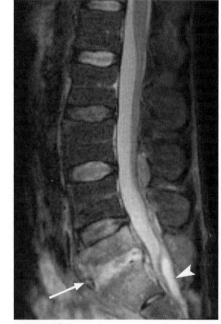

FIGURE 81B

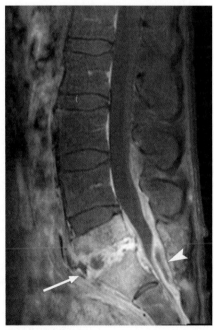

FIGURE 81C

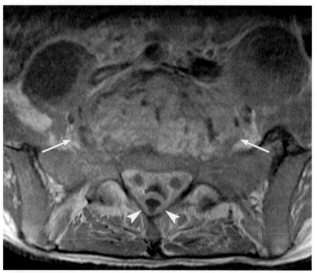

FIGURE 81D

FINDINGS: Figure 81A: Lateral radiograph of the lumbar spine demonstrates severe collapse of the L5–S1 intervertebral disk space (*arrow*) with erosion of the inferior L5 endplate and superior S1 endplate. Figure 81B: Sagittal STIR image demonstrates abnormal hyperintense signal within the disk space (*arrow*) and throughout the adjacent L5 and S1 vertebral bodies. There is also a lentiform fluid collection posterior to the thecal sac (*arrowhead*), which appears to displace the dura anteriorly. Figures 81C and 81D: Corresponding contrast-enhanced sagittal, fat-suppressed T1-weighted image (Fig. 81C), and contrast-enhanced axial T1-weighted image at L5–S1 (Fig. 81D) demonstrate enhancement of the L5–S1 disk space (*arrows*) and the adjacent vertebral bodies. In addition, there is abnormal enhancement in the epidural and prevertebral soft tissues, including portions of the psoas muscles. Also note enhancement along the periphery of the aforementioned epidural fluid collection (*arrowheads*) which is compressing the spinal canal.

DIFFERENTIAL DIAGNOSIS The imaging findings in this case are essentially pathognomonic for infectious spondylodiscitis, but it is useful in these cases to try to distinguish between pyogenic and nonpyogenic (usually tuberculous) spondylodiscitis. *Tuberculous (TB) spondylitis* most commonly involves the thoracic spine and tends to cause vertebral collapse with relative preservation of the disk space, which helps distinguish it from pyogenic discitis. Pyogenic discitis more commonly affects the lumbar spine and causes relatively greater degrees of disk space narrowing. In addition, subligamentous spread, which may span multiple vertebral segments, is more typically seen in tuberculous spondylitis. *Degenerative disk disease* may present with disk and endplate abnormalities, which have similar signal characteristics to infection on MRI but does not cause this degree of vertebral endplate destruction or soft tissue enhancement. In patients undergoing hemodialysis for chronic renal disease, a destructive spondyloarthropathy mimicking discitis on imaging can also be observed, and a similar arthropathy can also been seen in patients with neurogenic spine disorders. In *dialysis-related spondyloarthropathy*, decreased signal intensity in the disk and adjacent endplates on both T1-weighted and T2-weighted images often allows one to distinguish this entity from infection, but this entity can occasionally present with increased intervertebral disk and vertebral body signal on T2-weighted images, making differentiation from infectious spondylodiscitis impossible. *Neuropathic spondyloarthropathy* is more likely than infection to demonstrate vacuum disk phenomenon, facet involvement, and spondylolistheses. In this case, the presence of an epidural abscess essentially eliminates these two entities. *Vertebral metastases*, may involve multiple adjacent vertebral levels as well as the epidural space, but generally do not involve the intervening disk spaces.

DIAGNOSIS Pyogenic spondylodiscitis with epidural abscess.

DISCUSSION In the US, most instances of infectious spondylodiscitis are caused by pyogenic bacterial pathogens, and a single organism is identified in roughly two-thirds of these cases. *Staphylococcus aureus* is the most common causal organism, followed by gram-negative bacilli and streptococci/enterococci. Gram-negative bacilli are frequently seen in association with immunosuppression, diabetes, and IV drug use, and following procedures involving the gastrointestinal and genitourinary tracts, whereas infections complicating spine procedures are most commonly caused by *S. aureus*. Cases of spondylodiscitis attributable to atypical infections such as TB, brucellosis, or fungi are fairly uncommon in

the US; however, TB is becoming an increasingly prevalent cause of spine infection among patients who are immunosuppressed, homeless, or IV drug users. TB spondylitis is also seen in patients who have immigrated from endemic areas where TB can account for up to 46% of cases of infectious spondylodiscitis.

Infections of the spine develop via three routes: (1) hematogenous spread; (2) direct external inoculation; and (3) spread from contiguous tissues. Of these, the hematogenous route is the most common. In adult patients, hematogenous spondylodiscitis most commonly begins in the end arterioles adjacent to the vertebral body endplates posterior to the anterior longitudinal ligament. Infection then spreads from the vertebral body into the disk space and then to the adjacent endplate. In children, in whom arterial anastomoses and vascular channels still penetrate the intervertebral disk, organisms may directly inoculate the disk space and cause an isolated discitis. These anastomoses involute by approximately 13 years of age, at which time the disk becomes avascular.

The age distribution for pyogenic spondylodiscitis is bimodal, with peaks in early childhood and in the sixth decade. In addition to the conditions noted here, other risk factors for developing infectious spondylodiscitis include increasing age, alcoholism, and chronic conditions such as cirrhosis, malignancy, and renal failure. Patients most commonly present with back or neck pain that is classically not relieved by either rest or analgesics, and 60% to 70% of patients with pyogenic infections present with fever. Neurologic deficits occur in up to 50% of patients, but severe deficits such as paraplegia are uncommon. Symptom onset is usually insidious, and there is typically a delay in diagnosis of 2 to 6 months from initial symptom onset (even longer in cases of TB). Among patients with pyogenic discitis, the lumbar spine is most frequently affected (60%), followed by the thoracic spine (30%), and then the cervical spine (10%). Multilevel involvement occurs in 5% to 18% of patients with pyogenic infection and in more than 20% of patients with TB.

The imaging findings in this case are typical of advanced pyogenic spondylodiscitis with vertebral endplate destruction, abnormal marrow and disk signal and enhancement, and enhancement of the prevertebral and epidural soft tissues on MRI. Early discitis may be difficult to diagnose, but a fairly reliable sign of early discitis is loss of the internuclear cleft on T2WI. Epidural abscesses have been reported to complicate between 4% and 38% of cases of non-postoperative spondylodiscitis. The term epidural abscess is actually a misnomer, because any epidural process associated with infection presenting as either a fluid collection or a soft tissue mass is considered an epidural abscess. In this case, there was both extensive epidural phlegmon as well as a discrete fluid collection. The presence of an epidural abscess is generally considered as an indication for surgery.

Treatment of infectious spondylitis is targeted at the specific pathogen. Blood cultures are the simplest and most cost-effective means of identifying the causal organism, and they demonstrate an yield of between 40% and 60%. Biopsies are reserved for patients with negative blood cultures, but may be negative in up to 39% of cases.

Question for Further Thought

1. Why is the intervertebral disk space more likely to be spared in cases of TB spondylitis than in pyogenic spondylodiscitis?

Reporting Responsibilities

Findings of infectious spondylodiscitis should be communicated promptly to the referring clinician, and MRI should be suggested for any cases of suspected discitis, as it best demonstrates associated soft tissue abnormalities and compromise of the spinal canal. The official radiology report should include the level(s) of involvement, degree of vertebral collapse, presence of epidural or paraspinous abscesses, and the presence and degree of spinal canal compromise. In addition, if there are findings suggesting that the discitis may be caused by an atypical organism (e.g., tuberculosis), this should also be indicated.

What the Treating Physician Needs to Know

- Is the process most likely infectious or noninfectious in etiology? If infection is suspected, are there findings suggesting it is because of an atypical organism (e.g., TB, Brucella, or fungal)?
- Is there involvement of just one intervertebral disk level, or are multiple levels involved?
- Is there evidence of an abscess in the epidural space or in the adjacent paraspinous soft tissues?
- Is the significant compromise of the spinal canal?

Answer

1. The intervertebral disk space is more likely to be spared in cases of TB spondylitis because *Mycobacterium*, unlike typical pyogenic organisms, lack the proteolytic enzymes to digest the disk.

CLINICAL HISTORY *Motor vehicle crash.*

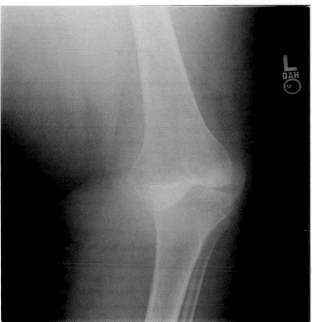

FIGURE 82A

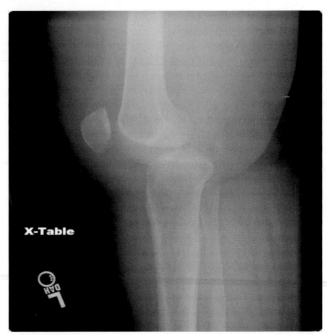

FIGURE 82B

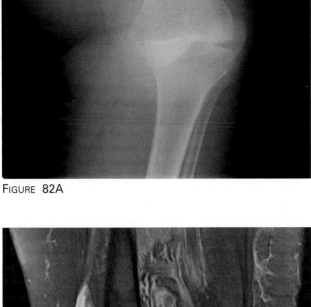

FIGURE 82C

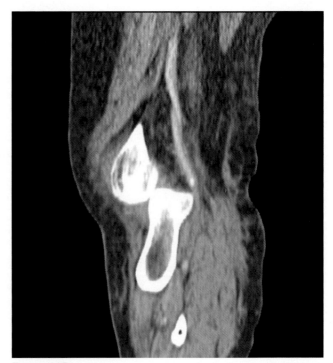

FIGURE 82D

FINDINGS Supine AP (Fig. 82A) and cross-table lateral (Fig. 82B) radiographs of the left knee demonstrate posterior and slight lateral displacement of the tibia relative to the femur with marked varus angulation. The patella is also displaced laterally. No fracture is seen. Sagittal MR image (Fig. 82C) demonstrates marked posterior displacement of the tibial plateau and completely torn anterior (*short arrow*) and posterior cruciate ligaments (*long arrow*); the femoral attachment of the fibular collateral ligament was also avulsed (not shown). Oblique sagittal reformatted image from a CT angiogram (Fig. 82D) of the popliteal fossa demonstrates an opacified popliteal artery to the level of the tibiofemoral joint beyond which it is unopacified, consistent with complete occlusion.

DIFFERENTIAL DIAGNOSIS Anterior, posterior, medial, lateral, or rotary knee dislocation with/without associated neurovascular injury.

DIAGNOSIS Posterior knee dislocation with associated ligamentous and popliteal artery injuries.

DISCUSSION Knee dislocations are rare, usually resulting from extreme trauma, and can be limb-threatening from associated neurovascular damage. The true frequency of knee dislocations is unknown because of the possibility of reduction, spontaneous or otherwise, prior to evaluation by a physician or because of other distracting injuries in the polytrauma setting. Unreduced dislocations usually present with obvious physical examination findings, but spontaneously reduced dislocations can lead to underestimation of the severity of injury, thereby risking the limb.

Knee dislocation, which implies disruption of the tibiofemoral articulation, requires either rupture of both anterior and posterior cruciate ligaments or rupture of at least three of the four major knee ligaments. Injuries resulting in either of these multiple ligament ruptures may be caused by motor vehicle collisions, contact sports, or even a fall from standing position in the setting of obesity, a range of settings involving various degrees of energy. High-energy traumatic dislocations are more likely to result in severe soft tissue, particularly neurovascular, damage; low-energy dislocations are not immune to neurovascular injury.

A number of methods of classifying knee dislocations exist with the goal of predicting prognosis and directing treatment. Anatomic classification describes the direction of the tibia in relation to the femur after dislocation: anterior (most common, because of hyperextension), posterior (second most common, because of direct impact on the proximal tibia), medial, lateral, and rotary (rare). An advantage of this approach is that the direction may be apparent on physical or radiographic examination. This approach is limited by the possibility of reduction prior to the assessment and limited ability to predict prognosis or treatment. Classification based on which of the knee ligaments are ruptured requires advanced imaging (MRI) and potentially examination under anesthesia, but is very good at predicting prognosis and treatment. In the acute setting, the classification is not very important, because recognizing that neurovascular injury is not just a possibility in any knee dislocation, but also that the risk is independent of the degree of energy involved in the traumatic event.

Popliteal artery injury occurs in 20% to 40% of knee dislocations secondary to direct trauma or secondary to stretch injury because of its relatively firm proximal attachment at the adductor hiatus and distally in the location where it penetrates the tendinous arch of the soleus. Stretch injury is most associated with dislocations in the sagittal plane (anterior or posterior). Injury to the popliteal artery secondary to direct trauma seems to occur most frequently in posterior dislocations. Injury to the peroneal nerve, which occurs in up to one-third of cases, is similarly caused by direct trauma (e.g., adjacent fibular neck fracture) or stretch injury resulting from tethering at the fibular neck.

If knee dislocation is suspected clinically, evaluation of limb perfusion is the first priority. If vascular injury is left untreated for more than 8 hours, the risk of amputation is 86%, versus an 11% chance if treated within 8 hours.[1] Overt lack of limb perfusion on physical examination requires immediate vascular surgery. Otherwise, immediate reduction, preferably closed, should be performed to prevent continued stretch/pressure injury on the neurovascular structures. Following reduction or if closed reduction cannot be achieved, the next step is a thorough vascular examination, including arterial phase imaging. Catheter angiography or CT angiography may be obtained as the first-line imaging assessment of the popliteal artery; choice depends on availability. CT is often more readily accessible than catheter angiography and has a lower radiation dose. If either of these modalities is not available, duplex ultrasonography and potentially ankle-brachial indices may provide useful information.[2] Types of vascular lesions include dissection, transection, and thrombosis. Intimal flaps may also be seen and may in some cases progress to dissection.

For the patient in whom knee dislocation is not initially suspected, tibiofemoral incongruity on the initial supine AP and cross-table radiographs may be the only radiographic clue that a dislocation has occurred. Although isolated cruciate ligament injuries are often associated with large knee effusions, rupture of the tibiofemoral joint capsule associated with knee dislocation may decompress the joint; the presence of an effusion cannot be relied upon to indicate an acute injury.

Questions for Further Thought

1. After reduction and reassessment of neurovascular status, what is the treatment of knee dislocation?
2. Other than arterial injury, what are some other complications of knee dislocation?

Reporting Responsibilities

Knee dislocation is an emergency; direct communication with the referring clinician is required.

What the Treating Physician Needs to Know

- Presence and description of knee dislocation.

- Potential for limb-threatening vascular injury (even in seemingly low-energy traumatic events) requiring imaging of the popliteal artery (CT or catheter angiography).
- Any associated fractures.

Answers

1. After the dislocated knee has been reduced and any vascular injury has been addressed, surgery to restore knee stability is performed. An MRI will allow detailed descriptions of the ligament injuries (midsubstance tears vs. avulsions), meniscal tears, and fractures. Outcomes after surgical restoration of knee stability are much more favorable than for nonoperative management; rates of long-term stiffness and return to preinjury function are much lower in those treated nonoperatively.

2. In the short term, knee dislocations may be complicated by acute compartment syndrome, nerve injury, and deep venous thrombosis. Given the risk of compartment syndrome, prophylactic fasciotomies of the four compartments of the leg are often performed if a vascular injury has occurred. The peroneal nerve may be stretched, contused, or overtly disrupted during the dislocation. Symptoms usually include motor deficits (e.g., foot drop) as well as sensory deficits. Peroneal nerve injuries, which are more fully characterized by nerve conduction studies, are difficult to treat and prognosis is poor. In general, surgical exploration is performed if there is no evidence of recovery by 3 to 6 months after the injury, although some advocate exploration at the time of ligament reconstruction, which is similar to the situation for most peripheral nerve injuries. Deep venous thrombosis is a risk after all orthopedic operations, but particularly in the setting of a knee dislocation with an associated vascular injury.

CLINICAL HISTORY *Close-range gunshot wound.*

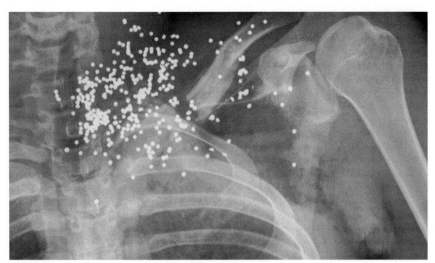

FIGURE 83A

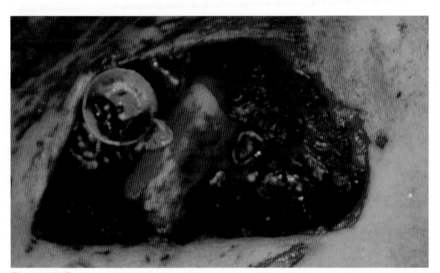

FIGURE 83B

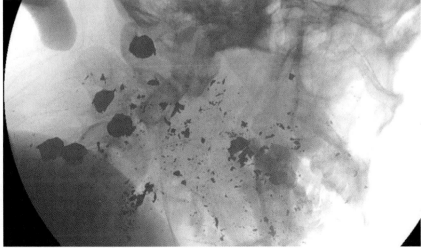

FIGURE 83C

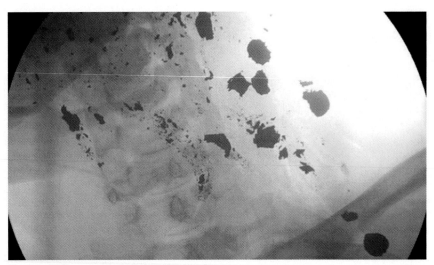

Figure 83D

FINDINGS Postmortem AP radiograph of the left upper chest (Fig. 83A) reveals a comminuted midshaft clavicle fracture and numerous tiny, rounded metallic densities clustered about the clavicle, but mostly in the supraclavicular region. Note the relative size of the metallic densities in relation to the clavicular shaft; they are much smaller. Postmortem radiograph of the anterior upper chest centered on a large skin defect (Fig. 83B) reveals a piece of bone from the underlying comminuted clavicle fracture and a round, grayish appearing structure with central impression consistent with the wad from a shotgun shell. Lateral (Fig. 83C) and AP (Fig. 83D) fluoroscopic spot images from a postmortem examination of another patient reveal numerous large metallic densities clustered in the lateral left neck. The largest fragments are similar in size to the clavicular shaft (best seen in Fig. 83D). On the AP view much smaller fragments of metal density are noted along near-linear tracks adjacent to the larger metal density structures, much like a comet.

DIFFERENTIAL DIAGNOSIS Low-energy hand gun injury, high-power hunting rifle injury, close-range shotgun injury, long-range shotgun injury.

DIAGNOSIS Close-range shotgun blast with birdshot (Figs. 83A and B). Close-range shotgun blast with buckshot (Figs. 83C and D).

DISCUSSION Shotguns are a form of firearm designed to fire "shot," which are pellets of various sizes, and are considered low-to-moderate energy firearms as compared to hunting and military rifles. The shotgun pellets are collected in a shotgun shell, which is composed of an outer plastic shell, a metal (brass) head, a primer (located in the head), the powder charge, and a (usually plastic) wad that contains the pellets. Pellets are typically made of lead, though if used for hunting migratory fowl, must be made of a nonlead material, often steel. When fired, both the wad and the pellets are propelled forward; the wad usually drops off in the first few meters. Although shotguns have long barrels, similar to rifles, they are not rifled as this would cause more rapid spread of the shot. The gauge of a shotgun refers to the weight of a round lead ball that just fits into the bore of the barrel in fractions of a pound: a 12-gauge shotgun has a larger bore than a 20-gauge shotgun.

Shot comes in two general types: birdshot and buckshot. Birdshot comes in a range of sizes from 0.16 to 0.23 inches. Buckshot sizes range from 0.24 to 0.6 inches. The vast majority of shotgun injuries involve birdshot. All buckshot pellets have a diameter on par with many handgun and rifle bullets. The number of pellets is inversely related to the gauge of the shotgun shell. Single-pellet slugs are also available. A detailed description of shotgun shells and specifics of shot are beyond the scope of this discussion.

The destructive potential of a shotgun blast varies tremendously based on range. Shotgun pellets tend to be clustered within the target with the degree of spread roughly corresponding to increasing range. Close-range wounds will result in massive soft tissue defects because the pellets tend to act as one larger mass. At longer ranges, each pellet is more likely to act as an individual projectile resulting in numerous penetrating skin wounds. Bartlett described the degrees of possible soft tissue injury and general management principles based on the likely range increment for birdshot:[1]

- Type III—less than 3 m (point blank); extreme soft tissue damage, wadding may be in the wound; aggressive, long-term in-hospital treatment owing to high probability of major fractures, vascular injury, nerve injury, and infection.

- Type II—3 to 7 m; severe soft tissue damage, no wadding in the wound; management similar to type III injuries.

- Type I—greater than 7 m; damage of the subcutaneous tissues and deep fascia similar to low-energy projectile wounds; managed as multiple low-energy wounds.

- Type 0—7 to 20 m; skin penetration only; managed as multiple low-energy wounds.

At ranges greater than 40 to 50 m, skin penetration becomes much less likely. Because of the much greater mass of the individual pellets in buckshot, effective ranges are much higher and can result in devastating injury at up to 135 m.

Radiography is an essential component in the evaluation of gunshot wounds both for evaluation of the osseous and soft tissue trauma, but also for localization. Establishing the type of projectile is useful, but should be done with caution on radiographs. The minimum buckshot size is 0.24 inches or 6 mm. As most pellets are much smaller than 6 mm, one can usually identify birdshot (as a group) without difficulty. Determination of the exact type requires knowledge of the degree of magnification, which requires knowledge of the distance from the detector to the object, and a precise measurement of its diameter. Determination of these two parameters is sufficiently difficult to achieve to arrive at an accurate estimate of pellet size; pellet diameters vary by only a few percent. Measurement of the pellet diameter on CT is limited by beam-hardening/photon starvation artifact. Lead shot may deform on contact with bone whereas shot made out of other metals will not. The wad, when present, is radiolucent.

Buckshot is designed to deliver the maximum amount of energy to the target. This is achieved by its round shape and lack of a jacket, as is seen with many bullets. This allows the pellet to fragment on impact, each fragment subsequently acting as a projectile in its own right. When lead projectiles fragment, they can leave a comet-shaped track of lead debris, sometimes called a "lead snowstorm." This phenomenon is most often described for high-velocity hunting rifles using partially jacketed lead bullets.

Questions for Further Thought

1. What is the billiard ball effect?
2. A solitary pellet projects over the right lung base, far removed from the cluster of pellets in the left thigh. How did this happen?

Reporting Responsibilities

The presence of shotgun pellets per se is not an emergency; a timely report is required.

What the Treating Physician Needs to Know

- Location of pellets.
- Relative size (birdshot vs. buckshot).

Answers

1. In short-range shotgun wounds the leading edge of the closely clustered mass of shot meets high-resistance upon contact with the body resulting in a massive decrease in speed in relation to pellets at the rear of the shot mass. The shot coming in behind contacts the much slower moving shot already in the wound and disperses the pellets, much like a cue ball disperses a racked set of billiard balls. As a result of this billiard ball effect, a short-range wound can artifactually appear to be the result of a longer-range shotgun blast.
2. Pellets occasionally migrate into the vascular system and may end up in the pulmonary and cerebral vasculature. Although often asymptomatic, they have been implicated in pulmonary infarcts, cerebral stroke, and myocardial infarction.[2]

CLINICAL HISTORY *26-year-old fell on an outstretched hand.*

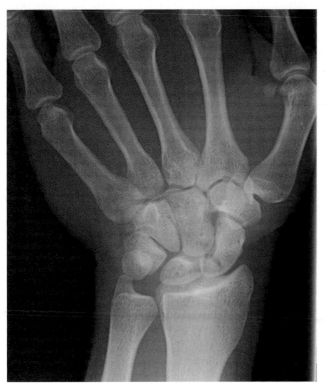

FIGURE 84A

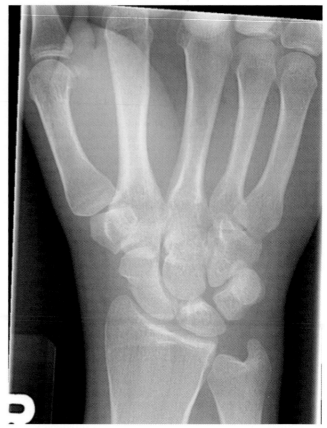

FIGURE 84B

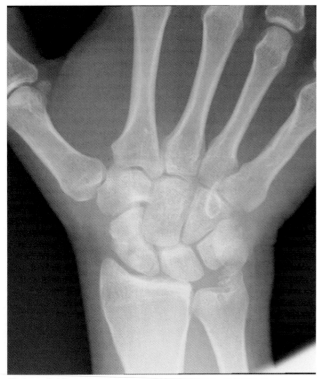

FIGURE 84C

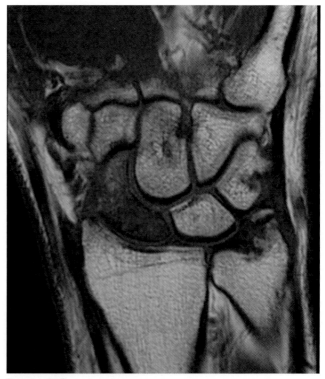

FIGURE 84D

FINDINGS An ulnar-deviated PA radiograph of the left wrist (Fig. 84A) demonstrates an oblique, nondisplaced fracture of the proximal scaphoid pole. A clenched-fist PA radiograph of the right wrist in a second patient (Fig. 84B) demonstrates a transverse, nondisplaced fracture of the scaphoid waist. In a third patient, indeterminate wrist radiographs, represented here by an ulnar-deviated PA view (Fig. 84C), revealed mixed sclerosis and possible lucency in the mid and proximal scaphoid. Subsequent MRI of the wrist, represented here by a coronal T1-weighted image (Fig. 84D), reveals a near-transverse complete fracture of the proximal scaphoid pole and extensive bone marrow edema localized to the scaphoid.

DIFFERENTIAL DIAGNOSIS Radial styloid fracture, scaphoid fracture, lunate dislocation.

DIAGNOSIS Scaphoid fracture.

DISCUSSION Scaphoid fractures most commonly occur in active young people, typically males in their 20s, and account for the majority of carpal bone fractures. Scaphoid fractures are frequently associated with a fall on an outstretched hand that result in forced dorsiflexion of the wrist. In this position, the scaphoid becomes trapped against the dorsal lip of the distal radius while being held in place by the strong ligamentous support of the scaphoid leading to high tensile stress on the concave volar aspect of the scaphoid. The most common location of scaphoid fractures in descending order is the waist, proximal pole, distal pole, and the tubercle (distal volar prominence). Symptoms commonly include radial wrist pain ("anatomic snuff box pain") with minimal swelling and possible decreased range of motion.

Several classification systems for scaphoid fractures exist. The most widely used is the Herbert classification system[1], which classifies both acute and chronic scaphoid fractures:

- Type A:
  - A1—tubercle; A2—nondisplaced crack in scaphoid waist.
- Type B:
  - B1—oblique, distal one-third; B2—displaced fracture of the waist; B3—proximal pole; B4—associated fracture-dislocation; B5—comminuted fracture.
- Type C: Delayed union.
- Type D: Established nonunion.

In this classification system, proximal pole and oblique distal scaphoid fractures are always unstable, but waist fractures are only considered unstable if they are displaced. An unstable fracture is suggested by the following: greater than 1 mm displacement or associated with a carpal derangement, including scapholunate dissociation. In the latter case, findings of capitolunate angulation greater than 15° on a lateral radiograph and scapholunate angulation (measurement made in relation to the distal fracture fragment) greater than 70° on a lateral radiograph are signs of instability.

Radiographs are an excellent first-line imaging modality, capturing the diagnosis in the majority of cases. The typical radiographic series for the evaluation of the scaphoid includes the usual PA, lateral, and pronated oblique views augmented by the scaphoid view. The scaphoid view is a PA view taken in ulnar deviation, which results in dorsal rotation of the scaphoid elongating its profile on the PA view and increased stress at the scapholunate articulation. Although it is not routine practice, Herbert recommended obtaining bilateral wrist radiographs in all patients with suspected scaphoid fracture emphasizing the value of comparison to the contralateral side.[1] Although scaphoid fractures can often be diagnosed on radiographs, they are not perfect: initial radiographs have a sensitivity ranging between 65% and 85%[2]; up to 20% of cases of suspected scaphoid fracture with negative radiographs will subsequently be found to have a scaphoid fracture. In the setting of negative radiographs, three advanced imaging options are available: CT, MRI, and radionuclide bone scintigraphy. According to a recent meta-analysis, these modalities have sensitivities of 85.2%, 97.7%, and 97.8%, respectively, and specificities of 99.5%, 99.8%, and 93.5%, respectively.[4] The data on sensitivity of follow-up radiographs is extremely heterogeneous ranging from extremely low sensitivities to high sensitivities and a wide range of follow-up intervals.[4] On MRI, the fracture line in acute fractures is characterized by a usually very hypointense curvilinear signal abnormality on T1-weighted images and often with corresponding hypointense or hyperintense signal abnormality on fluid-sensitive sequences. The adjacent bone marrow edema is characterized by low signal intensity on T1-weighted images and hyperintensity on fluid-sensitive sequences. The fracture line may be subtle, even on MRI; the extensive associated bone marrow edema is the feature leading to MRI's high sensitivity for fracture. In general, the imaging algorithm for suspected scaphoid fractures begins with radiographs. If negative, immediate MRI should be considered. Alternatively, splinting and repeat radiographs after at least 2 weeks should be obtained.

Determination of displacement is not a small matter. Displaced fractures go on to nonunion at a much higher rate (46%) than nondisplaced fractures (6%).[2] Radiographs are only able to make this distinction 20% of the time; CT can be helpful in assessment of displacement.[3]

Stable, nondisplaced scaphoid fractures are treated with a splint or short arm cast for 2 to 3 months. Unstable fractures are treated with surgical intervention, usually with closed reduction, percutaneous fixation or open reduction, internal fixation. This is usually achieved with a screw that has a variable thread pitch—low pitch distally (wide spacing between threads) and high pitch proximally; a single turn of the screw results in a small amount of linear movement proximally, but a larger amount of linear movement distally. Since the proximal aspect of the screw is locked in the proximal fracture fragment, the distal fragment must move toward the proximal fragment encouraging abutment and impaction at the fracture site. Distal pole fractures usually heal with cast treatment within 2 months.

A high rate of osteonecrosis occurs with this injury; when present, surgery with bone grafting is required. As a large portion of the scaphoid is covered in articular cartilage, there are only two entry sites for the scaphoid blood supply—one near the waist (dorsal branch of the radial artery) and one distally (volar branch of the radial artery). The proximal two-thirds of the scaphoid are entirely dependent on retrograde interosseous blood flow from the dorsal arterial branches. Thus when a proximal fracture cuts off the only arterial supply, osteonecrosis may result. Osteonecrosis is diagnosed by identifying a sclerotic scaphoid on radiograph or low signal on MRI. Whether one can reliably detect early osteonecrosis using dynamic contrast-enhanced MRI, for example, is a matter of debate. Scaphoid malunion and nonunion are also complications as with most fractures and result in decreased grip strength and degenerative changes.

Question for Further Thought

1. What is a "Humpback" deformity?

Reporting Responsibilities

Scaphoid fractures are not emergencies; a timely dictation is required.

What the Treating Physician Needs to Know

- Fracture location.
- Displacement: if indeterminate, CT should be considered.
- Associated carpal derangements (e.g., scapholunate dissociation, perilunate dislocation).
- Negative radiographs do not exclude scaphoid fracture; immediate MRI or clinical and radiographic follow-up should be obtained.

Answer

1. A humpback deformity results when the proximal scaphoid fracture fragment maintains alignment with the lunate and the distal fragment flexes and is volarly rotated, increasing the intrascaphoid angle. An angle greater than 45° is associated with a poor outcome. This is the most common scaphoid fracture malunion.

CLINICAL HISTORY *37-year-old male presents with new onset of extreme leg weakness and memory issues.*

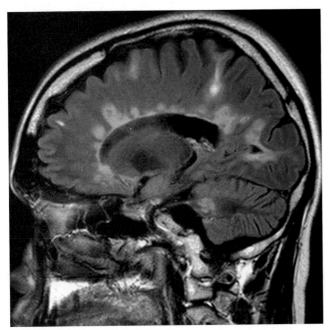

FIGURE 85A

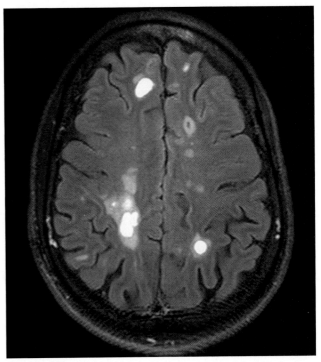

FIGURE 85B

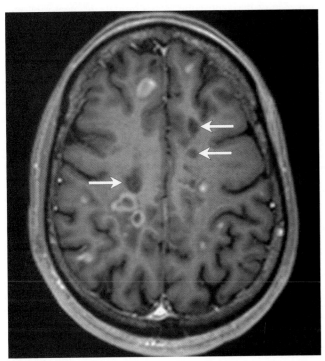

FIGURE 85C

FINDINGS Figure 85A: Sagittal FLAIR image slightly to the left of midline demonstrates numerous hyperintense white matter lesions, many of which are adjacent to the lateral ventricle and oriented perpendicular to the callosal–septal margin. There is prominence of the sulci compatible

with cerebral volume loss. Figure 85B: Axial FLAIR image just superior to the lateral ventricles demonstrates extensive hyperintense lesions within the centrum semiovale and juxtacortical white matter. Figure 85C: Axial postcontrast T1 image demonstrates both peripheral and solid enhancement of a number of the white matter lesions. Notice that the enhancing lesions correspond to some of the most brightly hyperintense lesions on FLAIR imaging. Note also the hypointense lesions within the bilateral frontal lobes (*arrows*) consistent with "black holes," indicating myelin/axonal loss.

DIFFERENTIAL DIAGNOSIS The findings in this case are characteristic of an acute flare of multiple sclerosis (MS), but a number of other entities can produce white matter lesions on imaging. On the benign end of the spectrum, *chronic leukoaraiosis* and *migraine headaches* could be included in the differential for MS. Leukoaraiosis is typically seen in older patients, often in association with long-standing hypertension, and the lesions in this entity do not enhance. Patients younger than 40 years suffering from migraines may demonstrate T2 hyperintense foci, predominantly within the subcortical white matter. These lesions have a frontal and parietal lobe predilection and are stable over time. *Virchow–Robin (VR)* spaces are dilated perivascular spaces containing CSF. Common locations for VR spaces include the basal ganglia, centrum semiovale, and corona radiata. They may simulate MS plaques on MR in that they will demonstrate T1 hypointensity and T2 hyperintensity, but will appear hypointense on FLAIR imaging because of CSF within these spaces, which differentiates them from MS plaques. In the setting of multiple enhancing lesions, one might consider multiple *brain metastases*. Generally most metastases will enhance, whereas only active plaques will enhance in multiple sclerosis. In addition, brain metastases tend to demonstrate varying degrees of peripheral vasogenic edema, whereas MS plaques do not. *Acute disseminated encephalomyelitis (ADEM)* may also be in the differential of multiple T2 hyperintense lesions within the white matter. Lesions in ADEM range from punctate to quite large and typically do not involve the callosal–septal interface. ADEM occurs most commonly in children and typically follows a minor viral infection or immunization.

DIAGNOSIS Multiple sclerosis with acute exacerbation.

DISCUSSION Multiple sclerosis (MS) is the most common demyelinating disease in the Western world, and affects up to 350,000 Americans. The etiology of this chronic inflammatory condition is currently unknown, although it is currently thought to be autoimmune. In young and middle-aged adults, MS is the foremost cause of nontraumatic neurologic disability. Demographically, MS classically affects young women, with a peak age of approximately 30 years. In spite of a young female predominance, MS may affect patients of any age or gender.

Multiple sclerosis remains a clinical diagnosis with imaging serving as an adjunct in the initial diagnostic process, and later as a means of evaluating progression. Clinical presentation is variable, ranging from vague neurologic complaints such as weakness, paresthesias, and impaired vision to loss of sphincter control, blindness, and dementia in the worst cases. Cranial nerve palsies may be present.

MRI is the imaging modality of choice for evaluation of MS patients. The classic findings are multiple T2/FLAIR ovoid hyperintense lesions within the periventricular white matter oriented perpendicular to the corpus callosum seen best on sagittal imaging. These lesions, originating from the callosal–septal margin, are termed "Dawson's Fingers." T2 hyperintense lesions are also commonly present in the subcortical white matter, corpus callosum, cerebellum, optic nerve, and spinal cord. These T2 hyperintense plaques demonstrate corresponding T1 hypointensity. MS plaques that demonstrate profound T1 hypointensity, below that of normal-appearing gray matter, have been termed "black holes", which are indicative of permanent myelin or axon loss and may correlate with patient disability/clinical symptoms. FLAIR imaging is excellent at detecting lesions in the supratentorial brain, but does not perform as well as T2WI at detecting lesions in the posterior fossa, brain stem, and spinal cord. Postcontrast T1W imaging may demonstrate nodular, ring, or arc enhancement within active plaques. The sensitivity of enhancing lesions for detecting disease activity is greater than clinical examination. Enhancement within an MS plaque generally lasts from 2 to 8 weeks, but may be present for more than 6 months. As the condition progresses, global cerebral atrophy, spinal cord atrophy, and volume loss of the corpus callosum may be seen.

Currently, therapies for MS center around controlling disease progression. Such therapies include interferon, steroids, and monoclonal antibodies. Although many of these therapies demonstrate at least moderate degrees of efficacy at controlling the disease, they are not without side effects. Several of these immune-suppressing medications have been shown to cause progressive multifocal leukoencephalopathy (PML) from activation of the JC virus within the central nervous system. Typical findings of PML on MRI include confluent T2/FLAIR hyperintensity within the subcortical and periventricular white matter with no contrast enhancement.

Question for Further Thought

1. Why are classic MS plaques oriented perpendicular to the callosal–septal margin?

Reporting Responsibilities

On an initial workup, the radiology report should include the number of T2 hyperintense white matter lesions, as well as the locations of these lesions (with specific note made of the presence of periventricular, juxtacortical, infratentorial, and spinal cord lesions). Initial and follow-up reports should also include the location(s) of any new or enhancing lesions, as these tend to correlate with disease progression. The number and location of chronic plaques on T1 imaging should also be described, because these lesions correlate with patient debility. The degree of cerebral and corpus callosal volume loss should also be reported. The one scenario that should be reported immediately and directly to the referring physician are findings suggesting the development of PML in patients who are being treated with natalizumab.

What the Treating Physician Needs to Know

- If the patient does not have a preexisting diagnosis, is the distribution of lesions suggestive of multiple sclerosis?
- Are there any enhancing plaques? Are there any T1 "black holes?"
- What is the degree, if any, of cerebral volume loss? Corpus callosal volume loss?
- Are there findings to suggest development of PML?

Answer

1. The appearance of Dawson's fingers, which are MS plaques oriented perpendicularly to the callosal–septal margin, is attributed to inflammatory changes and demyelination focused along the course of the periventricular medullary veins.

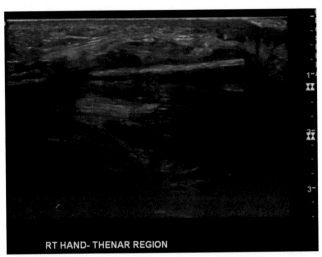

FIGURE 86A

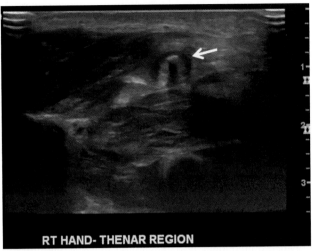

FIGURE 86B

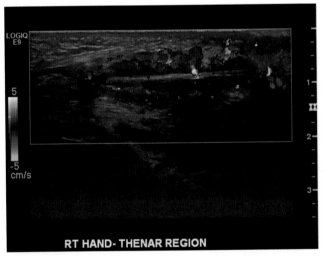

FIGURE 86C

FINDINGS Long (Fig. 86A) and short (Fig. 86B) axis sonographic images of the thenar eminence of the right hand demonstrate a 2.8-cm long, linear, echogenic structure (*arrow* on short-axis image) surrounded by a halo of hypoechogenicity located nearly 1 cm deep to the skin surface. There is posterior acoustic shadowing with comet-like hyperechogenicity projecting deep to the structure at the edges. Doppler evaluation (Fig. 86C) reveals marked surrounding vascularity.

DIFFERENTIAL DIAGNOSIS Foreign body, soft tissue calcification, or soft tissue tumor.

DIAGNOSIS Foreign body (wood splinter) with surrounding edema and inflammation.

DISCUSSION Retained foreign bodies can result from any penetrating trauma, commonly motor vehicle accidents or industrial accidents. Metal, wood, and glass foreign bodies are most common. Foreign bodies are easily missed; 38% of foreign bodies are missed on initial evaluation.[1] Early detection is important, as retained foreign bodies act as a nidus for infection or granulomatous reactions.

Radiographs will demonstrate foreign bodies only if the difference in densities between the foreign body and surrounding soft tissues is sufficiently high to make detection possible. Although glass is nearly universally detectable radiographically in the extremities,[2] for wood foreign bodies the difference in density is often too small to be appreciated on radiographs. Ultrasonography is the preferred imaging modality for suspected superficial foreign bodies because of its ease of use, low cost, and lack of ionizing radiation. Ultrasonography can also be used to facilitate foreign body removal.

A high-frequency ultrasound transducer, which provides excellent near-field resolution, is preferred because most retained foreign bodies are located in the superficial soft tissues. Modern transducers have excellent near-field imaging characteristics; a standoff pad is usually not required, but could be considered especially if dermal involvement is suspected. The sonographic appearance of foreign bodies depends on the acoustic properties of the foreign material; however, all foreign bodies so far studied appear echogenic.[3] Posterior acoustic shadowing depends on the surface of the foreign body with flat surfaces producing dirty shadows and reverberation artifact because of multiple backscattered echoes detected by the transducer, while irregular surfaces produce clean shadowing because of ultrasound waves being scattered at different angle causing loss of signal to the transducer.[3] Hyperechoic or hypoechoic streaks may be observed at the edges of a retained foreign body. Edema surrounding a foreign body can produce a hypoechoic halo. Doppler interrogation will reveal adjacent hyperemia in proportion to the degree of associated inflammation. A recent meta-analysis of 17 studies showed a pooled sensitivity of 72% and specificity of 92% for the sonographic detection of any soft tissue foreign body and a pooled sensitivity of 96.7% and specificity of 84.2% in a subgroup analysis for the detection of radiolucent foreign bodies including wood.[4] Cadaver studies have demonstrated a sensitivity of 87% and specificity of 97% for the sonographic detection of 2.5 mm long wooden foreign bodies with increased sensitivity with increased size.[5] Potential false-positive findings include gas, soft tissue calcifications including bone fragments, and granulomas.

Management usually includes removal of the foreign body and treatment of associated infection, if any. Early detection of foreign bodies is important to prevent infectious or inflammatory complications such as cellulitis or abscess. In cases of penetrating trauma, possible injuries to nerve, muscle, and tendon should also be evaluated, although these complications are much less likely compared to infectious complications.[4] Retained foreign bodies increase the risk of infection by an adjusted odds ratio of 2.6.[5]

Questions for Further Thought

1. What percentage of glass is detectable with radiography?
2. What is the role of cross-sectional imaging in the evaluation of retained foreign bodies?
3. Does depth of foreign body affect its detectability?

Reporting Responsibilities

Foreign bodies are not emergencies; a timley report is required.

What the Treating Physician Needs to Know

- Size, shape, and detailed location of the foreign body.

- If radiography does not reveal a suspected foreign body, ultrasonography should be considered.

Answers

1. Glass has variable density depending on its composition; however, all glass is radiopaque to some degree. Just as is the case for sonography, sensitivity of radiography is size-dependent: sensitivity for detection of glass foreign bodies ≥2 mm is close to 100%, but drops to a low of 61% for glass foreign bodies on the order of 0.5 mm in size.[6]

2. CT is an excellent modality for the detection of foreign bodies because of its ability to detect subtle (in comparison to radiography) density differences. Wood, poorly detectable on radiography, can usually be identified on CT with wide windowing.[7] MR is not an ideal imaging technique to identify foreign bodies. Signal characteristics of foreign bodies are not unique and can mimic calcification or tendon. Ferromagnetic foreign bodies also cause significant artifacts in MR images, which limit the evaluation of the foreign body. A study using phantom foreign bodies also demonstrated that many types of foreign bodies are not visible on MR, making it an insensitive technique.[7] The increased radiation exposure and cost limit the use of CT for routine evaluation of extremity foreign bodies.

3. Increasing depth of foreign bodies has been shown to decrease the sensitivity of radiography for normally radiopaque foreign bodies.[8] Although this is not generally an issue for extremity foreign bodies, it may be an issue in the proximal thigh, pelvis, and trunk and in obese individuals. Sonographic evaluation is also limited at increasing depth as a large drop in signal quality occurs rapidly with the use of the high frequencies needed for extremity evaluation. Decreasing the frequency allows visualization of deeper structures, but likely at the expense of missing small foreign bodies.

CLINICAL HISTORY *36-year-old male with a psychiatric disorder and recurrent history of foreign body placement presented with dysuria and hematuria.*

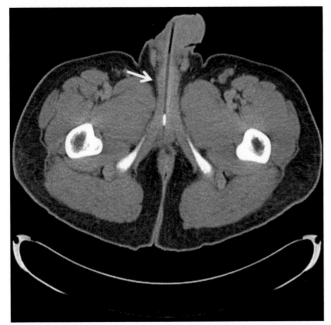

FIGURE 87A

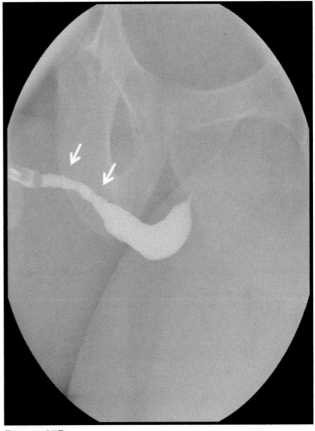

FIGURE 87B

FINDINGS Figure 87A: Axial CT scan of the pelvis shows a cartridge of a pen with a proximal metallic component and an air- and ink-filled lumen of the rest of the foreign body (*arrow*). A pen was removed and a portion of a plastic spoon was also removed from the urethra. Figure 87B: A retrograde urethrogram performed after the foreign body removal demonstrates mild narrowing and irregular lumen of the mid and distal penile urethra (*arrows*), compatible with recurrent history of foreign body placement.

DIFFERENTIAL DIAGNOSIS Urethral foreign body, infection.

DIAGNOSIS Foreign body in the urethra.

DISCUSSION Foreign bodies in the lower genitourinary tract are not common and are usually related to self-insertion via the urethral meatus, either related to sexual practices or psychometric issues.[1] These retained foreign bodies can proceed to cause severe localized pain and hematuria, especially if they result in obstruction and infection. Diagnosis often relies on clinical history and is confirmed on cystoscopic retrieval of the foreign body.

The role of imaging mainly determines the presence of foreign bodies, and if not already clinically certain, the size and shape. The location of a deeply inserted object should be identified as it allows alternative approach, such as via cystotomy. The mobility of these objects, however, cannot be assessed on imaging, and the degree of involvement into the urethral or bladder wall are often a rough estimate. Presence of sharp ends is relevant as there is a higher risk of urethral injury.

Radiographs and computed tomography (CT) can be performed to evaluate for radiopaque foreign bodies, with the plain radiograph being easier and faster, while CT being more sensitive for plastic objects and more accurate in localization. Foreign bodies inserted into the urethra are typically radiopaque on plain radiograph and CT, as a rigid form is often necessary to allow placement through the penile shaft. Plain radiograph is usually sufficient in most cases. Ultrasound can be technically challenging and relies on the availability of the expertise. Larger objects typically demonstrate shapes that are geometric and artificial, such as a straight linear pen. A smaller object may not show an obvious geometrical shape, but its focal appearance and very high attenuation may render easy identification. Metallic objects with sharp margins often demonstrate streak artifacts, which are not seen in calcifications.

Discontinuity of the urethral wall, adjacent fluid collections, and other complications can occasionally be identified by CT and retrograde urethrogram. The most common complications were mucosal tears of the urethra and false passages.[2] Further complications such as obstruction, strictures, infection, gangrene, fistula, and diverticula formation can occur if such foreign bodies are not promptly removed.[3]

The treatment is determined by the size, number, location, and shape of the intra-urethral foreign body. Treatment often requires endoscopic removal and/or surgery, if the former fails.

Question for Further Thought

1. If urethral stricture or rupture is suspected, what study should be performed?

Reporting Responsibilities

Foreign bodies in the urethra should be immediately reported to the referring clinician. Early detection of a foreign body will help for successful endoscopic removal, and less complications.

What the Treating Physician Needs to Know

- The type, size, number, shape, and location of the foreign body, especially the estimated length of the distal and proximal ends from the meatus.
- Presence of periurethral fluid collection should raise the concern of a perforation.

Answer

1. If urethral stricture or rupture is suspected, fluoroscopic retrograde urethrogram should be performed instead of CT. Both CT and MRI are limited in the assessment of the location and size of the perforation site, and are better evaluated on fluoroscopic urethrogram.

CLINICAL HISTORY *43-year-old female with a history of lupus treated with steroids, presents with developing left knee pain, swelling, and fevers.*

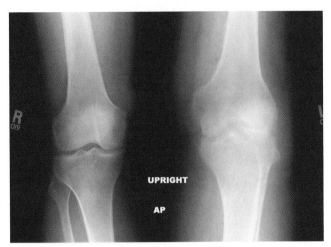

FIGURE 88A

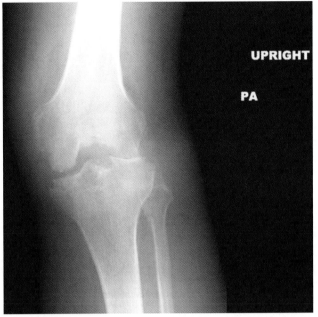

FIGURE 88B

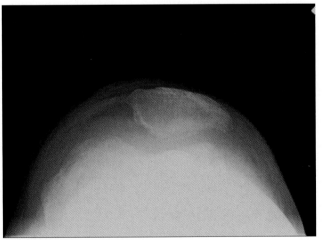

FIGURE 88C

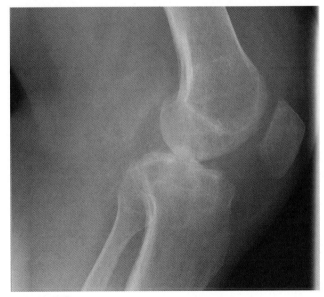

FIGURE 88D

FINDINGS Radiographs of the left knee reveal an erosive process involving the tibiofemoral and patellofemoral joints with an associated effusion and subcutaneous soft tissue edema. Comparison to the normal knee is seen in the standing AP radiographs of both knees (Fig. 88A). The erosive disease, mostly characterized by pitting and indistinctness of the subchondral bone, is best appreciated on the flexed PA radiograph (Fig. 88B) and the tangential patellar radiograph

(Fig. 88C); an overt marginal erosion is seen in the medial aspect of the medial tibial plateau. The effusion and soft tissue swelling are best appreciated on the lateral (Fig. 88D) and tangential patellar radiographs.

DIFFERENTIAL DIAGNOSIS Rheumatoid arthritis, septic arthritis, seronegative spondyloarthropathy, or crystal deposition disease.

DIAGNOSIS Septic arthritis.

DISCUSSION Septic arthritis—inflammatory arthritis of a joint because of infection—is a potentially devastating condition. Joint destruction from septic arthritis results in irreversible loss of joint function in 25% to 50% of patients, and 75% of survivors develop a significant functional disability of the involved joint. The fatality rate from septic arthritis is on the order of 5% to 15%,[1] which reflects the serious nature of the disease, and need for prompt intervention.

Septic arthritis most commonly results from hematogenous spread of infection, such as from intravenous drug use, endocarditis, indwelling catheter, or distant spread from a remote source, such as pneumonia or distant wound infection. It can also originate from direct inoculation, such as from surgery, trauma, or penetrating foreign body. Local spread of infection is another mechanism for inoculating a joint, a mechanism particularly associated with diabetic patients; the synovium lacks a protective basement membrane increasing its relative permeability to infectious organisms. Septic arthritis leads to rapid destruction of cartilage because of influx of acute inflammatory cells, release of proteolytic enzymes, inflammatory cytokines, and pressure necrosis from the accumulation of purulent synovial fluid.

Classification of septic arthritis is differentiated by pyogenic (bacterial) versus nonpyogenic organisms, such as viral, mycobacterial, fungal, and parasitic. The most common causative organisms for pyogenic arthritis, with their relative frequency, include *Staphylococcus aureus* (64%), *Streptococcus pneumonia* (20%), *Escherichia coli* (10%), *Haemophilus/Klebsiella/Pseudomonas* (4%), Group B *Streptococci*, and *Neisseria gonorrhoeae* (2%).[2] Intravenous drug users are more likely to have unusual causative species, such as *Mycobacterium avium*, *Pseudomonas*, and *Enterobacter* species.

Radiographs are the first-line imaging examination in suspected septic arthritis. Early in the course of septic arthritis, however, radiographs are normal. The first radiographic manifestation is a joint effusion, which can easily be visualized in joints where the joint capsule is bordered by fat on a standard projection, such as the knees, elbows, and ankles. Visualization of effusions in other joints, such as the glenohumeral joint, is problematic because the joint capsule is not bordered by fat on a standard projection or there are overlapping shadows; joint space widening or subluxation may be the first clue to an underlying effusion in these joints. As the disease progresses, joint space loss may be seen secondary to cartilage loss, cortical bone becomes indistinct, marginal erosions may develop, and signs of osteomyelitis may develop. The development of periarticular osteoporosis resulting from hyperemia is a late finding, also usually seen with more indolent infections, such as tuberculous infections. Sclerotic host reaction can become evident in long-standing bacterial infection. Eventually, joint ankylosis can be seen, which is rare, and more frequent in tuberculous than in pyogenic arthritis.

Ultrasonography is excellent at visualizing effusions in accessible joints, and is therefore the method of choice to identify and subsequently aspirate effusions. However, there are no reliable sonographic features that allow one to distinguish a bland from a septic effusion. Secondary sonographic signs of bone involvement include the presence of periosteal reaction and erosions.

MRI is a useful tool early in the course of disease when the clinical and radiographic findings may be indeterminate. MRI is more sensitive (100%), and more specific (77%) than other imaging modalities, and abnormal findings are evident within 24 hours of onset.[2] Precontrast T1-weighted images demonstrate decreased marrow signal within subchondral bone *on both sides of joint*. Fluid-sensitive sequences enable visualization of effusions, subchondral marrow edema, and perisynovial soft tissue edema—all manifested by increased signal. Postcontrast T1-weighted imaging demonstrates avidly enhancing thickened synovium, subchondral bone enhancement, and, in the case of direct spread of infection to the joint, adjacent soft tissue enhancement, possibly with an associated abscess. The relative frequency of MRI findings in septic arthritis is as follows: synovial enhancement (98%), marrow bare area changes (86%), abnormal T2 marrow signal (84%), abnormal enhancement (81%), abnormal T1 marrow signal (66%), perisynovial edema (84%), and joint effusion (70%) (almost one-third lack effusion, and joints of hand or foot are most common to be without appreciable effusion).[2]

Diagnosis of septic arthritis is confirmed by abnormal laboratory results from joint aspiration, either by culturing the causative organism or by inference in the setting of markedly elevated leukocyte count within the joint fluid. Upon confirmation that septic arthritis is present, surgical drainage and lavage is often necessary. Appropriate antibiotics are administered as soon as the diagnosis is confirmed or if there is a delay in obtaining the joint aspirate.

Question for Further Thought

1. Why would a radiologist performing a joint aspiration for suspected septic arthritis be careful to avoid injecting lidocaine into the joint before obtaining a sample?

Reporting Responsibilities

Septic arthritis is an emergency; a phone call to the referring clinician is essential.

What the Treating Physician Needs to Know

- Joint aspiration is the definitive diagnostic procedure.
- If the diagnosis is suspected, treatment with antibiotics should be started without delay.
- Early in the course of disease, radiographs are negative. MRI and ultrasonography may be obtained if the diagnosis remains in doubt.

Answer

1. Lidocaine is bacteriostatic and will diminish the ability to culture the causative organism from the joint aspirate. Older iodinated contrast media also had inhibitory effects on bacterial growth, but most are no longer in use.

CLINICAL HISTORY *18-year-old male pedestrian struck by a car traveling 55 mph and thrown 100 feet. The patient suffered a pulseless electrical activity arrest in the field and now presents with fixed and dilated pupils and no neurologic responses.*

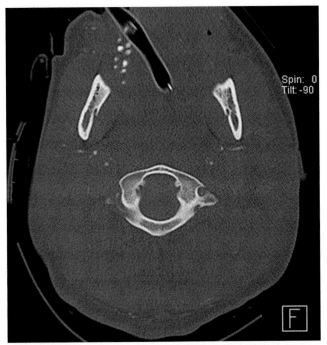

FIGURE 89A

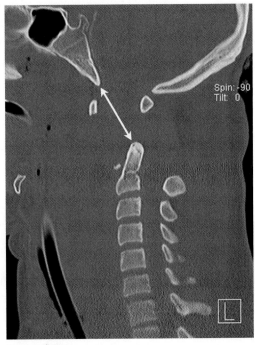

FIGURE 89B

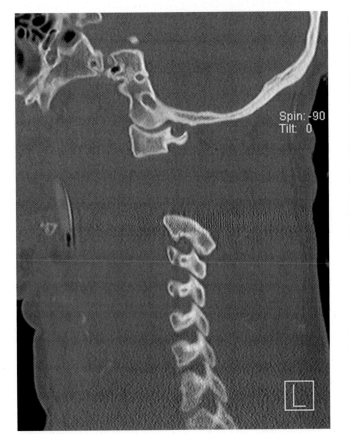

FIGURE 89C

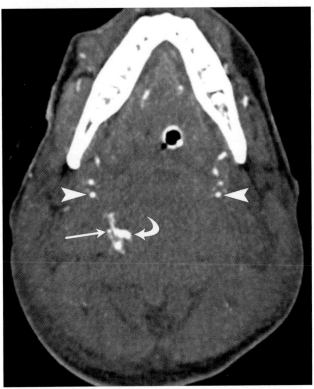

FIGURE 89D

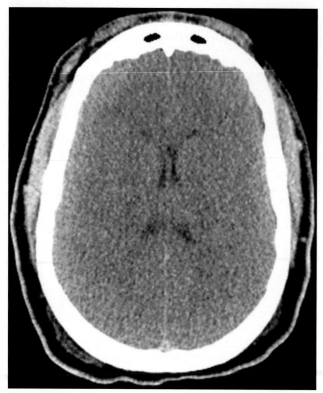

FIGURE 89E

FINDINGS
Figure 89A: Axial bone window CT image at the level of C1 demonstrates an intact C1 ring; however, the dens is not visualized in its normal position behind the anterior C1 arch. Figures 89B and 89C: Sagittal bone window CT images through the cervical spine demonstrate complete craniocervical dissociation, evidenced by marked widening of the dens-basion interval (*double arrow*), along with widening of the C1–C2 interspinous distance on the midsagittal image (Fig. 89B). A small avulsed bone fragment arising from the inferior aspect of the anterior C1 arch remains in normal position anterior to the dens; however, the remainder of C1 is superiorly distracted. On the parasagittal image (Fig. 89C) there is a large gap between the lateral masses of C1 and C2, while the atlantooccipital joint remains located. Figure 89D: Axial image from a CTA of the neck demonstrates extravasated contrast (*curved arrow*) adjacent to a small, opacified right vertebral artery (*thin arrow*). The left vertebral artery is not seen. Note also, the markedly diminished caliber of the internal carotid arteries (*arrowheads*). Figure 89E: Axial unenhanced head CT image demonstrates diffuse brain edema with complete loss of gray–white matter differentiation.

DIFFERENTIAL DIAGNOSIS
This is a clear case of *craniocervical dissociation (CCD)*, and no differential need be given. When evaluating craniocervical trauma, the most common injuries to keep in mind, in addition to CCD, are occipital condyle fractures, C1 and C2 fractures, atlantoaxial instability, C1–C2 rotatory subluxation, C1 Jefferson fractures, and odontoid fractures.

DIAGNOSIS
Craniocervical (atlantoaxial) dissociation with vertebral artery transection and anoxic brain injury.

DISCUSSION
CCD is a cervical spine injury in which there is complete disruption of the stabilizing ligaments between the occiput and C2 resulting in separation of the skull from the cervical spine. These injuries are usually the result of high-speed motor vehicle accidents, but certain conditions, such as rheumatoid arthritis and Down syndrome, can predispose to ligamentous injury in relatively low-speed collisions. The vast majority of cases of CCD are fatal, with older morgue studies estimating survival at less than 1%; however, as the emergency management of trauma victims has improved over time, the number of patients surviving CCD has increased, and patients may present with less-severe injuries to some but not all of the ligamentous structures at the craniocervical junction; these injuries are still considered unstable.

CT is the first-line imaging tool for assessing in traumatic neck injuries to assess for fracture and/or misalignment. A number of radiographic parameters have been proposed to assess the integrity and alignment of the craniocervical junction. These include:

- Wackenheim line—straight projection from the posterior aspect of the clivus, which should normally fall within 1 to 2 mm of the odontoid tip.
- Basion-axis interval (BAI)—distance from the basion to a line projecting cranially from the posterior cortex of the C2 body, normally 4 to 12 mm.
- Atlanto-dens interval (ADI)—distance between the anterior odontoid cortex and the posterior cortex of the anterior arch of C1, normally <3 mm.
- Basion-dens interval (BDI)—distance from the basion to the tip of the clivus, normally <12 mm.
- Atlanto-axial articulation—distance between the articular surfaces of the lateral masses of C1 and C2, normally <3 mm.
- Atlanto-occipital interval (AOI)—distance between the articular surface of the occipital condyle and lateral C1 mass, normally <1.4 mm.
- Powers ratio—ratio of the distance between the basion to the spinolaminar line at C1 to the distance between the opisthion to the midpoint of the posterior aspect of the anterior arch of C1, normally <1.0.

Abnormalities in any of these on CT should raise concern for craniocervical junction injury and should prompt a cervical spine MRI.

Various patterns of injury can be observed in patients with CCD, including occiput–C1 distraction, C1–C2 distraction, or combined occiput–C1 and C1–C2 distraction. This case demonstrated primarily C1–C2 distraction, which is the least common pattern of injury. Unfortunately, findings of CCD on plain radiographs and CT can be extremely subtle. In one study, only 23% of CCD cases were diagnosed on initial evaluation with CT or plain radiography. Therefore, even if initial evaluation with CT imaging is negative, MRI should be performed, if craniocervical junction injury is suspected on clinical grounds, so long as the patient is stable enough to undergo evaluation. In this case, given the patient's poor neurologic status and prognosis, MRI was not felt to be warranted. T2-weighted or STIR sequences are most sensitive for demonstrating ligamentous injury, cord injury, and edema. Increased signal on T2WI within and around the ligamentous structures should the integrity of those structures.

Patients with CCD are at significant risk for associated adverse neurologic outcomes, including spinal cord injuries producing complete tetraplegia, various cervicomedullary syndromes, and cranial nerve injuries; so MR examinations should also be closely scrutinized for injuries to the spinal cord and brainstem. Delay in surgical stabilization is associated with a greater neurologic risk than if early stabilization is performed. Therefore, early diagnosis and stabilization is critical to prevent or minimize significant neurologic morbidity. In addition, patients with CCD should be screened for cerebrovascular injuries, particularly injury to the vertebral arteries, which were evident in the patient presented.

Questions for Further Thought

1. Why are children more prone to craniocervical junction injuries than adults?
2. What are the prognosis and treatment for CCD?

Reporting Responsibilities

The diagnosis of ligamentous injury is critical to ensure early stabilization and avoid life-threatening spinal cord injury and complications. Therefore, suspicion of CCD should be promptly reported to the ordering physician to ensure that the neck is immobilized, and there should be a low threshold for ordering an MRI if the mechanism of injury, CT findings, or patient's symptoms are at all suspicious.

What the Treating Physician Needs to Know
CT:

- Is there evidence for misalignment of the craniocervical junction, including significant distraction or widening of important craniocervical measurements (e.g., BAI, ADI, BDI, or AOI)?
- Is there a fracture?
- Is there significant prevertebral soft tissue swelling (>7 mm at C2–C3)?

MRI:

- Is there an associated epidural hemorrhage causing canal stenosis?
- Which ligaments are disrupted and is there evidence of spinal cord injury or compression?

Other:

- Are there associated intracranial abnormalities?
- Is there evidence of a vascular injury?

Answers

1. The craniocervical junction is thought to be less stable in children than it is in adults for a number of reasons. First, the occipital condyles and atlas facets are smaller, and the atlantooccipital joint is more horizontally oriented in children than they are in adults. In addition, the large head size of children relative to the rest of the body combined with increased laxity of the neck ligaments in children also contribute to increased vulnerability to injury at the craniocervical junction.

2. Definitive treatment requires surgical stabilization with fusion from the occiput to at least C2.

CLINICAL HISTORY *40-year-old female with minor blunt trauma to the left chest presents with chest pain and shortness of breath.*

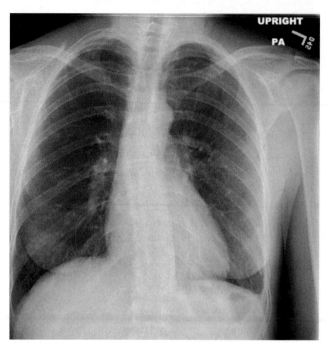

FIGURE 90A

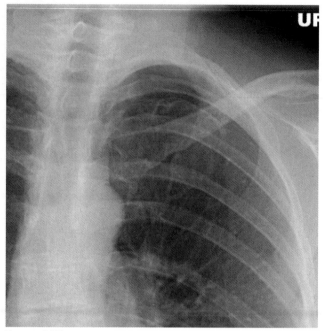

FIGURE 90B

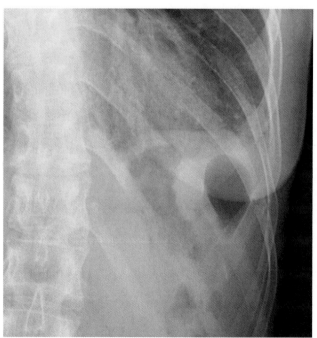

FIGURE 90C

FINDINGS PA radiograph of the chest (Fig. 90A) reveals a left apical pneumothorax, a small left pleural effusion, and a left lateral ninth rib fracture. Figure 90B is a magnified PA view of the left apical pneumothorax shown in Figure 90A. AP view of the lower ribs (Fig. 90C) again demonstrates the minimally displaced left lateral ninth rib fracture and small left pleural effusion.

DIFFERENTIAL DIAGNOSIS Pneumothorax, hemothorax, traumatic rib fracture, stress rib fracture, pathologic rib fracture.

DIAGNOSIS Traumatic rib fracture with pneumothorax and pleural effusion (hemopneumothorax).

DISCUSSION Rib fractures are the most common thoracic injury; they occur in 10% of total traumatic injuries overall and in nearly 40% of severe blunt trauma cases (motor vehicle collisions, falls, industrial accidents).[1] Rib fractures occur in isolation only 6% to 13% of the time.[2] Rib fractures are uncommon in penetrating trauma. The fifth to ninth ribs are the most frequently fractured. Fractures of the superior ribs are usually only seen in high-energy trauma; considerable force is required to break these ribs because of shielding by the scapula and clavicle. Fracture of the inferior ribs may be less common due to being less rigidly fixed. Rib fractures may also cause secondary complications including pneumothorax, hemothorax, pulmonary contusion, pulmonary laceration, and pain leading to abnormal pulmonary mechanics. First and second rib fractures are associated with great arch vascular and brachial plexus injuries. Lower rib fractures are associated with lacerations of the liver, spleen, and kidneys. Overall trauma morbidity and mortality correlates with increasing number of rib fractures, particularly in the elderly, given lower cardiopulmonary reserve.

Pneumothorax and hemothorax alone and in combination are the most common acute complications. Pneumothorax results from laceration of the underlying pleura and lung parenchyma with the edges of fractured ribs. Hemothorax, presenting as an ipsilateral pleural effusion, results from bleeding secondary to laceration of underlying lung and/or adjacent intercostal or chest wall vessels. In patients with isolated rib fractures, pneumothorax and hemothorax may not be evident at the time of presentation, but may be delayed up to 48 hours; this was observed more frequently in patients with three or more rib fractures.[2] The pain associated with rib fractures can lead to respiratory splinting, abnormal pulmonary mechanics with decreased ventilation, and impaired clearance of secretions, which predisposes to atelectasis and pneumonia.

The correlation between higher numbers of rib fractures and higher morbidity and mortality may in part be due to rib fractures serving as a sentinel sign for increasing severity of underlying cardiothoracic, neurologic, and abdominopelvic injury. This association is exaggerated in the elderly population, particularly in those aged 65 years and older.[1] The elderly are predisposed to increasing numbers of rib fractures with a lesser degree of trauma due to intrinsically decreased bone strength. The number of rib fractures may be used as part of a number of trauma scoring systems, and may affect the decision to hospitalize or place in an intensive care setting. Some sources suggest three or more rib fractures as a reference point at which to consider hospitalization, even in isolated rib trauma, to avoid the morbidity and mortality related to the aforementioned complications.[2]

Radiography and physical examination are the first steps in the evaluation of clinically suspected rib injury after minor blunt trauma. Although rib fractures cause morbidity in terms of pain, the secondary complications (pneumothorax and hemothorax) are of much greater clinical significance. Even though chest radiography has a low (50%) sensitivity for rib fractures,[3] chest radiography has excellent sensitivity for pneumothorax and hemothorax. Identification of these complications necessitates close monitoring (and potentially an intervention), whereas the absence of these findings will result in conservative therapy to manage the patient's pain regardless of whether a rib fracture is detected or not. As a result, imaging should begin with an upright PA chest radiograph.[1] If associated acute complications are excluded with chest radiography, the pursuit of additional imaging to identify/quantify fractures is usually not necessary. Dedicated rib radiographs (AP and oblique views of the upper and lower ribs with bone technique) can be obtained if documentation of a rib fracture is needed for a specific indication or circumstance, such as an elderly patient with poor pulmonary reserve, and quantification of rib fractures is needed to determine the need for hospitalization. CT is more sensitive than radiography for detection of rib fractures, but usually only obtained in the setting of high-energy trauma. Ultrasonography has also been shown to be more sensitive than radiography for detection of rib fracture with the potential to evaluate the ribs, costal cartilage, and costochondral junction.

Isolated rib fractures may be treated with NSAIDS or narcotics. Hospitalized patients may undergo a pain regimen including nerve block and/or epidural, and pulmonary toilet also plays an important role. Pneumothorax or hemothorax may be treated with tube thoracostomy, or, possibly, thoracotomy if there is persistent bleeding.

Questions for Further Thought

1. What is flail chest?
2. Who gets rib stress fractures?

Reporting Responsibilities

Isolated rib fractures are not emergencies; a timely report is required. The presence of a secondary complication (especially a pneumothorax) is a potential emergency; direct communication with the referring physician is required.

What the Treating Physician Needs to Know

- Presence of pneumothorax and hemothorax.
- Location of visualized rib fractures. Superior rib fractures imply high-energy trauma. Lower rib fractures are associated with abdominal organ injury.
- Number of rib fractures. The presence of three or more rib fractures in an elderly patient is associated with increased morbidity and mortality.

Answers

1. Flail chest results from three or more segmental fractures (same rib broken in two separate places) within consecutive ribs or fractures of more than five consecutive ribs. Assessment for this condition should be made in every person suffering major thoracic trauma and occurs in approximately 5% of high-energy thoracic trauma patients.[2] Flail chest can cause paradoxical movement with respiration resulting in decreased respiration and ventilation; however, this effect can be masked by positive pressure ventilation. Flail chest is associated with higher mortality, perhaps because it serves as a marker for more severe thoracic injury; these patients will be placed in an ICU setting and given pain control. Chronic chest pain may be a long-term complication.

2. Stress rib fractures are an uncommon injury mostly affecting athletes and elderly patients with chronic cough.[1] Repetitive strong contractions of the chest wall muscles or the diaphragm leads to this form of rib injury. Thus, athletes who frequently activate these muscles—for example,

baseball pitchers (specifically first rib) and batters, golfers, rowers (lower ribs), weight lifters, and swimmers—are prone to this injury. Clinical presentation may include localized pain, point tenderness, or localized soft tissue swelling. Like stress fractures elsewhere, if the ribs are rested from activity, they will likely heal without complication. If not, they may evolve into a complete fracture. Given the often subtle nature of stress fractures, cross-sectional imaging may be needed to confirm this diagnosis.

CLINICAL HISTORY *6-week-old male who presented with projectile, nonbloody, and nonbilious vomiting after every feed for 4 days.*

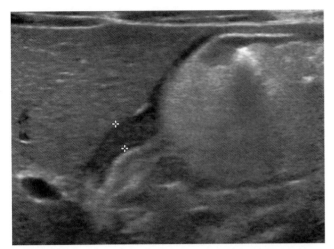

FIGURE 91A

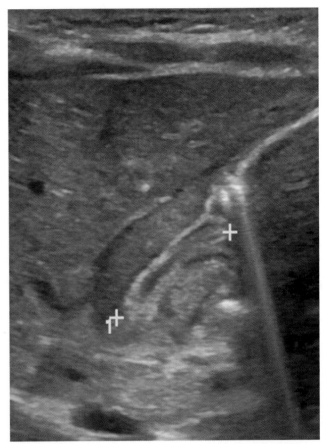

FIGURE 91B

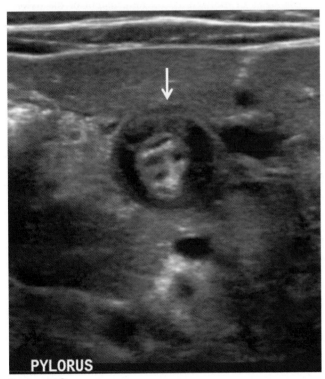

PYLORUS

FIGURE 91C

DIFFERENTIAL DIAGNOSIS Pylorospasm, gastroesophageal reflux, midgut volvulus, duodenal web/stenosis, annular pancreas, and hypertrophic pyloric stenosis.

DIAGNOSIS Hypertrophic pyloric stenosis.

DISCUSSION Pyloric stenosis occurs when hypertrophy and hyperplasia of the muscular layers of the pylorus leads to narrowing of the gastric pylorus causing gastric outlet obstruction. The cause of pyloric stenosis remains unknown, but both environmental and hereditary factors are thought to contribute to this disorder. Pyloric stenosis has a male predilection (4:1) and is more commonly seen in Caucasians.

Infants diagnosed with pyloric stenosis are clinically normal at birth. Within the first 4 to 6 weeks of life, the patient begins to experience emesis eventually progressing until the classic projectile, nonbilious emesis is seen. As the frequency of vomiting increases, the infant will begin to experience weight loss. Most patients diagnosed with pyloric stenosis are between the ages of 3 and 12 weeks. On physical examination, a nontender, mobile, hard pylorus termed "an olive" can be felt in the right upper quadrant. Another physical examination finding is the prominent gastric peristaltic

FINDINGS Figure 91A: Longitudinal ultrasound image of the pylorus demonstrates a thickened pyloric muscle measuring 4.1 mm (between *cursors*). Figure 91B: Longitudinal ultrasound image of the pylorus shows a markedly thickened, hypoechoic gastric pyloric muscle with an elongated pyloric canal length measuring 17 mm (between *cursors*). Figure 91C: Transverse US image of the pyloric channel shows the target sign of pyloric stenosis (*arrow*) because of circumferential hypertrophied hypoechoic muscle surrounding echogenic mucosa.

wave, known as succussion splash, which can be observed in a distended stomach because of gastric outlet obstruction. However, with the rise of imaging, both of these physical examination findings have become less important in the diagnosis. Laboratory tests may show hypokalemic, hypochloremic metabolic alkalosis with possible early prerenal failure caused by dehydration. Based on a combination of history, physical examination findings, and these laboratory values, the clinician may suspect the diagnosis of pyloric stenosis.

Ultrasound (US) is the modality of choice in diagnosing pyloric stenosis. Ultrasound allows for real-time and direct visualization of hypertrophied pyloric muscle without ionizing radiation, in comparison to an upper gastrointestinal tract fluoroscopic examination (UGI) that was the standard diagnostic imaging modality previously. Ultrasound findings diagnostic of pyloric stenosis are a thickened and elongated pyloric muscle. Exact measurements of what constitutes pyloric stenosis are a subject of some debate, but generally accepted measurements are a thickness of greater than 3 mm (measuring only the hypoechoic muscle) and a pyloric channel of greater than 15 mm. In addition, the pylorus should be observed for at least 10 to 15 minutes to see if gastric contents pass through the pylorus. This real-time imaging helps differentiate true pyloric stenosis from pylorospasm. While observing the pylorus, the patient is typically given a liquid glucose solution, such as Pedialyte. Secondary signs that can be helpful in the diagnosis include the "nipple sign" when the thickened pyloric mucosa protrudes into the distended gastric antrum. The "target sign" of pyloric stenosis is seen on a transverse image of the pyloric channel because of circumferential hypertrophied hypoechoic muscle surrounding echogenic mucosa.

Rarely, UGI can be used as an adjunct. This examination is infrequently performed today because of lack of direct visualization of the hypertrophied muscle and the use of ionizing radiation. The UGI examination can infer the diagnosis of pyloric stenosis rather than directly visualize the hypertrophied muscle. Delayed gastric emptying and elongated pylorus with a narrow lumen outlined with contrast (string sign), which can appear duplicated (double-track sign) are common UGI findings. In addition, the thickened pylorus indents the contrast-filled antrum (shoulder sign) or base of the duodenal bulb (mushroom sign) with the pylorus appearing beak-shaped. Despite the lack of common use of UGI in diagnosing pyloric stenosis, it should be noted that an UGI examination is crucial in the diagnosis of other serious illnesses, such as midgut volvulus in the pediatric population.

Surgical treatment includes pyloromyotomy, which is a curative procedure for pyloric stenosis.

Questions for Further Thought

1. What is the role of UGI examination in the diagnosis of pyloric stenosis?
2. How does pyloric stenosis differ from pylorospasm?

Reporting Responsibilities

Pyloric stenosis should be urgently reported to the ordering physician. However, unlike midgut volvulus, this is not an emergent condition, and the patient can be treated with supportive care until an operating room becomes available.

What the Treating Physician Needs to Know

- Thickness of the pylorus >3 mm, length of the pyloric channel > 15 mm, and failure of the pylorus to open are the criteria for the diagnosis of pyloric stenosis on ultrasound.
- If the ultrasound or clinical findings are equivocal, then the patient can undergo an UGI examination to rule out other serious obstructive etiologies, such as midgut volvulus.

Answers

1. UGI examination is an adjunct diagnostic tool in cases of pyloric stenosis when other imaging findings are inconclusive, or when the clinical presentation is atypical and other potentially serious obstructive etiologies need to be ruled out.
2. Pylorospasm is the failure of relaxation of the pylorus. In contrast to pyloric stenosis, opening of the pylorus and passage of fluid can be seen eventually with prolonged observation. There is a theory that pylorospasm in some patients may progress to overt pyloric stenosis. Because of this, if the patient's clinical symptoms progress or do not resolve, an ultrasound can be repeated at 24-hour increments to see if pyloric stenosis has developed.

CLINICAL HISTORY *39-year-old male presents with right hip pain following a front-end motor vehicle collision.*

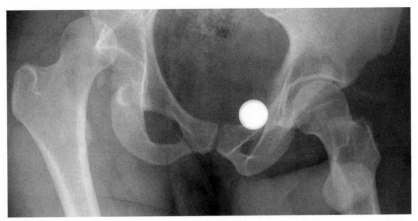

FIGURE 92A

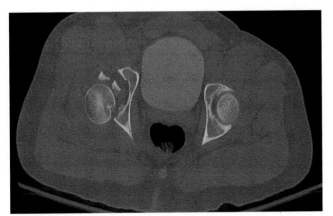

FIGURE 92B

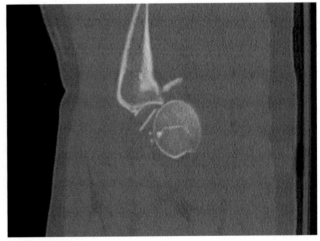

FIGURE 92C

FINDINGS Supine AP radiograph of the pelvis (Fig. 92A) demonstrates a dislocated right hip, with marked superior displacement of the femoral head; the right femur is internally rotated relative to the left. There is a vertically oriented fracture of the posterior acetabular wall. Axial CT image of the pelvis at the level of the right femoral head following attempted reduction (Fig. 92B) demonstrates partial reduction with persistent posterior and superior subluxation. Two large intra-articular osseous bodies are present. Sagittal CT image through the right hip (Fig. 92C) demonstrates posterior subluxation of the femoral head and both intra- and extra-articular bone fragments.

DIFFERENTIAL DIAGNOSIS Hip dislocation (anterior or posterior) with or without acetabular fracture or femoral head fracture.

DIAGNOSIS Traumatic posterior hip dislocation with post-reduction intra-articular fracture fragments.

DISCUSSION Posterior hip dislocations outnumber anterior hip dislocations by approximately 9:1. Hip dislocation occurs most often in the setting of high-energy trauma, such as in motor vehicle collisions when the hip is flexed and adducted and the knee is pushed dorsally by impact with the dashboard. Injuries that are commonly associated with posterior hip dislocation include fracture of the posterior acetabular wall, injury of the acetabular labrum, sciatic nerve injury, and injury to the ipsilateral knee. The degree of hip flexion and adduction at the time of injury correlates with the subsequent injury pattern. Increasing flexion and adduction inversely correlates with the size of the posterior wall fracture fragment (i.e., the more adducted the hip, the smaller the fragment), with even greater flexion and adduction favoring pure dislocation injury without a fracture component. When the posterior acetabular wall is fractured, fragments may remain within the intra-articular space following reduction. In one case series, intra-articular fragments were found in 43 out of 109 cases of posterior hip dislocation with acetabular fracture (39%).[1]

193

In general, AP pelvis radiographs are sufficient to diagnose a hip dislocation. It can be difficult to determine anterior from posterior hip dislocations on a single AP image, but there are few indicators. First, a posteriorly dislocated hip is often internally rotated while an anteriorly dislocated hip is often externally rotated. Second, in a well-centered nonrotated image, a posteriorly dislocated femoral head will appear smaller than the contralateral side secondary to geometric magnification. Alternatively, Judet views can be obtained to better delineate anterior from posterior dislocation. Evaluation for acetabular fracture or intra-articular fragments usually requires additional images after the initial screening AP pelvis radiograph. Getting follow-up radiographs in multiple projections on a patient with recent trauma may not completely define the extent of injury or be feasible secondary to difficulty with patient positioning. Therefore, full assessment is best performed with CT. CT is also recommended for preoperative planning and can be repeated postoperatively to ensure that all intra-articular fragments have been removed.

Two interventions have an impact on long-term prognosis. First, reduction of the hip dislocation should be performed urgently in order to reduce the risk of avascular necrosis (AVN) of the femoral head. When reduced within 24 hours of injury, the incidence of AVN has been reported to be 6%, while the rate of AVN is 28% when reduction is delayed >24 hours.[2] Second, evaluation for and removal of intra-articular fracture fragments should be performed as early as possible because intra-articular fragments may prevent complete reduction of the dislocation and will cause cartilage damage with subsequent osteoarthrosis if not removed.

Question for Further Thought

1. What types of acetabular fractures are most commonly seen with hip dislocation?

Reporting Responsibilities

Posterior hip dislocation is an emergency, but is often evident clinically; direct communication with the referring clinician is recommended. The presence of intra-articular fragments on a post-reduction study should prompt a phone call if the patient is not already in the care of an orthopedic surgeon.

What the Treating Physician Needs to Know?

- Presence of hip dislocation (recommend follow-up CT after reduction).
- Presence of intra-articular fragments.
- Other osseous injuries (femoral head, femoral neck, pelvic ring).
- Any soft tissue injuries on cross-sectional imaging (e.g., bladder injury, intramuscular hematoma, etc.).

Answer

1. Judet and Letournel developed a classification system for acetabular fractures based on three elementary types of fractures: column fractures, wall fractures, and transverse fractures. The most common fracture types are isolated posterior wall and combined posterior wall with transverse fractures. Combined, these two types account for approximately 47% of acetabular fractures. Posterior wall fractures are most commonly associated with posterior hip dislocation. Posterior wall fractures are deemed unstable when >40% of the posterior wall is involved.

CLINICAL HISTORY *8-month-old female who presented with acute onset of lethargy and weakness. No significant medical history other than a mild upper respiratory infection a few weeks prior.*

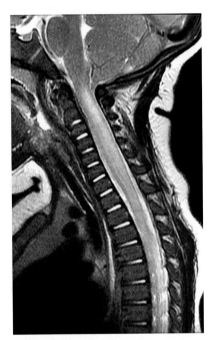

FIGURE 93A

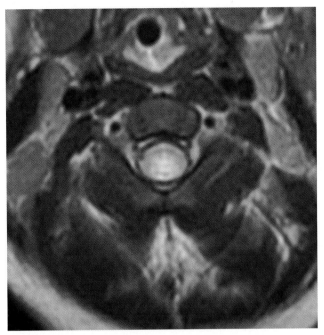

FIGURE 93B

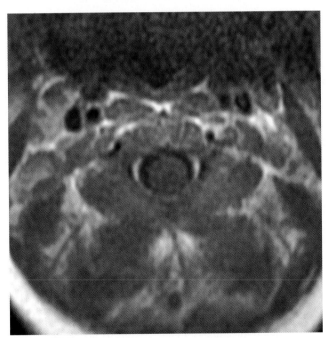

FIGURE 93C

FINDINGS Figure 93A: Sagittal T2WI through the cervical spine demonstrates a longitudinally extensive segment of abnormally increased signal within the cervical and upper thoracic spinal cord extending from roughly C1 through T2. The involved cervical cord also appears expanded. Figure 93B: Axial T2WI at the level of C3 demonstrates increased signal involving the entire cross-sectional area of the cord, which is difficult to distinguish from the surrounding CSF. Figure 93C: Corresponding axial contrast-enhanced T1WI demonstrates no abnormal enhancement within the involved cord. A concurrently obtained brain MRI (not shown) was normal.

DIFFERENTIAL DIAGNOSIS Differential considerations for an intramedullary T2 hyperintense lesion include *acute transverse myelitis (ATM)*, which can be idiopathic or associated with diseases such as multiple sclerosis, acute disseminated encephalomyelitis (ADEM), neuromyelitis optica (NMO), and various autoimmune disorders (e.g. systemic lupus erythematosus, Sjogren's syndrome, Behcet's disease, and antiphospholipid antibody syndrome). *Infectious myelitis*, which can be caused by a number of viral, bacterial, or parasitic pathogens, can be indistinguishable from ATM. *Intramedullary spinal tumors* such as astrocytomas and ependymomas may also present as expansile cord lesions. These frequently enhance and may demonstrate additional features such as hemorrhage or calcifications. In addition, symptoms due to spinal cord tumors typically develop over a protracted time period. *Vascular lesions* such as AVMs or dural arteriovenous fistulas (AVFs) can produce spinal cord swelling and edema, but these lesions usually also demonstrate prominent vessels in or on the surface of the spinal cord. They also present more insidiously unless they have acutely hemorrhaged. Furthermore, dural AVFs usually present in middle-aged and elderly men and involve the distal cord and conus. *Spinal cord ischemia* is typically a disease of older adults with a history of severe atherosclerotic disease, and may demonstrate signal abnormality isolated to the anterior gray matter horns of the spinal cord.

DIAGNOSIS   Acute transverse myelitis.

DISCUSSION   Acute transverse myelitis (ATM) refers to a spinal cord syndrome that presents abruptly with motor, sensory, and autonomic symptoms. Approximately 20% of ATM cases occur in children, with two peaks of incidence observed in the pediatric population—the first being between 0 and 2 years and the second between 5 and 17 years of age. The diagnosis of transverse myelitis is one of exclusion, as a number of conditions can produce a myelopathy with symptoms similar to those of ATM. These include spinal compression, infection, ischemia, intramedullary tumors, vascular malformations, toxic and metabolic processes such as vitamin B_{12} deficiency, and prior spinal radiation. If these conditions are excluded, a patient can be presumed to have a diagnosis of ATM, and further attempts are then typically made to determine whether the condition is arising in association with an underlying disease or is idiopathic in nature.

Most pediatric cases of ATM fall into the idiopathic category, which accounts for 89% of ATM diagnoses in children, compared to only 36% in adults. Diseases associated with pediatric ATM include acute disseminated encephalomyelitis (ADEM), multiple sclerosis (MS), neuromyelitis optica (NMO), and connective tissue diseases such as systemic lupus erythematosus.

In most cases of pediatric ATM, the onset of myelopathy is preceded by a mild illness occurring in the 3 weeks prior to symptom onset, with additional factors such as recent vaccination or allergy shots also being potential provoking factors. Patients usually present initially with back pain, motor deficits, numbness, ataxic gait, or loss of bowel or bladder control. Weakness generally involves the lower extremities, but may also affect the torso and upper extremities. Sensory loss is typically noted in a band-like or transverse distribution, with decrease in sensation distally (hence the name "transverse" myelitis). Encephalopathy is not classically seen in isolated ATM, but may be present in cases associated with ADEM.

On axial T2WI, the lesions of ATM may involve just the central cord, with sparing of the periphery, or may involve the entire cross section of the cord. Enhancement following contrast administration is variable, but is absent in most cases. In addition to spinal MRI, which should be performed whenever a patient presents with acute myelopathy, evaluation of ATM should include imaging of the brain to identify additional CNS lesions; lumbar puncture with CSF evaluation for cell count and IgG index, oligoclonal bands, aquaporin 4 (AQP4) IgG, and viral and bacterial tests; and serum evaluation for infectious causes of myelitis, AQP4 IgG, and an autoimmune panel. Ophthalmologic evaluation should also be performed to assess for evidence of optic neuritis.

In this particular case, the patient presented with imaging findings of longitudinally extensive transverse myelitis (LETM), which is defined as intramedullary T2-hyperintense signal in the spinal cord that spans at least 3 vertebral

segments in craniocaudal extent. LETM is commonly observed in cases of idiopathic pediatric ATM as well as in cases of ATM associated with ADEM and NMO. On the other hand, spinal cord lesions due to MS typically involve fewer than 3 contiguous vertebral segments. Patients with ADEM should have evidence of one or more brain lesions on MRI, while NMO is associated with optic neuritis and positive serum or CSF assays for AQP4 IgG. Although this patient's presentation was suggestive of ADEM (given her encephalopathic presentation), the negative brain MRI effectively ruled out the diagnosis. Furthermore, serum studies were negative for AQP4 IgG, and her autoimmune panel was normal. She was therefore given a final diagnosis of idiopathic ATM.

Certain lesion locations warrant close monitoring for respiratory or cardiac complications in patients with ATM. High cervical and medullary lesions can affect the lower cranial nerves, which may result in loss of ability to protect the airway and maintain airway patency. Cervical lesions above C5 can affect the diaphragm, resulting in loss of inspiratory diaphragmatic excursion and, ultimately, respiratory compromise. Finally, thoracic lesions above T6 can cause autonomic dysreflexia.

The initial treatment for suspected ATM is intravenous steroids, along with supportive therapy to maintain respiratory and circulatory function. If symptoms fail to improve or worsen within 24 to 48 hours, plasma exchange therapy should be considered. There is also some evidence suggesting a benefit from administration of intravenous immunoglobulin and cyclophosphamide. In most cases, symptoms of ATM begin to progress over the first few days before plateauing at approximately 1 week. The time from symptom onset to initial recovery averages 9 days.

Questions for Further Thought

1. What percentage of patients with ADEM demonstrate spinal cord involvement?
2. What is the prognosis for children with ATM? What is the prognosis in adults?

Reporting Responsibilities

If a diagnosis of ATM is suspected based on the findings of spinal MRI, further evaluation with a dedicated contrast-enhanced brain MRI should be suggested to help establish if the myelitis is associated with an underlying disease. In addition, lesions in critical locations, including the upper cervical cord and lower brainstem, should be promptly communicated to the requesting clinician, as lesions in these locations are potentially life threatening because of the possibility of respiratory compromise.

What the Treating Physician Needs to Know?

- Are the spinal imaging findings compatible with the diagnosis of ATM? If not, are there alternate findings to explain myelopathy?
- What spinal cord levels are involved? Does the lesion involve ≥3 vertebral segments or <3 vertebral segments?

- Are there lesions evident in the brain?
- Are there imaging findings to suggest optic neuritis?

Answers

1. Approximately 30% of patients diagnosed with ADEM demonstrate spinal cord lesions on MR imaging.

2. Roughly 33% to 50% of children with ATM recover completely. 10% to 20% will have poor outcomes, while the remainder will be left with milder residual deficits. In adult patients with ATM, it has historically been reported that approximately one-third have a good outcome, one-third have a fair outcome, and one-third have a poor outcome.

CLINICAL HISTORY *36-year-old male with acute onset calf pain while playing tennis.*

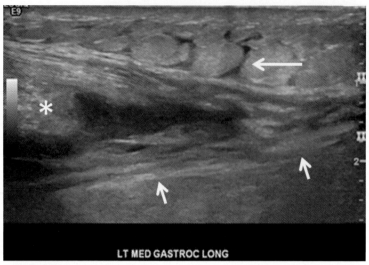

FIGURE 94A

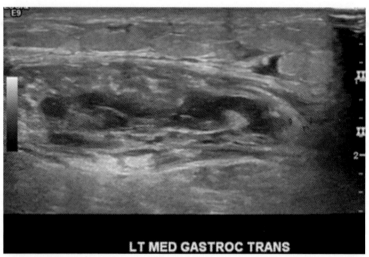

FIGURE 94B

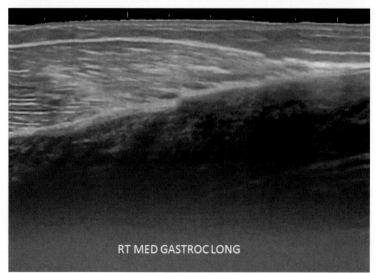

FIGURE 94C

FINDINGS Long/sagittal (Fig. 94A) and short/transverse (Fig. 94B) axis gray-scale sonographic images of the left medial head of gastrocnemius demonstrate a moderate- to large-sized near-triangular-shaped hypoechoic defect at the distal myotendinous junction. The heterogeneity seen on the short-axis image is consistent with a hematoma. Intact fibers are seen on the left side of the image. The *asterisk* indicates the retracted portion of the muscle. The *short arrows* point to the Achilles tendon/myotendinous junction that separates the gastrocnemius (superficial) from the soleus (deep). Interdigitating free fluid within the subcutaneous tissues (*long arrow*) consistent with edema is present. Long-axis view of the contralateral leg (Fig. 94C) shows the myofibrils making contact with the myotendinous junction. Note how the more distal (right side of image) fibrillar pattern appears smudged and more hyperechoic than the more proximal (left side of image) fibrillar pattern.

DIFFERENTIAL DIAGNOSIS Medial head of gastrocnemius muscle tear, plantaris rupture, proximal Achilles tendon tear, ruptured popliteal cyst, intramuscular abscess, deep vein thrombosis.

DIAGNOSIS Large left medial head of gastrocnemius partial tear (Figs. 94A and 94B), low-grade right medial head of gastrocnemius strain (Fig. 94C).

DISCUSSION The gastrocnemius muscle is located in the superficial posterior compartment of the leg and predominantly provides plantar flexion at the ankle. There are two heads of the gastrocnemius, medial and lateral, which originate at the femoral condyles and unite to form the Achilles tendon along with the soleus. The gastrocnemius crosses the knee, ankle, and subtalar joints before inserting on the calcaneus. The gastrocnemius is thought to be more susceptible to injury compared with other leg muscles because of crossing the knee and ankle joints; nearly all calf muscle strain injuries involve the medial head. The medial head of gastrocnemius is larger than the lateral head and contains proportionally more "fast twitch" muscle fibers. The increased number of fast twitch fibers correlates with the medial head's importance in running and jumping activities.[1] Hyperextension of the knee in conjunction with forced dorsiflexion causes increased strain at the myotendinous junction relative to a muscle crossing only a single joint (e.g., the soleus) because of the large amount of stretch in this position. Muscle strain injuries typically occur during eccentric contraction where the muscle is contracting while lengthening; strain injuries occur only when muscle fibers are longer than the resting muscle length, which is more likely to occur with muscles crossing two joints.[1] Although muscles with increased proportion of fast twitch fibers are more frequently injured and while it seems plausible that the ability to rapidly produce a contraction can exceed the strain limit of the muscle especially during an eccentric contraction, this has not been proven. Tears of the medial head of the gastrocnemius are usually sports-related injuries, commonly affecting middle-aged persons and sometimes referred to as "tennis leg," given its association with tennis and other racquet sports. The severity of the strain injury can range from microscopic tears to complete dissociation of the myotendinous junction and nearly always occurs at the distal myotendinous junction. Onset of pain and swelling in the calf is immediate. Ecchymosis may be present.

No validated grading system for muscle strain injuries exists. Many classify muscle strain injuries as low grade, moderate grade, and high grade, but exact definitions differ among practitioners. Low-grade injuries are associated with microtears without formation of a detectable confluent fluid collection. High-grade tears are characterized by complete disruption of the myotendinous junction and complete loss of muscle function. Moderate-grade tears represent a relatively large spectrum of partial tears at the myotendinous junction, but all with an identifiable fluid collection; an estimate of the percentage of fiber disruption at the myotendinous junction is needed to make this grade useful. Moderate-grade tears are associated with pain and diminished, but not absent muscle function.

Imaging in the setting of a suspected medial head of gastrocnemius tear is performed to determine severity of injury (complete or partial tear) and exclusion of alternative pathology. Radiographs are usually normal, but may show nonspecific soft tissue swelling. Both ultrasonography and MRI provide adequate soft tissue contrast to establish and characterize a muscle tear. Sonographic examination should be considered as a first-line imaging modality because of the short examination duration and low relative cost. Sonographic findings include loss of the normal fibrillar muscle pattern on long-axis images as it inserts onto the myotendinous junction of the proximal Achilles tendon to overt fiber disruption with fluid collections interposed between the torn muscle fibers and the myotendinous junction. Low-grade strains will be characterized by mild hyperechogenicity of the muscle fibers with indistinctness of the normal fibrillar echotexture. Partial and complete tears will be characterized by muscle fiber retraction. Often adjacent subcutaneous soft tissue swelling with wisps of interdigitating linear hypoechogenicity indicating edema will be present. If the injury is severe, these findings will be present in the overlying subcutaneous tissues. A retrospective US study of 141 patients with a clinical diagnosis of "tennis leg" demonstrated partial medial head of gastrocnemius tears at the myotendinous junction in 66.7% of patients. In patients with a partial gastrocnemius tear, a fluid collection between the medial head of gastrocnemius and soleus muscles was identified in 62.8%.[2] Similar findings can be expected on MRI, which can also document low-grade strains by the presence of diffuse muscle edema without confluent fluid. Ultrasonography can also document healing progress in follow-up patients.[3] MRI is preferred in instances of diagnostic uncertainty or suspected alternative pathology such as an underlying mass lesion.

Complications of medial head of gastrocnemius injuries include leg muscle herniation, myositis ossificans, scarring, contracture, functional impairment, and, uncommonly, compartment syndrome. Treatment options include supportive management and compression. Union of medial head of gastrocnemius with soleus muscle was more rapid in a statistically significant number of patients who received compression after injury.[4] Treatment with compression is also associated with decreased hemorrhage and early ambulation.

Questions for Further Thought

1. Are medial head of gastrocnemius tears ever treated surgically?
2. What other calf soft tissue injuries can present with acute medial calf pain?

Reporting Responsibilities

Medial head of gastrocnemius muscle tear is not an emergency; a timely report is required.

What the Treating Physician Needs to Know

- Tear location.
- Partial versus complete tear.
- Size of associated hematoma/fluid collection for future comparison.
- Integrity of the Achilles tendon, plantaris tendon, and soleus.

Answers

1. Surgical intervention is usually reserved for treatment of resulting compartment syndrome in the posterior compartment of the calf. Primary repair of the gastrocnemius is also occasionally considered if persistent complete loss of muscle function or anatomic defect is seen in the gastrocnemius.[5]
2. Acute onset calf pain during athletic activity is not always due to medial head of gastrocnemius tear. Plantaris tendon rupture can mimic gastrocnemius injury and presents with a fluid collection between the medial head of gastrocnemius and soleus; the gastrocnemius myotendinous junction will be intact on imaging. Disruption of the tendon needs to be documented for this diagnosis as spontaneous fluid collections without tendon rupture can also occur in this region. Acute onset of pain and swelling in the calf can also be suggestive of a thrombosed lower extremity vein. Thus, evaluating the adjacent popliteal and calf veins for patency is helpful in excluding venous thrombosis. In the US study of 141 patients with a diagnosis of "tennis leg" mentioned above, the other findings in the posterior calf included fluid collection without tendon or myotendinous rupture (30%), plantaris tendon rupture (1.4%), soleus partial rupture (0.7%), and deep vein thrombosis (10%).[2]

CLINICAL HISTORY *50-year-old patient with 48 hours of worsening left-sided chest pain, persistent nausea, and vomiting.*

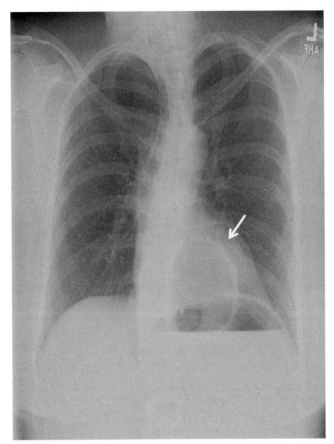

FIGURE 95A

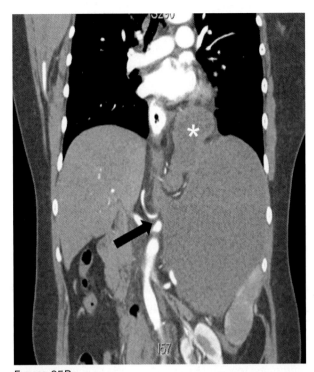

FIGURE 95B

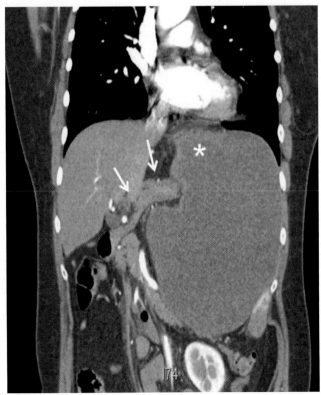

FIGURE 95C

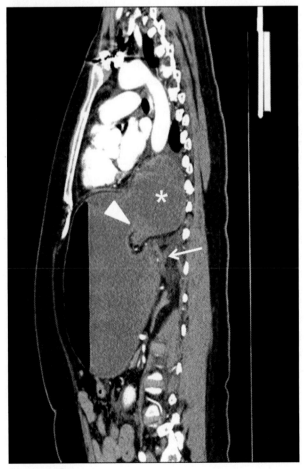

FIGURE 95D

FINDINGS Figure 95A: Plain radiograph of the chest shows a retrocardiac air-filled mass, corresponding to the gastric antrum above the diaphragm (*arrow*). Figure 95B: Coronal contrast-enhanced CT image of the upper abdomen demonstrates a distended stomach with abnormal orientation. The gastroesophageal (GE) junction (*black arrow*) lies inferior to the left diaphragm and below the gastric antrum (*asterisk*), representing a mesenteroaxial volvulus. The greater curvature remains to the left of the lesser curvature. Figure 95C: Coronal CT image of the upper abdomen anterior to Figure 95B demonstrates the gastric antrum (*asterisk*) in the left upper abdomen and nondilated proximal duodenum (*arrows*) superior to the gastric fundus. Figure 95D: Sagittal CT image of the abdomen shows herniation of the dilated gastric antrum (*asterisk*) into the thorax. The gastric antrum and pylorus (*arrowhead*) is located superior to the GE junction (*arrow*), compatible with a mesenteroaxial volvulus. Gastric fluid-filled distention was related to gastric outlet obstruction.

DIFFERENTIAL DIAGNOSIS Sliding hiatal hernia, paraesophageal hernia, gastric volvulus.

DIAGNOSIS Mesenteroaxial gastric volvulus.

DISCUSSION Gastric volvulus refers to abnormal orientation of the stomach. This may vary from being completely asymptomatic to vague chronic dyspepsia to acute or recurring severe epigastric pain. Majority (up to 90%) of gastric volvulus are chronic, and may be due to congenital or traumatic etiologies or can be seen with hiatal hernia. Other risk factors may include left diaphragmatic hernia, pyloric stenosis, and adhesions. This is most common in the fifth decade of life, but can be seen in any age group. Patients with acute volvulus may present with Borchardt triad, which includes severe abdominal pain, intractable retching without vomiting, and inability to pass a nasogastric tube into the stomach.

The stomach is normally held by the gastrophrenic, gastrosplenic, gastrohepatic, and gastrocolic ligaments, but retains a certain degree of mobility. Agenesis or laxity of the ligaments or loss of ligamentous support, especially in atypical spaces (intrathoracic herniation), along with gastric peristalsis and abnormal attachments from adhesions (surgery or ulcer), can lead to an abnormal position and rotation. This can potentially cause luminal obstruction or compromise the vascular supply.

Abnormal rotation of the stomach more commonly occurs along the long axis of the organ, called organoaxial volvulus, with the greater curvature located superior to the lesser curvature. The stomach can twist on its short axis, called mesenteroaxial volvulus, causing the gastric antrum to be displaced above the gastroesophageal junction. Mesenteroaxial volvulus is more readily appreciated, given that the two landmarks of the gastroesophageal junction and gastric antrum are easily identified, especially on a coronal CT image.

Imaging is important to identify abnormal rotation and to evaluate for incomplete or complete gastric outlet obstruction. The latter of which is more likely to occur if there is more than 180° of rotation. This can cause the stomach to become dilated and fluid filled. If the stomach is large enough, it can herniate into the thorax and cause cardiorespiratory compromise.

Imaging of gastric volvulus includes radiography, fluoroscopy, and computed tomography (CT). Chest radiograph can demonstrate a retrocardiac air-filled mass, corresponding to the stomach above the diaphragm. An abdominal radiograph can demonstrate increased soft tissue density in the upper abdomen, corresponding to distended fluid-filled stomach or two air-fluid levels, corresponding to the fundus and antrum of the stomach. An upper gastrointestinal (UGI) fluoroscopic study can be performed to evaluate for rotation of the stomach and to detect the passage of ingested oral contrast material into the duodenum. CT is performed in the acute setting of epigastric pain and vomiting to identify the rotation of the herniated stomach and transition point.

Patients with chronic gastric volvulus can be managed conservatively. However, acute gastric volvulus requires surgical intervention.

Question for Further Thought

1. What would be the modality of choice for suspected chronic gastric volvulus?

Reporting Responsibilities

Acute gastric volvulus is a surgical emergency, and the referring clinician should be notified immediately.

What the Treating Physician Needs to Know?

- Identifying the site, cause, and axis of rotation of a gastric volvulus.
- Identifying the complications of gastric volvulus, most commonly gastric outlet obstruction and rarely devascularization and ischemia.

Answer

1. Upper gastrointestinal (UGI) series is the preferred choice for chronic volvulus as the projection can be optimized to allow visualization of the course of the esophagus, stomach, and duodenum. In the acute setting, CT is the preferred modality to better assess for perforation and other causes of pain or obstruction.

CLINICAL HISTORY *38-year-old with knee pain while playing basketball.*

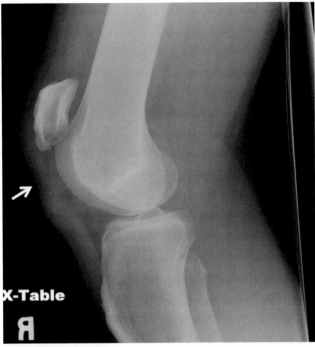

FIGURE 96A

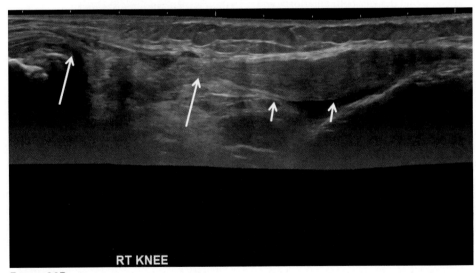

FIGURE 96B

FINDINGS Lateral radiograph of the right knee (Fig. 96A) demonstrates patella alta and focal deficiency (*arrow*) in the proximal patellar tendon; distal patellar tendon is somewhat wavy. Long-axis gray-scale sonographic image of the right knee (Fig. 96B) demonstrates complete loss of continuity of the normal fibrillar echotexture of the proximal patellar tendon. *Long arrows* depict the tear edges. *Short arrows* depict intact tendon, which appears somewhat thickened and wavy because of loss of normal tensile stress; an element of tendinosis may also be present.

DIAGNOSIS Patellar tendon rupture.

DISCUSSION Acute injuries of the knee extensor mechanism composed of the quadriceps tendon, the patella, and the patellar tendon most commonly result in patellar fracture followed in incidence by quadriceps tendon rupture; patellar tendon rupture is the least common of these extensor mechanism injuries. Patellar tendon rupture occurs most often in physically active men under the age of 40, but may also occur in older patients with underlying systemic disease. The proximal patellar tendon is injured with sports injuries, and other sites (midsubstance or distal tendon) are usually torn with underlying medical conditions. The normal patellar tendon is able to withstand extremely large tensile stresses, the equivalent of 17.5 times normal body weight.[1] As a result, a preexisting pathologic condition is necessary before rupture can occur. Most commonly, this condition is patellar tendinosis, a lesion resulting from repetitive microtrauma. Systemic conditions such as gout, rheumatoid arthritis, renal failure, diabetes mellitus, systemic lupus erythematosus, and medication (corticosteroids and fluoroquinolones) have also been implicated in patellar tendon rupture.

The typical mechanism of injury is a forceful contraction of the quadriceps muscle in the setting of a flexed knee, a situation that may arise with an abrupt deceleration while running or jumping. In the elderly, a common mechanism is a fall on a flexed knee. Signs and symptoms include high-riding patella, swelling, tenderness, cramping, and complete inability to extend the knee.

Although physical examination is usually sufficient to diagnose a patellar tendon rupture, confirmation with imaging is sometimes necessary. Regardless of imaging modality, the patellar and quadriceps tendons are taut when the knee is imaged in any degree of flexion and have well-defined anterior and posterior margins; any deviation is concerning for tendon pathology. The patellar tendon itself demonstrates homogenous soft tissue density on radiographs that is visible because it is bordered by fat density both anteriorly and posteriorly, homogeneous low signal on both T1- and T2-weighted MR images, and a fibrillar echotexture along the long axis of the tendon on ultrasonography. Waviness of either the patellar or quadriceps tendon is concerning for a tear. A lateral radiograph is usually sufficient to confirm the diagnosis of a patellar tendon rupture especially when proximal displacement of the patella (patella alta), redundant quadriceps tendon, and focal attenuation of the patellar tendon are seen. A partial tear or tendinosis is more likely if either the anterior or posterior (most common) interface is blurred or there is focal enlargement without patella alta; radiographs are unable to make this distinction. MRI and ultrasonography are equally capable of diagnosing and characterizing patellar tendon ruptures. Sagittal fluid-sensitive images (MRI) or long-axis images (ultrasonography) through the patellar tendon are usually sufficient for diagnosis of a tear. A full-thickness tear will often, but not always, have a clearly definable gap between the torn ends of the tendon. Axial or short-axis images may be needed to assess the size of a partial tear. Signs of a tear include a transverse full-thickness or partial-thickness, fluid-filled defect. On MRI, this fluid-filled defect will be a fluid bright cleft in an otherwise intermediate- to dark-appearing tendon. Sonographically, patellar tendon tears may appear as nearly anechoic clefts (fluid) or heterogeneously hyperechoic material (interposed fat from Hoffa's fat pad) displaced into the tear. The quadriceps tendon may be redundant because of lack of tensile stress. In cases where there is uncertainty regarding the extent of the tear, dynamic sonography can be performed to document the presence of tear enlargement with either attempted active knee extension or passive knee flexion. As most tears occur in the presence of tendinosis, thickening of the tendon and elevated, but not fluid bright, signal will likely be seen adjacent to the tear on MRI, and thickened, hypoechoic tendon demonstrating loss of the normal fibrillar echotexture will be noted on ultrasonography.

Management for small, partial tears includes immobilization with a brace to facilitate holding the knee straight through the healing period. Crutches with knee locked in extension and physical therapy are also usually required. Complete tears require surgery with transpatellar bone tunnels. Chronic complete tear following total knee arthroplasty may require using an allograft, synthetic mesh, or an autograft. After surgery, many report stiffness, but regain nearly equal motion compared to the uninjured leg. Complications are few but include knee stiffness, quadriceps atrophy, and a second rupture. Acute repairs are associated with excellent outcomes.

Questions for Further Thought

1. What is jumper's knee?
2. What is an apophyseal sleeve avulsion?

Reporting Responsibilities

Patellar tendon rupture is not an emergency; a timely report is required.

What the Treating Physician Needs To Know?

- Location of tear.
- Full-thickness versus partial-thickness; percentage involvement with partial tears.

Answers

1. Jumper's knee refers to tendinosis of the proximal patellar tendon. Repetitive strong quadriceps contractions in the setting of a flexed knee, as may be seen in jumping sports such as basketball, in excess of the tensile strength of the tendon and at a rate greater than the tendon's normal ability to heal itself result in a dysregulated healing response, that ultimately lead to derangement of the normal fibrillar architecture of the tendon. For reasons that are poorly understood, this almost always occurs at the proximal end of the tendon and begins at the deep border of the tendon. Paralleling the progression of tendinosis, tears begin at the deep border of the tendon. The pediatric version of jumper's knee is Sinding–Larsen–Johansson syndrome, which is characterized by repetitive microtrauma to the proximal patellar tendon in the setting of a still partially cartilaginous inferior patellar pole; this condition typically occurs in active 10- to 15-year-olds.[2] The usual findings of tendinosis are present with additional intratendinous ossifications possibly representing small avulsed fragments from the inferior patellar pole.

2. Patellar sleeve avulsion is most commonly seen in 8- to 12-year-olds and involves avulsion of an arc of articular cartilage (deep aspect) and cartilage plus periosteum

(superficial aspect) from the inferior pole of the patella.[3] As there may be no mineralized bone involved, there may be no radiographic indication of an avulsion injury other than patella alta. Sagittal MR images will differentiate Sinding–Larsen–Johansson syndrome from patellar sleeve avulsion. Findings of proximal patellar tendinosis with possible intratendinous ossifications with preserved articular cartilage will be seen in Sinding–Larsen–Johansson syndrome, while cartilaginous injury with osseous deformity will be seen with patellar sleeve avulsion. Treatment differs between these two entities: Sinding–Larsen–Johannson syndrome, an overuse syndrome, is treated nonoperatively, while patellar sleeve avulsion, an acute fracture equivalent, is treated with open reduction and possible internal fixation with potential reconstruction of the extensor mechanism.

CLINICAL HISTORY *56-year-old male with a history of end-stage renal disease and hypertension, found unresponsive, and unable to move his right arm and leg.*

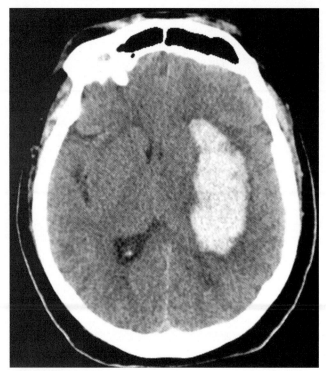

FIGURE 97A

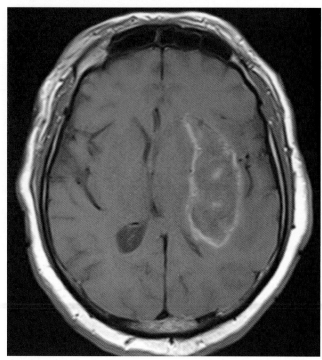

FIGURE 97B

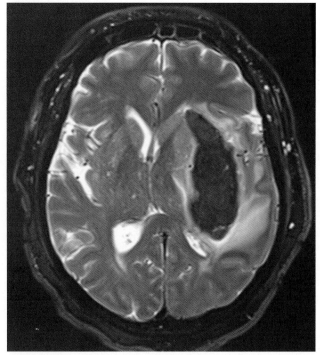

FIGURE 97C

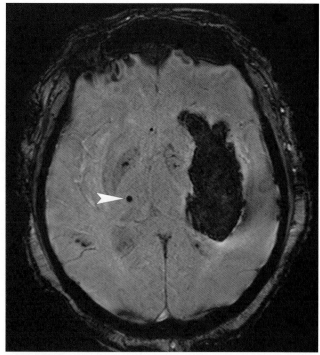

FIGURE 97D

FINDINGS Figure 97A: Axial noncontrast CT image demonstrates a large, hyperdense hematoma centered in the lateral aspect of the left lentiform nucleus, compressing the left lateral ventricle and producing left to right midline shift. Figures 97B and 97C: Corresponding axial noncontrast T1W (Fig. 97B) and T2W (Fig. 97C) images demonstrate the hemorrhage to be predominately isointense to brain on T1WI and hypointense on T2WI centrally, indicative of deoxyhemoglobin. The periphery of the lesion demonstrates T1 shortening, indicating localized breakdown of hemoglobin into methemoglobin. The T2WI also demonstrates vasogenic edema around the hemorrhage. Though not shown, MRA did not demonstrate evidence of an aneurysm or arteriovenous malformation. Figure 97D: Axial SWI image demonstrates signal void throughout the hematoma. In addition, there is a small focus of signal dropout in the right thalamus (*arrowhead*), compatible with a remote microhemorrhage. Similar foci of signal dropout, suggestive of remote microhemorrhages, were also evident in the bilateral dentate nuclei (not shown).

DIFFERENTIAL DIAGNOSIS A hemorrhagic lesion centered in the basal ganglia may be seen in numerous conditions. The most common cause of spontaneous hemorrhage arising in the basal ganglia or thalami is *hypertensive hemorrhage*. Additional imaging features suggestive of the diagnosis include evidence of prior hemorrhages in characteristic locations such as the deep gray matter nuclei (as is seen in this case), dentate nuclei, and brainstem, as well as leukoaraiosis commonly seen in patients with long-standing hypertension. *Amyloid angiopathy* characteristically presents with lobar hemorrhage, and SWI may demonstrate evidence of remote, peripherally distributed hemorrhages elsewhere. Furthermore, hemorrhages due to amyloid angiopathy usually occur in patients over the age of 60. *Deep venous infarction* in the internal cerebral veins can present with hypodensities in the thalami, which may simulate a resolving hypertensive hemorrhage. Patients who are coagulopathic may also present with hemorrhage in the deep gray structures. *Hemorrhagic neoplasms* can present in the basal ganglia. A contrast-enhanced MRI study is indicated to look for the presence of tumoral enhancement. Given the high prevalence of metastatic tumors to the brain compared to primary brain neoplasm, most hemorrhagic tumors are extracranial in origin. Underlying *vascular malformations*, including arteriovenous malformations (AVMs) and cavernous malformations, can also present with hemorrhage. AVMs demonstrate a tangled collection of vessels in or adjacent to the hemorrhage on CTA or MRA, while cavernous malformations can demonstrate "popcorn like" calcifications on CT and a hemosiderin ring on MRI from recurrent hemorrhage.

DIAGNOSIS Hypertensive hemorrhage.

DISCUSSION Hypertensive intracranial hemorrhage is defined as acute nontraumatic hemorrhage secondary to systemic hypertension, and is the most common cause of intracranial hemorrhage in the adult population. About 50% of nontraumatic intracranial hemorrhages are attributed to hypertension. Patients with hypertensive hemorrhage often have a history of long-standing and poorly controlled hypertension, which is hypothesized to lead to atherosclerosis and fibrinoid necrosis of the intracranial vessels. The vessels that are most commonly affected are perforating small vessels. Microaneurysms of these perforating arteries, termed *Charcot–Bouchard aneurysms*, are thought to be responsible for the hemorrhages. The small penetrating vessels involved are predominately found in the lenticulostriate regions, with a small percentage also found in the pons and cerebellum. As a result, these locations represent the most common sites of hypertensive hemorrhage, with the basal ganglia and thalami being the most commonly involved (80%), followed by the pons and cerebellum (10%). Approximately 5% to 10% of patients will have a lobar hemorrhage.

Hypertensive intracranial hemorrhage most commonly occurs in the middle-aged to elderly patients and in males. African Americans are affected more frequently, which likely reflects the high prevalence of hypertension in this population. About 20% of patients presenting with acute neurologic deficits have hypertensive intracranial hemorrhage, and large hypertensive hemorrhages may lead to impaired consciousness and sensorimotor deficits as was the case in the presented patient.

The imaging findings in this case are typical for hypertensive hemorrhage in the basal ganglia. The large left to right midline shift and compression of the bilateral lateral ventricles are mass effect complications that may result from a large hematoma. Intraventricular extension of the hematoma with associated hydrocephalus can occur and portends a poor prognosis. Treatment of hypertensive intracranial hemorrhage is mostly nonsurgical. Evacuation of the hematoma itself has no associated benefit in most cases. Symptomatic management of the mass effect and decreasing intracranial pressure by medical management and ventricular shunting is the mainstay of treatment.

Question for Further Thought

1. What is the typical timeline for patients with hypertensive hemorrhage to deteriorate?

Reporting Responsibilities

Findings of hypertensive hemorrhage should be communicated promptly to the referring physician, and MRI should be suggested in stable patients to exclude the possibility of an underlying mass or vascular malformation. The official radiology report should include the site of the hemorrhage, age of the hemorrhage (best detected on MRI), intraventricular extension, hydrocephalus, and the presence of mass effect, including herniation syndromes.

What the Treating Physician Needs to Know?

- Is the location typical for hypertensive hemorrhage, or is it more suggestive of an alternative diagnosis such as amyloid angiopathy?
- Are there other findings to support the diagnosis of hypertensive hemorrhage (e.g., remote microhemorrhages in characteristic locations or advanced leukoaraiosis)?

- Is there mass effect (midline shift or herniation)?
- Is there intraventricular extension of hemorrhage or hydrocephalus?
- Is there be an underling mass or vascular malformation?

Answer

1. Increasing mass effect from the expansion of the hematoma potentially results in herniation or hydrocephalus peak in the first 48 hours. Therefore, patients should be closely monitored during this time frame.

CLINICAL HISTORY *80-year-old female presenting with gradual onset of mental status changes.*

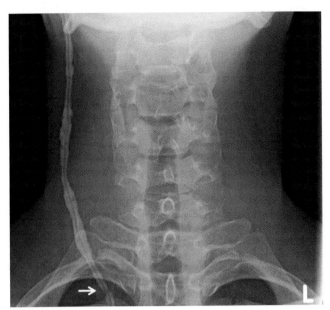

FIGURE 98A

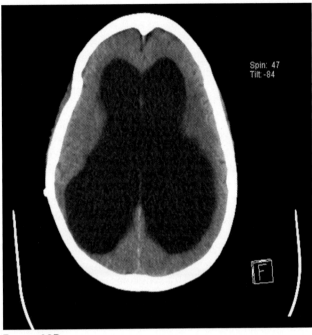

FIGURE 98B

FINDINGS AP radiograph of the neck (Fig. 98A) demonstrates extensive calcification about the ventriculoperitoneal shunt tubing that overlies the right neck. A focal discontinuity is present where the tubing overlies the right lung apex (*arrow*). Axial CT image in brain window (Fig. 98B) reveals severe dilatation of the lateral ventricles.

DIFFERENTIAL DIAGNOSIS Hydrocephalus ex vacuo, ventriculoperitoneal shunt discontinuity, intact ventriculoperitoneal shunt with concretions.

DIAGNOSIS Ventriculoperitoneal shunt discontinuity with hydrocephalus.

DISCUSSION Ventriculoperitoneal (VP) shunts are a highly effective treatment for hydrocephalus. Unfortunately, shunt malfunction is common, occurring in up to 40% of cases at 1 year and 70% of cases at 10 years.[1] Clinical presentation in the setting of shunt failure is highly variable; headache, nausea, and vomiting are frequently reported, all of which can be attributed to elevated intracranial pressure. Delayed diagnosis and treatment can lead to cranial nerve palsies, seizures, decreased level of consciousness, and coma.

Modern day ventriculoperitoneal shunts are composed of a proximal catheter, reservoir, valve regulator, and distal catheter. The reservoir is located in the subcutaneous tissues over the skull and feeds a one-way valve. The proximal catheter extends from the reservoir intracranially and typically terminates in the frontal horn of either lateral ventricle, while the distal catheter extends caudally through the subcutaneous tissues of the neck, anterior chest, and anterior abdomen, ultimately terminating in the peritoneal cavity. Mechanical complications, including shunt obstruction, disconnection, fracture, and migration, are the most common causes of shunt malfunction. Obstruction of the proximal shunt catheter is the most common cause of shunt malfunction in the first 2 years, often shortly after placement from postoperative debris and blood products. Other common causes of obstruction include shunt kinking, choroid plexus ingrowth at the proximal tip, and pseudocyst formation at the distal tip. Pseudocysts are loculated collections of CSF caused by peritoneal adhesions or covering of the catheter tip by the greater omentum. Shunt disconnection typically occurs soon after placement because of improper surgical technique or defective shunt components. Repeated mechanical stress can lead to shunt weakening and fracture, most often in the neck. Over time, dystrophic calcifications (sometimes called concretions) may develop around the shunt tubing, predisposing them to fracture. Additional complications include infection, ventricular loculations, overdrainage, and ascites.

When ventriculoperitoneal shunt failure is suspected, imaging is obtained to identify a mechanical cause and search for secondary signs of shunt malfunction. A radiographic shunt series composed of AP and lateral radiographs from the skull to the distal end of the shunt is the mainstay of evaluation of shunt integrity. Shunt disconnection, fracture, migration, and calcification are typically readily identified on radiographs. An unenhanced head CT is often ordered in conjunction with the radiographic shunt series to evaluate for ventricular enlargement. Close comparison with prior studies is important, as changes in ventricular size may be subtle. Transependymal flow of CSF, edema along the shunt catheter, and subgaleal fluid collections are secondary signs of shunt failure.[1] Continued concern for shunt malfunction after normal or indeterminate radiographs and head CT are usually followed by radionuclide shunt scintigraphy to document the passage, or lack thereof, of radiotracer through the shunt.

Management of shunt malfunction varies based on etiology. Shunt fracture and migration require shunt revision. Obstruction, depending on the cause, may require replacement or repositioning. In cases of shunt disconnection, existing components may be able to be reconnected. Infection can be confirmed by aspiration of CSF from the shunt reservoir, and antibiotic therapy can be tailored accordingly. Ventricular loculations are managed by fenestration or placement of multiple shunts. Overdrainage is common and clinically insignificant in the absence of symptoms or elevated intraventricular pressure.

Questions for Further Thought

1. What other types of ventricular shunts are there? What are their complications?
2. Are VP shunts MRI safe?

Reporting Responsibilities

Clinical presentation, not imaging findings, determines the need for emergent neurosurgical evaluation. Imaging findings of shunt malfunction without associated symptoms is not an emergency; a timely report is required.

What the Treating Physician Needs to Know?

- Presence of a clear mechanical cause of shunt malfunction such as disconnect, fracture, or migration.

- Presence of potential mechanical causes of shunt malfunction such as suboptimal shunt positioning or shunt calcification.
- Secondary signs of shunt malfunction: changes in ventricle size, transependymal flow of CSF, fluid collections.

Answers

1. Less common ventricular shunts include ventriculoatrial and ventriculopleural shunts, with the distal catheter tip terminating in the right atrium or pleural space, respectively. Ventriculopleural shunts are typically used for temporary ventricular decompression prior to resection of an obstructing tumor or placement/revision of a ventriculoperitoneal shunt. Ventriculopleural shunt complications include empyema from infection and subcutaneous edema if the distal tip erodes through the chest wall. Ventriculoatrial shunts are typically placed when ventriculoperitoneal shunting has failed or there is a contraindication, such as peritoneal or intraperitoneal infection. Ventriculoatrial shunts can migrate within the right atrium or through a patent foramen ovale, resulting in reduced drainage. Migration within the right atrium may cause arrhythmias. Infection of a ventriculoatrial shunt can result in endocarditis and septic emboli. Cases have been reported of catheter erosion through the right ventricular free wall, resulting in pericardial effusion. Erosion through the interatrial or interventricular septum creates a communication between the right and left heart, placing the patient at risk for paradoxical emboli.[1]

2. VP shunts are MRI safe in that they are not associated with abnormal heating or movement. The shunt valve, which controls the rate at which fluid is drained from the ventricles, is controlled by magnets, which may be affected by MRI. Obtaining radiographs of the valve before and after MRI will allow documentation of any shunt valve change and allow for correction. Some modern shunt valves are not affected by the magnetic field in current 1.5T and 3T scanners.

CLINICAL HISTORY *40-year-old female who presents with acute right upper quadrant abdominal pain, nausea, and vomiting.*

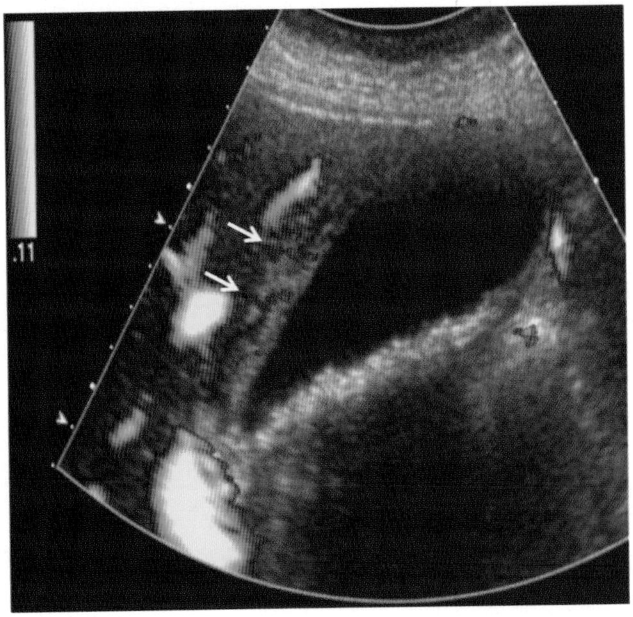

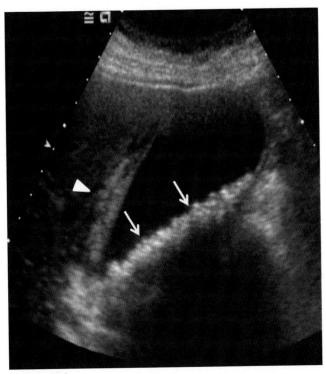

FIGURE 99A

FIGURE 99B

FINDINGS Figure 99A: Longitudinal ultrasound image of the gallbladder demonstrates multiple small shadowing gallstones (*arrows*) and thickened gallbladder wall measuring up to 1 cm (*arrowhead*). The sonographic Murphy's sign was positive. Figure 99B: Longitudinal power Doppler ultrasound image of the gallbladder shows thickened, hyperemic gallbladder wall (*arrows*). Findings compatible with acute cholecystitis.

DIFFERENTIAL DIAGNOSIS Chronic cholecystitis, acute hepatitis, hypoproteinemia, adenomyomatosis, pancreatitis.

DIAGNOSIS Acute calculous cholecystitis.

DISCUSSION Acute cholecystitis represents acute inflammation of the gallbladder. It is primarily caused by cholelithiasis obstructing the gallbladder neck or cystic duct. The obstruction leads to inflammation of the mucosa due to chemical injury from bile salts and/or superimposed infection. The inflammation causes reactive mucus production, which leads to distention and increased intraluminal pressure. The intraluminal distention restricts blood flow to the gallbladder wall, leading to wall thickening. Eventually, the gallbladder can become necrotic from prolonged ischemia. Complications of untreated cholecystitis include gangrenous cholecystitis, emphysematous cholecystitis, hemorrhagic cholecystitis, and eventually gallbladder perforation. In

emphysematous cholecystitis, gas produced by gas-forming bacteria is identified in the wall and lumen of the gallbladder. Because of its rapid progression to gangrene and perforation, emphysematous cholecystitis is a surgical emergency. In gangrenous cholecystitis, the gallbladder wall becomes necrotic with linear echogenicities in the gallbladder lumen, representing sloughed membranes. Small abscesses or hemorrhage in the gallbladder wall may develop. Perforation of the gallbladder can occur in prolonged inflammation with a small defect in the gallbladder wall and adjacent pericholecystic fluid collection/abscess.

Ultrasound is the preferred modality of choice in the initial workup of right upper quadrant pain. The most sensitive ultrasound findings of acute cholecystitis are gallstones and presence of a sonographic Murphy's sign. A positive sonographic Murphy's sign is when the patient feels maximal abdominal tenderness from the pressure of the ultrasound probe over the gallbladder area while in deep inspiration. However, the sonographic Murphy's sign cannot be assessed if the patient has been given analgesics prior to the ultrasound exam. Other secondary signs include distended gallbladder, thickened gallbladder wall >3mm, hyperemic gallbladder wall, and pericholecystic fluid. These are less specific and can be present in other entities such as hepatitis, congestive heart failure, pancreatitis, cirrhosis, and hypoalbuminemia.

If the findings of ultrasound are inconclusive for acute cholecystitis, a cholescintigraphy with hepato-iminodiacetic acid (HIDA) can be performed. Lack of visualization of the gallbladder on a HIDA scan is diagnostic of acute cholecystitis. HIDA scan is typically reserved for sonographically equivocal cases of acute cholecystitis, since it is unable to identify complications of acute cholecystitis or alternative causes of right upper quadrant pain. Computed tomography (CT) findings of acute cholecystitis include gallstones, gallbladder distention, gallbladder wall thickening, mucosal hyperenhancement, pericholecystic fluid/fat stranding, and sludge. However, CT is less sensitive than ultrasound.

Treatment for acute cholecystitis is typically cholecystectomy. However, in patients who are unstable, percutaneous transhepatic cholecystostomy drainage may be appropriate with antibiotics. Gallbladder ischemia, infection, and perforation can occur if acute cholecystitis is left untreated.

Questions for Further Thought

1. What is the test of choice in the setting of equivocal ultrasound findings of acute cholecystitis?
2. What are the causes of thickened gallbladder wall other than cholecystitis?

Reporting Responsibilities

Findings of acute cholecystitis should be emergently reported to the referring clinician.

What the Treating Physician Needs to Know?

- Presence of gallstones and other findings of acute cholecystitis.
- Presence of emphysematous cholecystitis, gangrenous cholecystitis, and perforation.

Answers

1. Scintigraphy using Technetium-99m-labeled iminodiacetic acid (HIDA) is the test of choice in the setting of equivocal ultrasound findings of acute cholecystitis.
2. There are many causes of gallbladder wall thickening, including biliary and nonbiliary causes. A few examples include cirrhosis, hepatitis, congestive heart failure, hypoalbuminemia, acute pancreatitis, perforated duodenal ulcer, and gallbladder carcinoma.

CLINICAL HISTORY *53-year-old male with history of type 2 diabetes mellitus presents with a non-healing ulcer on the plantar surface of his right foot at the base of the great toe. He also complains of fevers and diffuse erythema of the right foot.*

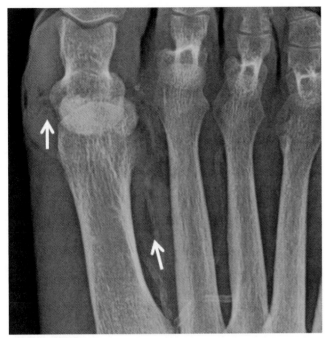

FIGURE 100A

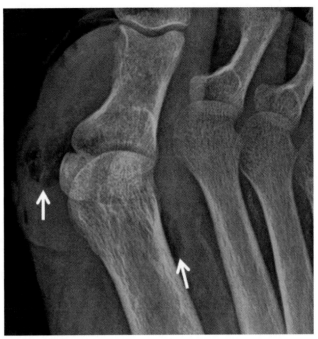

FIGURE 100B

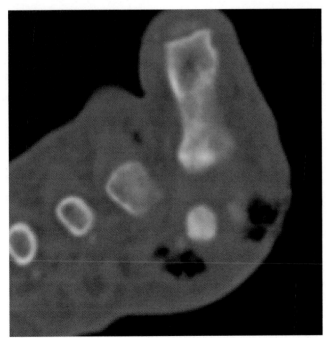

FIGURE 100C

FINDINGS AP and oblique radiographs of the right foot (Figs. 100A and 100B) demonstrate soft tissue edema and subcutaneous gas in the soft tissues about the first metatarsophalangeal (MTP) joint, which also tracks along the first and second metatarsals. The oblique view demonstrates a soft tissue defect subjacent to the first MTP joint. Axial CT of the right foot (Fig. 100C) at the level of the metatarsal heads reveals soft tissue gas about the first MTP joint with an associated superficial cutaneous defect.

DIFFERENTIAL DIAGNOSIS Gas-forming soft tissue infection, recent debridement, penetrating trauma, osteomyelitis.

DIAGNOSIS Soft tissue infection with gas-forming organism.

DISCUSSION Soft tissue infection of the feet with cutaneous ulceration is a common complication for patients with diabetes mellitus. The neuropathy (sensory, motor, and autonomic) and arterial insufficiency of advanced diabetes result in impaired pain response to injury with an associated impaired healing response that leads to the chronic skin ulcerations common in the diabetic foot. Although infection with gas-forming organisms is not common in this setting, it heralds a more severe, usually polymicrobial infection instead of the more typical infection with *Staphylococcus aureus*. Organisms commonly cultured from polymicrobial soft tissue infections in this setting include *Clostridium, Proteus, E. coli, Bacteroides,* and *Enterobacteriaceae.*

Initial evaluation of the diabetic foot is performed with the standard three-view radiographic series (dorsal-plantar, oblique, and lateral views) that may be supplemented with additional oblique views. Soft tissue swelling and edema may be the only signs of infection. Bone infection may be present, which is characterized by focal areas of osteopenia or overt erosions. If soft tissue gas is present, it is important to determine whether there has been recent debridement or other surgical intervention that could account for its presence. Soft tissue gas secondary to infection is often characterized by numerous small locules of gas that may be clustered together. CT is much more sensitive for soft tissue gas than radiographs, though CT is rarely obtained for the sole purpose of identifying soft tissue gas in the setting of diabetic foot infection. MRI is relatively insensitive to soft tissue gas, though large collections will appear as signal voids on T1- and T2-weighted sequences. With its excellent soft tissue contrast, MRI excels at identifying abnormalities of bone and deep soft tissue structures and may be used not just for diagnosis, but also for preoperative planning. MRI, however, is not very specific; reactive inflammation may appear identical to septic inflammation. Ultrasonography is an excellent modality for the identification of soft tissue gas, which appears as mobile tiny echogenic reflectors either tracking along a fascial plane (necrotizing fasciitis) or within a focal region of necrosis (gas gangrene). These reflectors can block the sound waves from penetrating beyond the gas, making assessment of the anatomy deep to the gas extremely difficult. Radionuclide bone scintigraphy is very sensitive, but quite nonspecific; its use is limited to those in whom MRI is contraindicated or if multifocal disease needs to be documented.

Soft tissue gas secondary to infection is an indication for urgent debridement or amputation, depending on the extent of infection. Patients often require multiple debridements in order to establish aseptic healing tissue. This is followed by long-term intravenous antibiotic therapy.

Question for Further Thought

1. What foot deformities play a role in diabetic foot infections?

Reporting Responsibilities

The presence of soft tissue gas in the setting of infection is a surgical emergency; a phone call to the referring clinician is required.

What the Treating Physician Needs to Know

- The presence, location, and extent of soft tissue gas and edema; in the absence of penetrating trauma, this represents infection with a gas-forming infection.
- The presence of cortical irregularities, periosteal reaction, or focal osteopenia; signs of infectious osteitis/osteomyelitis.
- If the radiographs are equivocal for soft tissue gas and infection with a gas-forming organism is suspected, then CT should be considered for further evaluation.

Answer

1. Structural abnormalities of the foot, such as pes planus, hallux valgus, claw toes, and neuropathic (Charcot) arthropathy, lead to abnormal plantar pressures. Altered plantar pressures in the setting of neuropathy and peripheral arterial disease predispose to ulceration and soft tissue infection.

HEMORRHAGIC VENOUS SINUS THROMBOSIS
Case 1

1. Leach JL, Fortuna RB, Jones BV, et al. Imaging of cerebral venous thrombosis: current techniques, spectrum of findings, and diagnostic pitfalls. *Radiographics.* 2006;26(suppl 1):S19–S41.

2. Poon CS, Chang JK, Swarnkar A, et al. Radiologic diagnosis of cerebral venous thrombosis: pictorial review. *AJR Am J Roentgenol.* 2007;189(6)(suppl):S64–S75.

3. Saposnik G, Barinagarrementeria F, Brown RD Jr, et al. Diagnosis and management of cerebral venous thrombosis: a statement for healthcare professionals from the American Heart Association/American Stroke Association. *Stroke.* 2011;42(4):1158–1192.

ADENOCARCINOMA MIMICKING PNEUMONIA
Case 2

1. Austin JHM, Garg K, Aberle D, et al. Radiologic implications of the 2011 classification of adenocarcinoma of the lung. *Radiology.* 2013;266(1):62–71.

2. Popat N, Raghavan N, McIvor RA. Severe bronchorrhea in a patient with bronchioloalveolar carcinoma. *Chest.* 2012;141(2):513–514.

BLADDER RUPTURE
Case 3

1. Vaccaro JP, Brody JM. CT cystography in the evaluation of major bladder trauma. *Radiographics.* 2000;20:1373–1381.

2. Sandler CM, Hall JT, Rodriguez MB, et al. Bladder injury in blunt pelvic trauma. *Radiology.* 1986;158:633–638.

OPEN BOOK PELVIS WITH ARTERIAL EXTRAVASATION
Case 4

1. Khurana B, Sheehan SE, Sodickson AD, et al. Pelvic ring fractures: what the orthopedic surgeon wants to know. *Radiographics.* 2014;34(5):1317–1333. doi:10.1148/rg.345135113.

2. Theumann NH, Verdon JP, Mouhsine E, et al. Traumatic injuries: imaging of pelvic fractures. *Eur Radiol.* 2002;12(6):1312–1330. doi:10.1007/s00330-002-1446-7.

MASTOIDITIS
Case 5

1. Vasquez E, Castellote A, Piqueras J, et al. Imaging of complications of acute mastoiditis in children. *Radiographics.* 2003;23(2):359–372.

INFECTED AORTIC STENT GRAFT WITH AORTITIS
Case 6

1. Hsu RB, Tsay YG, Wang SS, et al. Surgical treatment for primary infected aneurysm of the descending thoracic aorta, abdominal aorta, and iliac arteries. *J Vasc Surg.* 2002;36:746–750.

2. Kahlberg A, Melissano G, Tshomba Y, et al. Strategies to treat thoracic aortitis and infected aortic grafts. *J Cardiovasc Surg (Torino).* 2015;56(2):269–280.

3. Macedo TA, Stanson AW, Oderich GS, et al. Infected aortic aneurysms: imaging findings. *Radiology.* 2004;231(1):250–257.

ADRENAL HEMORRHAGE
Case 7

1. Johnson PT, Horton KM, Fishman EK. Adrenal imaging with MDCT: nonneoplastic disease. *AJR Am J Roentgenol.* 2009;193:1128–1135.

2. Jordan E, Poder L, Courtier J, et al. Imaging of nontraumatic adrenal hemorrhage. *AJR Am J Roentgenol.* 2012;199:W91–W98.

3. Murphy BJ, Casillas J, Yrizarry JM. Traumatic adrenal hemorrhage: radiologic findings. *Radiology.* 1988;169:701–703.

RADIOGRAPHIC SIGNS OF ACL TEAR
Case 8

1. Bollen SR, Scott BW. Rupture of the anterior cruciate ligament—a quiet epidemic? *Injury.* 1996;27(6):407–409.

2. Campos JC, Chung CB, Lektrakul N, et al. Pathogenesis of the Segond fracture: anatomic and MR imaging evidence of an iliotibial tract or anterior oblique band avulsion. *Radiology.* 2001;219(2):381–386.

3. Grimberg A, Shirazian H, Torshizy H, et al. Deep lateral notch sign and double notch sign in complete tears of the anterior cruciate ligament: MR imaging evaluation. *Skeletal Radiol.* 2015;44(3):385–391.

4. Yu JS, Bosch E, Pathria MN, et al. Deep lateral femoral sulcus: study of 124 patients with anterior cruciate ligament tear. *Emerg Radiol.* 1995;2(3):129–134.

JUMPED FACETS
Case 9

1. Agus H, Kayali C, Arslantas M. Nonoperative treatment of burst-type thoracolumbar vertebra fractures: clinical and radiological results of 29 patients. *Eur Spine J.* 2004;14:536–540.

2. Denis F. The three column spine and its significance in the classification of acute thoracolumbar spinal injuries. *Spine.* 1983;8:817–831.

3. Ferguson R, Allen B Jr. A mechanistic classification of thoracolumbar spine fractures. *Clin Orhtop Relat Res.* 1984;189:77–88.

4. Lee JY, Vaccaro AR, Lim MR, et al. Thoracolumbar injury classification and severity score: a new paradigm

for the treatment of thoracolumbar spine trauma. *J Orthop Sci.* 2005;10:671–675.

5. Mcafee PC, Yuan HA, Fredrickson BE, et al. The value of computed tomography in thoracolumbar fractures. An analysis of one hundred consecutive cases and a new classification. *J Bone Joint Surg Am.* 1983;65:461–473.

6. Parthia MN, Petersilge CA. Spinal trauma. *Radiol Clin North Am.* 1991;29:847–865.

7. Patel AA, Dailey A, Brodke DS, et al. Thoracolumbar spine trauma classification: the Thoracolumbar Injury Classification and Severity Score system and case examples. *J Neurosurg Spine.* 2009;10:201–206.

8. Vaccaro AR, Zeiller SC, Hulbert RJ, et al. The thoracolumbar injury severity score: a proposed treatment algorithm. *J Spinal Disord Tech.* 2005;18:209–215.

BRONCHIECTASIS CAUSED BY ASPIRATION
Case 10

1. Cantin L, Bankier AA, Eisenberg RL. Bronchiectasis. *AJR Am J Roentgenol.* 2009;193:W158–W171.

2. Lee AL, Button BM, Denehy L, et al. Gastro-oesophageal reflux in noncystic fibrosis bronchiectasis. *Pulm Med.* 2011;2011:395020.

3. Parr DG, Guest PG, Reynolds JH, et al. Prevalence and impact of bronchiectasis in alpha1-antitrypsin deficiency. *Am J Respir Crit Care Med.* 2007;176(12):1215–1221.

DUODENAL PERFORATION
Case 11

1. Heller MT, Haarer KA, Itri JN, et al. Duodenum: MDCT of acute conditions. *Clin Radiol.* 2014;69:e48–e55.

2. Jayaraman MV, Mayo-Smith WW, Movson JS, et al. CT of the duodenum: an overlooked segment gets its due. *Radiographics.* 2001;21:S147–S160.

INFECTED HIP PROSTHESIS
Case 12

1. Awan O, Chen L, Resnik CS. Imaging evaluation of complications of hip arthroplasty: review of current concepts and imaging findings. *Can Assoc Radiol J.* 2013;64(4):306–313. doi:10.1016/j.carj.2012.08.003.

2. Johnson AJ, Zywiel MG, Jones LC, et al. Reduced reinfection rates with postoperative oral antibiotics after two-stage revision hip arthroplasty. *BMC Musculoskelet Disord.* 2013;14(1):123. doi:10.1186/1471-2474-14-123.

3. Mulcahy H, Chew FS. Current concepts of hip arthroplasty for radiologists. Part II: revisions and complications. *AJR Am J Roentgenol.* 2012;199(3):570–580. doi:10.2214/AJR.12.8844.

CEREBRAL METASTASES
Case 13

1. Fink KR, Fink JR. Imaging of brain metastases. *Surg Neurol Int.* 2013;4(suppl 4):S209–S219.

2. Garg RK, Sinha MK. Multiple ring-enhancing lesions of the brain. *J Postgrad Med.* 2010;56(4):307–316.

3. Nabors LB, Ammirati M, Bierman PJ, et al. Central nervous system cancers: clinical practice guidelines in oncology. *J Natl Compr Canc Netw.* 2013;11(9):1114–1151.

4. Smirniotopoulos JG, Murphy FM, Rushing EJ, et al. Patterns of contrast enhancement in the brain and meninges. *Radiographics.* 2007;27(2):525–551.

ECTOPIC PREGNANCY
Case 15

1. Barash JH, Buchanan EM, Hillson C. Diagnosis and management of ectopic pregnancy. *Am Fam Physician.* 2014;90:34–40.

2. Bryan-Rest LL, Scoutt LM. Ectopic pregnancy. In: Fielding JR, Brown DL, Thurmond AS, eds. *Gynecologic Imaging.* 1st ed. Philadelphia, PA: Elsevier Saunders; 2011:330–355.

3. Doubilet PM, Benson CB, Bourne T, et al. Diagnostic criteria for nonviable pregnancy early in the first trimester. *N Engl J Med.* 2013;369:1443–1451.

4. Doubilet PM. Ultrasound evaluation of the first trimester. *Radiol Clin North Am.* 2014;52:1191–1199.

5. Lin EP, Bhatt S, Dogra VS. Diagnostic clues to ectopic pregnancy. *Radiographics.* 2008;28:1661–1671.

MEDIAL EPICONDYLE AVULSION
Case 16

1. Gottschalk HP, Eisner E, Hosalkar HS. Medial epicondyle fractures in the pediatric population. *J Am Acad Orthop Surg.* 2012;20(4):223–232.

CAUDA EQUINA SYNDROME SECONDARY TO LUMBAR DISK EXTRUSION
Case 17

1. Chou R, Qaseem A, Snow V, et al. Diagnosis and treatment of low back pain: a joint clinical practice guideline from the American College of Physicians and the American Pain Society. *Ann Intern Med.* 2007;147:478–491.

2. Gregory DS, Seto CK, Wortley GC, et al. Acute lumbar disc pain: navigating evaluation and treatment choices. *Am Fam Physician.* 2008;78(7):835–842.

3. Lin M, Bory K. Musculoskeletal back pain. In: Marx JA, Hockberger RS, Walls RM, eds. *Rosen's Emergency Medicine.* 8th ed. Philadelphia, PA: Elsevier Saunders; 2014:643–655.

4. Small SA, Perron AD, Brady WJ. Orthopedic pitfalls: cauda equina syndrome. *Am J Emerg Med.* 2005;23(2):159–163.

5. Spector LR, Madigan L, Rhyne A, et al. Cauda equina syndrome. *J Am Acad Orthop Surg.* 2008;16:471–479.

TRAUMATIC BRONCHIAL INJURY
Case 18

1. Collins J, Stern E. *Chest Radiology: The Essentials*. Philadelphia, PA: Lippincott Williams & Wilkins; 2015.
2. Hippargi H. Traumatic bronchial rupture: an unusual case of tension pneumothorax. *Int J Emerg Med*. 2010;3:193–195.
3. Savas R, Alper H. Fallen lung sign: radiographic findings. *Diagn Interv Radiol*. 2008;14:120–121.
4. Tack D, Defrance P, Delcour C, et al. The CT fallen-lung sign. *Eur Radiol*. 2000;10(5):719–721.
5. Unger JM, Schuchmann GG, Grossman JE, et al. Tears of the trachea and main bronchi caused by blunt trauma: radiologic findings. *AJR Am J Roentgenol*. 1989; 153(6):1175–1180.

RECTUS SHEATH HEMATOMA
Case 19

1. Kapan S, Turhan AN, Alis H, et al. Rectus sheath hematoma: three case reports. *J Med Case Rep*. 2008;2:22.
2. Rimola J, Perendreu J, Falco J, et al. Percutaneous arterial embolization in the management of rectus sheath hematoma. *AJR Am J Roentgenol*. 2007;188:W497–W502.

LATERAL PROCESS OF TALUS FRACTURE
Case 20

1. Funk J, Srinivasan S, Crandall J. Snowboarder's talus fractures experimentally produced by eversion and dorsiflexion. *Am J Sports Med*. 2003;31(6):921–928.
2. Jibri Z, Mukherjee K, Kamath S, et al. Frequently missed findings in acute ankle injury. *Semin Musculoskelet Radiol*. 2013;17(4):416–428. doi:10.1055/s-0033-1356471.
3. Perera A, Baker JF, Lui DF, et al. The management and outcome of lateral process fracture of the talus. *Foot Ankle Surg*. 2010;16(1):15–20. doi:10.1016/j.fas.2009.03.004.

ZMC FRACTURE
Case 21

1. Alcala-Galiano A, Arribas-Garcia IJ, Martin-Perez MA, et al. Pediatric facial trauma: children are not just small adults. *Radiographics*. 2008;28:441–461.
2. Hopper R, Salemy S, Sze R. Diagnosis of midface fractures with CT: what the surgeon needs to know. *Radiographics*. 2006;26:783–793.
3. Ukisu R, Funaki S, Matsunari K, et al. Facial and orbital fractures revisited with MDCT. *European Society of Radiology*. ECR 2011 Poster # C-2195.

EMPYEMA
Case 22

1. Collins J, Stern EJ. *Chest Radiology: The Essentials*. Philadelphia, PA: Lippincott Williams & Wilkins; 2007.
2. Diacon AH, Theron J, Schuurmans MM, et al. Intrapleural streptokinase for empyema and complicated parapneumonic effusions. *Am J Respir Crit Care Med*. 2004;170(1):49–53.
3. Light RW. Diseases of the pleura, mediastinum, chest wall, and diaphragm. In: George RB, Light RW, Matthew MA, et al., eds. *Chest Medicine*. Baltimore, MD: Williams & Wilkins; 1990:318–412.
4. Stark DD, Federle MP, Goodman PC, et al. Differentiating lung abscess and empyema: radiography and computed tomography. *AJR Am J Roentgenol*. 1983;141(1):163–167.
5. Wozniak CJ, Paull DE, Moezzi JE, et al. Choice of first intervention is related to outcomes in the management of empyema. *Ann Thorac Surg*. 2009;87(5):1525–1530; discussion 1530–1521.

CECAL VOLVULUS
Case 23

1. Delabrousse E, Sarliève P, Sailley N, et al. Cecal volvulus: CT findings and correlation with pathophysiology. *Emerg Radiol*. 2007;14(6):411–415.
2. Peterson CM, Anderson JS, Hara AK, et al. Volvulus of the gastrointestinal tract: appearances at multimodality imaging. *Radiographics*. 2009;29(5):1281–1293.

POSTERIOR SHOULDER DISLOCATION
Case 24

1. Jacobs RC, Meredyth NA, Michelson JD. Posterior shoulder dislocations. *BMJ*. 2015;350:h75. doi:10.1136/bmj.h75.
2. Kowalsky MS, Levine WN. Traumatic posterior glenohumeral dislocation: classification, pathoanatomy, diagnosis, and treatment. *Orthop Clin North Am*. 2008;39(4): 519–533. doi:10.1016/j.ocl.2008.05.008.
3. Tannenbaum EP, Sekiya JK. Posterior shoulder instability in the contact athlete. *Clin Sports Med*. 2013;32:781–796. doi:10.1016/j.csm.2013.07.011.

HYPOXIC ISCHEMIC BRAIN INJURY
Case 25

1. Don CW, Longstreth WT, Maynard C, et al. Active surface cooling protocol to induce mild therapeutic hypothermia after out-of-hospital cardiac arrest: a retrospective before-and-after comparison in a single hospital. *Crit Care Med*. 2009;37(12):3062–3069.
2. Huang BY, Castillo M. Hypoxic-ischemic brain injury: imaging findings from birth to adulthood. *Radiographics*. 2008;28(2):417–439.
3. Meissner B, Kallenberg K, Sanchez-Juan P, et al. Isolated cortical signal increase on MR imaging as a frequent lesion pattern in sporadic Creutzfeldt–Jakob disease. *AJNR Am J Neuroradiol*. 2008;29(8):1519–1524.
4. Yousem DM, Grossman RI. Anoxia, hypoxia, and brain death. In: Yousem DM, Grossman RI, eds. *Neuroradiology: The Requisites*. St. Louis, MO: Mosby; 2010:133.

FLAIL CHEST
Case 26

1. Clark GC, Schecter WP, Trunkey DD. Variables affecting outcome in blunt chest trauma: flail chest vs. pulmonary contusion. *J Trauma*. 1988;28(3):298–304.

2. Collins J. Chest wall trauma. *J Thorac Imaging.* 2000; 15(2):112–119.

3. Kilic D, Findikcioglu A, Akin S, et al. Factors affecting morbidity and mortality in flail chest: comparison of anterior and lateral location. *Thorac Cardiovasc Surg.* 2011;59(1):45–48.

4. Lomoschitz FM, Eisenhuber E, Linnau KF, et al. Imaging of chest trauma: radiological patterns of injury and diagnostic algorithms. *Eur J Radiol.* 2003;48(1):61–70.

HANGMAN FRACTURE
Case 27

1. Ding T, Maltenfort M, Yang H, et al. Correlation of C2 fractures and vertebral artery injury. *Spine.* 2010;35(12):E520–E524.

2. Dreizin D, Letzing M, Sliker C, et al. Multidetector CT of blunt cervical spine trauma in adults. *Radiographics.* 2014;34:1842–1865.

3. Levine AM, Edwards CC. The management of traumatic spondylolisthesis of the axis. *J Bone Joint Surg Am.* 1985;67(2):217–226.

4. Li XF, Dai LY, Lu H, et al. A systematic review of the management of hangman's fractures. *Eur Spine J.* 2006;15:257–269.

5. Schleicher P, Scholz M, Pingel A, et al. Traumatic spondylolisthesis of the axis vertebra in adults. *Global Spine J.* 2015;5:346–358.

TRIMALLEOLAR ANKLE FRACTURE
Case 28

1. Kaye JA, Jick H. Epidemiology of lower limb fractures in general practice in the United Kingdom. *Inj Prev.* 2004;10:368–374.

2. Singh R, Kamal T, Roulohamin N, et al. Ankle fractures: a literature review of current treatment methods. *Open J Orthop.* 2014;4:292–303.

3. Tiemstra J. Update on acute ankle sprains. *Am Fam Physician.* 2012;85(12):1170–1176.

LEMIERRE'S SYNDROME
Case 29

1. Karkos PD, Asrani S, Karkos CD, et al. Lemierre's syndrome: a systematic review. *Laryngoscope.* 2009;119(8):1552–1559.

2. Schubert AD, Hotz MA, Caversaccio MD, et al. Septic thrombosis of the internal jugular vein: Lemierre's syndrome revisited. *Laryngoscope.* 2015;125(4):863–868. doi:10.1002/lary.24995.

HYDROPNEUMOTHORAX
Case 30

1. Gupta A, Dutt N, Patel N. The different treatment modalities of pyopneumothorax—study of 50 cases. *Int J Med Sci Public Health.* 2000;2(3):609–612.

2. Khatib R, Siwik J. Pyopneumothorax: a complication of *Streptococcus pyogenes* pharyngitis. *Scand J Infect Dis.* 2000;32(5):564–565.

3. Raff MJ, Johnson JD, Nagar D, et al. Spontaneous clostridial empyema and pyopneumothorax. *Rev Infect Dis.* 1984;6(5):715–719.

4. Rassameehiran S, Klomjit S, Nugent K. Right-sided hydropneumothorax as a presenting symptom of Boerhaave's syndrome (spontaneous esophageal rupture). *Proc (Bayl Univ Med Cent).* 2015;28(3):344–346.

5. Samovsky M, Loberant N, Lemer J, et al. Tension pyopneumothorax. *Clin Imaging.* 2005;29(6):437–438.

TESTICULAR TORSION
Case 31

1. Bhatt S, Dogra VS. Role of US in testicular and scrotal trauma. *Radiographics.* 2008;28:1617–1629.

2. Dogra VS, Gottlieb RH, Oka M, et al. Sonography of the scrotum. *Radiology.* 2003;227:18–36.

3. Turgut AT, Bhatt S, Dogra VS. Acute painful scrotum. *Ultrasound Clin.* 2008;3:93–107.

PERILUNATE DISLOCATION
Case 32

1. Gilula LA. Carpal injuries: analytic approach and Case exercises. *AJR Am J Roentgenol.* 1979;133:503–517.

2. Herzberg G, Comtet JJ, Linscheid RL, et al. Perilunate dislocations and fracture-dislocations: a multi-center study. *J Hand Surg Am.* 1993;18(5):768–779.

3. Mayfield JK, Johnson RP, Kilcoyne RK. Carpal dislocations: pathomechanics and progressive perilunar instability. *J Hand Surg Am.* 1980;5(3):226–241.

4. Scalcione LR, Gimber LH, Ho AM, et al. Spectrum of carpal dislocations and fracture-dislocations: imaging and management. *AJR Am J Roentgenol.* 2014;203(3): 541–550.

5. Stanbury SJ, Elfar JC. Perilunate dislocation and perilunate fracture-dislocation. *J Am Acad Orthop Surg.* 2011; 19(9):554–562.

CHANCE FRACTURE
Case 33

1. Ball ST, Vaccaro AR, Albert TJ, et al. Injuries of the thoracolumbar spine associated with restraint use in head-on motor vehicle accidents. *J Spinal Disord.* 2000;13(4):297–304.

2. Bernstein MP, Mirvis SE, Shanmuganathan K. chance-type fractures of the thoracolumbar spine: imaging analysis in 53 patients. *AJR Am J Roentgenol.* 2006;187:859–868.

3. Le TV, Baaj AA, Deukmedjian A, et al. Chance fractures in the pediatric population. *J Neurosurg Pediatr.* 2011; 8:189–197.

4. Patel AA, Vaccaro AR. Thoracolumbar spine trauma classification. *J Am Acad Orthop Surg.* 2010;18:63–71.

ACUTE AORTIC INTRAMURAL HEMATOMA
Case 34

1. Birchard KR. Acute aortic syndrome and acute traumatic aortic injury. *Semin Roentgenol.* 2009;44(1):16–28.

INGESTED FOREIGN BODY
Case 35

1. Hunter TB, Taljanovic MS. Foreign bodies. *Radiographics.* 2003;23:731–757.
2. Kay M, Wyllie R. Pediatric foreign bodies and their management. *Curr Gastroenterol Rep.* 2005;7(3): 212–218.
3. Rodríguez-Hermosa JI, Codina-Cazador A, Sirvent JM, et al. Surgically treated perforations of the gastrointestinal tract caused by ingested foreign bodies. *Colorectal Dis.* 2008;10(7):701–707.

BOTH COLUMN ACETABULAR FRACTURE
Case 36

1. Geijer M, El-Khoury GY. Imaging of the acetabulum in the era of multidetector computed tomography. *Emerg Radiol.* 2007;14:271–287.
2. Lawrence DA, Menn K, Baumgaertner M, et al. Acetabular fractures: anatomic and clinical considerations. *AJR Am J Roentgenol.* 2013;201:W425–W436.

CEREBRAL CONTUSIONS
Case 37

1. Hardman JM, Manoukian A. Pathology of head trauma. *Neuroimaging Clin N Am.* 2002;12:175–187.
2. Provenzale J. CT and MR imaging of acute cranial trauma. *Emerg Radiol.* 2007;14:1–12.
3. Young RJ, Destian S. Imaging of traumatic intracranial hemorrhage. *Neuroimaging Clin N Am.* 2002;12:189–204.

LUNG ABSCESS
Case 38

1. Collins J, Stern E. *Chest Radiology: The Essentials.* Philadelphia, PA: Lippincott Williams & Wilkins; 2015.
2. Doherty GM. *Current Diagnosis and Treatment Surgery.* New York, NY: McGraw-Hill; 2010.
3. Hirshberg B, Sklair-Levi M, Nir-Paz R, et al. Factors predicting mortality of patients with lung abscess. *Chest.* 1999;115(3):746–750.

DUODENAL INJURY
Case 39

1. Linsenmaier U, Wirth S, Reiser M, et al. Diagnosis and classification of pancreatic and duodenal injuries in emergency radiology. *Radiographics.* 28(6):1591–1602.
2. Luchtman M, Steiner T, Faierman T, et al. Post-traumatic intramural duodenal hematoma in children. *Isr Med Assoc J.* 2006;8(2):95–97.

TIBIAL PLATEAU FRACTURE WITH MENISCAL ENTRAPMENT
Case 40

1. Albuquerque RP, Hara R, Prado J, et al. Epidemiological study on tibial plateau fractures at a level I trauma center. *Acta Ortop Bras.* 2013;21(2):109–115.
2. Berkson EM, Virkus WW. High-energy tibial plateau fractures. *J Am Acad Orthop Surg.* 2006;14:20–31.
3. Gardner MJ, Yacoubian S, Geller D, et al. The incidence of soft tissue injury in operative tibial plateau fractures: a magnetic resonance imaging analysis of 103 patients. *J Orthop Trauma.* 2005;19:79–84.
4. Markhardt BK, Gross JM, Monu JUV. Schatzker classification of tibial plateau fractures: use of CT and MR imaging improves assessment. *Radiographics.* 2009;29: 585–597.
5. Schatzker J. Compression in the surgical treatment of fractures of the tibia. *Clin Orthop Relat Res.* 1974;105: 220–239.

ORBITAL CELLULITIS, EPIDURAL ABSCESS, AND MENINGITIS
Case 41

1. Hauser A, Fogarasi S. Periorbital and orbital cellulitis. *Pediatr Rev.* 2010;31(6):242–249.
2. Hegde AN, Mohan S, Pandya A, et al. Imaging in infections of the head and neck. *Neuroimaging Clin N Am.* 2012;22(4):727–754.
3. LeBedis CA, Sakai O. Nontraumatic orbital conditions. Diagnosis with CT and MR imaging in the emergent setting. *Radiographics.* 2008;28:1741–1754.

MEDIASTINAL HEMATOMA
Case 42

1. Dyer DS, Moore EE, Ilke DN, et al. Thoracic aortic injury: how predictive is mechanism and is chest computed tomography a reliable screening tool? A prospective study of 1,561 patients. *J Trauma.* 2000;48:673–682.
2. Ellis JD, Mayo JR. Computed tomography evaluation of traumatic rupture of the thoracic aorta: an outcome study. *Can Assoc Radiol J.* 2007;58:22–26.
3. Miller FB, Richardson JD, Thomas HA, et al. Role of CT in diagnosis of major arterial injury after blunt thoracic trauma. *Surgery.* 1989;106:596–602.
4. Scaglione M, Pinto A, Pinto F, et al. Role of contrast-enhanced helical CT in the evaluation of acute thoracic aortic injuries after blunt chest trauma. *Eur Radiol.* 2001; 11:2444–2448.

OVARIAN TORSION
Case 43

1. Chang H, Bhatt S, Dogra V. Pearls and pitfalls in diagnosis of ovarian torsion. *Radiographics.* 2008;28:1355–1368.

2. Lee EJ, Kwon HC, Joo HJ, et al. Diagnosis of ovarian torsion with color Doppler sonography: depiction of twisted vascular pedicle. *J Ultrasound Med.* 1998;17(2):83–89.

LISFRANC FRACTURE-DISLOCATION
Case 44

1. Gupta RT, Wadhwa RP, Learch TJ, et al. Lisfranc injury: imaging findings for this important but often-missed diagnosis. *Curr Probl Diagn Radiol.* 2008;37(3):115–126.

2. Haapamaki VV, Kiuru MJ, Koskinen SK. Ankle and foot injuries: analysis of MDCT findings. *AJR Am J Roentgenol.* 2004;183(3):615–622.

3. Hardcastle PH, Reschauer R, Kutscha-Lissberg E, et al. Injuries to the tarsometatarsal joint: incidence, classification, and treatment. *J Bone Joint Surg Br.* 1982;64-B(3):349–356.

4. Myerson MS, Fisher RT, Burgess AR, et al. Fracture dislocations of the tarsometatarsal joints: end results correlated with pathology and treatment. *Foot Ankle.* 1986;6(5):225–242.

5. Welck MJ, Zinchenko R, Rudge B. Lisfranc injuries. *Injury.* 2015;46(4):536–541.

ACUTE RIGHT MCA OCCLUSION— "DENSE MCA" SIGN
Case 45

1. Chavhan GB, Shroff MM. Twenty classic signs in neuroradiology: a pictorial essay. *Indian J Radiol Imaging.* 2009;19(2):135–145.

2. Jensen-Kondering U, Riedel C, Jansen O. Hyperdense artery sign on computed tomography in acute ischemic stroke. *World J Radiol.* 2010;2(9):354–357.

3. Koo CK, Teasdale E, Muir KW. What constitutes a true hyperdense middle cerebral artery sign. *Cerebrovasc Dis.* 2000;10:419–423.

4. Moulin T, Cattin F, Crépin-Leblond T, et al. Early CT signs in acute middle cerebral artery infarction: predictive value for subsequent infarct locations and outcome. *Neurology.* 1996;47(2):366–375.

MYOCARDIAL ISCHEMIA
Case 46

1. Nagao M, Matsuoka H, Kawakami H, et al. Quantification of myocardial perfusion by contrast-enhanced 64-MDCT: characterization of ischemic myocardium. *AJR Am J Roentgenol.* 2008;191:19–25.

2. Tsai IC, Lee WL, Tsao CR, et al. Comprehensive evaluation of ischemic heart disease using MDCT. *AJR Am J Roentgenol.* 2008;191:64–72.

LIVER LACERATION
Case 47

1. Yoon W, Jeong YY, Kim JK, et al. CT in blunt liver trauma. *Radiographics.* 2005;25:87–104.

OBSCURED CERVICOTHORACIC JUNCTION WITH ANTEROLISTHESIS
Case 48

1. Daffner RH, Hackney DB. ACR appropriateness criteria on suspected spine trauma. *J Am Coll Radiol.* 2007;4:762–775.

2. Dreizen D, Letzing M, Sliker C, et al. Multidetector CT of blunt cervical spine trauma in adults. *Radiographics.* 2014;34(7):1842–1865. doi:10.1148/rg.347130094.

3. Rethnam U, Yesupalan RSU, Bastawrous SS. The Swimmer's view: does it really show what it is supposed to show? A retrospective study. *BMC Med Imaging.* 2008;8(1):2. doi:10.1186/1471-2342-8-2.

ACUTE SUBDURAL HEMATOMA
Case 49

1. Bradford R, Choudhary AK, Dias MS. Serial neuroimaging in infants with abusive head trauma: timing abusive injuries. *J Neurosurg Pediatr.* 2013;12(2):110–119.

2. Bullock MR, Chesnut R, Ghajar J, et al; Surgical Management of Traumatic Brain Injury Author Group. Surgical management of acute subdural hematomas. *Neurosurgery.* 2006;58(3)(suppl):S16–S24.

3. Chen JC, Levy ML. Causes, epidemiology, and risk factors of chronic subdural hematoma. *Neurosurg Clin N Am.* 2000;11:399–406.

4. Kloss BT, Lagace RE. Acute-on-chronic subdural hematoma. *Int J Emerg Med.* 2010;3:511–512.

5. Provenzale J. CT and MR imaging of acute cranial trauma. *Emerg Radiol.* 2007;14:1–12.

PERICARDITIS
Case 50

1. Bogaert J, Francone M. Pericardial disease: value of CT and MR imaging. *Radiology.* 2013;267(2):340–356.

2. Garcia MJ. *Noninvasive Cardiovascular Imaging: A Multimodality Approach.* Philadelphia, PA: Lippincott Williams & Wilkins; 2010.

3. Sun JS, Park KJ, Kang DK. CT findings in patients with pericardial effusion: differentiation of malignant and benign disease. *AJR Am J Roentgenol.* 2010;194:W489–W494.

MALGAIGNE FRACTURE
Case 51

1. Demetriades D, Karaiskakis M, Toutouzas K, et al. Pelvic fractures: epidemiology and predictors of associated abdominal injuries and outcomes. *J Am Coll Surg.* 2002;195(1):1–10.

2. Khurana B, Sheehan S, Sodickson A, et al. Pelvic ring fractures: what the orthopedic surgeon wants to know. *Radiographics.* 2010;34(5):1317–1333.

3. Yoon W, Kim J, Yeon J, et al. Pelvic arterial hemorrhage in patients with pelvic fractures: detection with

contrast-enhanced CT. *Radiographics*. 2004;24(6):1591–1605. doi:10.1148/rg.246045028.

PEDIATRIC SEPTIC HIP
Case 52

1. Cook PC. Transient synovitis, septic hip, and Legg-Calve-Perthes disease: an approach to the correct diagnosis. *Pediatr Clin North Am*. 2014;61(6):1109–1118.

CAROTID DISSECTION
Case 53

1. Fusco M, Harrigan M. Cerebrovascular dissections: a review. Part I: spontaneous dissections. *Neurosurgery*. 2011;68:242–257.

2. Fusco M, Harrigan M. Cerebrovascular dissections: a review. Part II: blunt cerebrovascular injury. *Neurosurgery*. 2011;68:517–530.

3. Patel R, Adam R, Maldjian C, et al. Cervical carotid artery dissection. *Cardiol Rev*. 2012;20:145–152.

4. Rodallec M, Marteau V, Gerber S, et al. Craniocervical arterial dissection: spectrum of imaging findings and differential diagnosis. *Radiographics*. 2008;28:1711–1728.

5. Thanvi B, Munshi SK, Dawson SL, et al. Carotid and vertebral artery dissection syndromes. *Postgrad Med J*. 2005;81:383–388.

PNEUMOCYSTIS JIROVECI PNEUMONIA
Case 54

1. Collins J, Stern E. *Chest Radiology: The Essentials*. Philadelphia, PA: Lippincott Williams & Wilkins; 2015.

2. Kanne JP, Yandow DR, Meyer CA. *Pneumocystis jiroveci* pneumonia: high-resolution CT findings in patients with and without HIV infection. *AJR Am J Roentgenol*. 2012;198:W555–W561.

MESENTERIC INJURY
Case 55

1. Atri M, Hanson JM, Grinblat L, et al. Surgically important bowel and/or mesenteric injury in blunt trauma: accuracy of multidetector CT for evaluation. *Radiology*. 2008;249:524–533.

2. Brofman N, Atri M, Epid D, et al. Evaluation of bowel and mesenteric blunt trauma with multidetector CT. *Radiographics*. 2006;26:1119–1131.

3. Dowe MF, Shanmuganathan K, Mirvis SE, et al. Findings of mesenteric injury after blunt trauma: implications for surgical intervention. *AJR Am J Roentgenol*. 1997;168:425–428.

MONTEGGIA FRACTURE
Case 56

1. Beutel BG. Monteggia fractures in pediatric and adult populations. *Orthopedics*. 2012;35(2):138–144.

2. Ring D. Monteggia fractures. *Orthop Clin North Am*. 2013;44(1):59–66.

RETROPHARYNGEAL ABSCESS
Case 57

1. Craig FW, Schunk JE. Retropharyngeal abscess in children: clinical presentation, utility of imaging, and current management. *Pediatrics*. 2003;111:1394–1398.

2. Hoang JK, Branstetter BF, Eastwood JD, et al. Multiplanar CT and MRI of collections in the retropharyngeal space: is it an abscess? *AJR Am J Roentgenol*. 2011;196:W426–W432.

PNEUMOTHORAX WITH DEEP SULCUS SIGN
Case 58

1. Kong A. The deep sulcus sign. *Radiology*. 2003;228(2):415–416.

PNEUMOPERITONEUM
Case 59

1. Braccini G, Lamacchia M, Boraschi P. Ultrasound versus plain film in the detection of pneumoperitoneum. *Abdom Imaging*. 1996;21(5):404–412.

2. Chui YH, Chen JD, Tiu CM, et al. Reappraisal of radiographic signs of pneumoperitoneum at emergency department. *Am J Emerg Med*. 2009;27:320–327.

3. Reeder MM, Felson B. *Reeder and Felson's Gamuts in Radiology, Comprehensive Lists of Roentgen Differential Diagnosis*. New York, NY: Springer-Verlag; 2003.

JEFFERSON FRACTURE
Case 60

1. Klimo P Jr, Ware ML, Gupta N, et al. Cervical spine trauma in the pediatric patient. *Neurosurg Clin N Am*. 2007;18(4):599–620.

2. Longo UG, Denaro L, Campi S, et al. Upper cervical spine injuries: indications and limits of the conservative management in halo vest. A systematic review of efficacy and safety. *Injury*. 2010;41(11):1127–1135.

ANEURYSMAL SUBARACHNOID HEMORRHAGE
Case 61

1. Conolly E, Rabinstein A, Carhuapoma J, et al. Guidelines for the management of aneurysmal subarachnoid hemorrhage: a guideline for healthcare professionals from the American Heart Association/American Stroke Association. *Stroke*. 2012;43(6):1711–1737.

2. Molyneux A, Kerr R, Stratton I, et al. International Subarachnoid Aneurysm Trial (ISAT) of neurosurgical clipping versus endovascular coiling in 2143 patients with ruptured intracranial aneurysms: a randomized trial. *Lancet*. 2002;360(9342):1267–1274.

3. Pierot L, Cognard C, Ricolfi F, et al. Immediate anatomic results after the endovascular treatment of ruptured intracranial aneurysms: analysis in the CLARITY series. *AJNR Am J Neuroradiol*. 2010;31(5):907–911.

4. van Rooij WJ, Sluzewski M, Beute GN, et al. Procedural complications of coiling of ruptured intracranial aneurysms:

incidence and risk factors in a consecutive series of 681 patients. *AJNR Am J Neuroradiol.* 2006;27(7):1498–1501.

POSTERIOR MEDIASTINAL HEMATOMA
Case 62

1. Creasy JD, Chiles C, Routh WD, et al. Overview of traumatic injury of the thoracic aorta. *Radiographics.* 1997;17:27–45.
2. Denis F. The three column spine and its significance in the classification of acute thoracolumbar spinal injuries. *Spine.* 1983;8:817–831.
3. Murakami R, Tajima H. Acute traumatic injury of the distal descending aorta associated with thoracic spine injury. *Eur Radiol.* 1998;8(1):60–62.

APPENDICITIS
Case 63

1. Leite NP, Pereira JM, Cunha R, et al. CT evaluation of appendicitis and its complications: imaging techniques and key diagnostic findings. *AJR Am J Roentgenol.* 2005;185:406–417.
2. Singh A, Danrad R, Hahn PF, et al. MR imaging of the acute abdomen and pelvis: acute appendicitis and beyond. *Radiographics.* 2007;27:1419–1431.
3. Spalluto LB, Woodfield CA, DeBenedectis CM, et al. MR imaging evaluation of abdominal pain during pregnancy: appendicitis and other nonobstetric causes. *Radiographics.* 2012;32:317–334.

BASE OF THUMB METACARPAL FRACTURE
Case 64

1. Soyer AD. Fractures of the base of the first metacarpal: current treatment options. *J Am Acad Orthop Surg.* 1999;7(6):403–412.

HEAD AND NECK SQUAMOUS CELL CANCER WITH NODAL METASTASES
Case 65

1. Crozier E, Sumer BD. Head and neck cancer. *Med Clin North Am.* 2010;94:1031–1046.
2. Hoang JK, Vanka J, Ludwig BJ, et al. Evaluation of cervical lymph nodes in head and neck cancer with CT and MRI: tips, traps, and a systematic approach. *AJR Am J Roentgenol.* 2013;200:W17–W25.
3. Mukherji SK, Armao D, Joshi VM. Cervical nodal metastases in squamous cell carcinoma of the head and neck: what to expect. *Head Neck.* 2001;23:995–1005.
4. Rosenberg TL, Brown JJ, Jefferson GD. Evaluating the adult patient with a neck mass. *Med Clin North Am.* 2010;94:1017–1029.

POST-PRIMARY TUBERCULOSIS
Case 66

1. Allen EA. Tuberculosis and other mycobacterial infections of the lung. In: Thurlbeck WM, Churlbeck AM, eds. *Pathology of the Lung.* 2nd ed. New York, NY: Thieme Medical; 1995:229–265.
2. Leung AN. Pulmonary tuberculosis: the essentials. *Radiology.* 1999;210:307–322.
3. Miller WT, Miller WT Jr. Tuberculosis in the normal host: radiological findings. *Semin Roentgenol.* 1993;28:109–118.

URETERAL INJURY
Case 67

1. Ortega SJ, Netto FS, Hamilton P, et al. CT scanning for diagnosing blunt ureteral and ureteropelvic junction injuries. *BMC Urol.* 2008;8:3–8.
2. Ramchandani P, Buckler PM. Imaging of genitourinary trauma. *AJR Am J Roentgenol.* 2009;192:1514–1523.

BASE OF FIFTH METATARSAL FRACTURE
Case 68

1. Theodorou DJ, Theodorou SJ, Kakitsubata Y, et al. Fractures of proximal portion of fifth metatarsal bone: anatomic and imaging evidence of a pathogenesis of avulsion of the plantar aponeurosis and the short peroneal muscle tendon. *Radiology.* 2003;226:857–865.
2. DeVries JG, Taefi E, Bussewitz BW, et al. The fifth metatarsal base: anatomic evaluation regarding fracture mechanism and treatment algorithms. *J Foot Ankle Surg.* 2015;54:94–98.

DIFFUSE AXONAL INJURY
Case 69

1. Adams JH, Jennett B, Mclellan DR, et al. The neuropathology of the vegetative state after head injury. *J Clin Pathol.* 1999;52(11):804–806.
2. Davis PC. Head trauma. *AJR Am J Neuroradiol.* 2007;28(8):1619–1621.
3. Gentry LR, Godersky JC, Thompson B, et al. Prospective comparative study of intermediate-field MR and CT in the evaluation of closed head trauma. *AJR Am J Roentgenol.* 1988;150(3):673–682.
4. Holshouser BA, Tong KA, Ashwal S. Proton MR spectroscopic imaging depicts diffuse axonal injury in children with traumatic brain injury. *AJNR Am J Neuroradiol.* 2005;26(5):1276–1285.
5. Matsukawa H, Shinoda M, Fujii M, et al. Intraventricular hemorrhage on computed tomography and corpus callosum injury on magnetic resonance imaging in patients with isolated blunt traumatic brain injury. *J Neurosurg.* 2012;117(2):334–339.
6. Medana IM, Esiri MM. Axonal damage: a key predictor of outcome in human CNS diseases. *Brain.* 2003; 126(Pt 3):515–530.
7. Mittl RL, Grossman RI, Hiehle JF, et al. Prevalence of MR evidence of diffuse axonal injury in patients with mild head injury and normal head CT findings. *AJNR Am J Neuroradiol.* 1994;15(8):1583–1589.

8. Saatman KE, Duhaime AC, Bullock R, et al. Classification of traumatic brain injury for targeted therapies. *J Neurotrauma*. 2008;25(7):719–738.

PULMONARY EDEMA (INTERSTITIAL)
Case 70

1. Collins J, Stern E. *Chest Radiology: The Essentials*. Philadelphia, PA: Lippincott Williams & Wilkins; 2015.
2. Goodman L. *Felson's Principles of Chest Roentgenology: A Programmed Text*. Philadelphia, PA: Saunders Elsevier; 2007.

ULCERATIVE PROCTOCOLITIS
Case 71

1. Jalan KN, Sircus W, Card WI, et al. An experience of ulcerative colitis. Toxic dilation in 55 cases. *Gastroenterology*. 1969;57:68–82.
2. Sheth SG, LaMont T. Toxic megacolon. *Lancet*. 1998;351:509–513.
3. Thoeni RF, Cello JP. CT imaging of colitis. *Radiology*. 2006;240(3):623–638.

NECROTIZING FASCIITIS—PEDIATRIC
Case 72

1. Chauhan A, Wigton MD, Palmer BA. Necrotizing fasciitis. *J Hand Surg Am*. 2014;39(8):1598–1601.
2. Jamal N, Teach SJ. Necrotizing fasciitis. *Pediatr Emerg Care*. 2011;27(12):1195–1199.

TEMPORAL BONE FRACTURE
Case 73

1. Aguilar EA III, Yeakley JW, Ghorayeb BY, et al. High resolution CT scan of temporal bone fractures: association of facial nerve paralysis with temporal bone fractures. *Head Neck Surg*. 1987;9(3):162–166.
2. Brodie HA. Management of temporal bone trauma. In: Flint PW, Haughey BH, Lund VJ, et al, eds. *Cummings Otolaryngology Head & Neck Surgery*. 5th ed. Philadelphia, PA: Mosby; 2010:2036–2048.
3. Brodie HA, Thompson TC. Management of complications from 820 temporal bone fractures. *Am J Otol*. 1997;18(2):188–197.
4. Cannon CR, Jahrsdoerfer RA. Temporal bone fractures. Review of 90 cases. *Arch Otolaryngol*. 1983;109(5):285–288.
5. Dahiya R, Keller JD, Litofsky NS, et al. Temporal bone fractures: otic capsule sparing versus otic capsule violating clinical and radiographic considerations. *J Trauma*. 1999;47(6):1079–1083.
6. Nageris B, Hansen MC, Lavelle WG, et al. Temporal bone fractures. *Am J Emerg Med*. 1995;13(2):211–214.
7. Parisier SC, Fayad JN, McGuirt WF. Injuries of the ear and temporal bone. In: Bluestone CD, Stool SE, Alper CM, et al, eds. *Pediatric Otolaryngology*. Vol 1. 4th ed. Philadelphia, PA: Saunders; 2003:829–860.

PULMONARY HEMORRHAGE DUE TO GRANULOMATOSIS WITH POLYANGIITIS
Case 74

1. Brown KK. Pulmonary vasculitis. *Proc Am Thorac Soc*. 2006;3:48–57.
2. Lohrmann C, Uhl M, Kotter E, et al. Pulmonary manifestations of wegener granulomatosis: CT findings in 57 patients and a review of the literature. *Eur J Radiol*. 2005;53:471–477.
3. Travis WD, Colby TV, Lombard C, et al. A clinicopathologic study of 34 cases of diffuse pulmonary hemorrhage with lung biopsy confirmation. *Am J Surg Pathol*. 1990;14:1112–1125.

CHOLEDOCHOLITHIASIS
Case 75

1. Kim YJ, Kim MJ, Kim KW, et al. Preoperative evaluation of common bile duct stones in patients with gallstone disease. *AJR Am J Roentgenol*. 2005;184(6):1854–1859.
2. Lee JT, Sagel SS, Stanley RJ, et al. *Computed Body Tomography with MRI Correlation*. 2nd ed. Philadelphia, PA: Lippincott-Raven; 2003.
3. Tonolini M, Ravelli A, Villa C, et al. Urgent MRI with MR cholangiopancreatography (MRCP) of acute cholecystitis and related complications: diagnostic role and spectrum of imaging findings. *Emerg Radiol*. 2012;19:341–348.

AC JOINT SEPARATION
Case 76

1. Melenevsky Y, Yablon CM, Ramappa A, et al. Clavicle and acromioclavicular joint injuries: a review of imaging, treatment, and complications. *Skeletal Radiol*. 2011;40:831–842.
2. Rockwood CA, Williams G, Young D. Disorders of the AC joint. In: *The Shoulder*. Vol 1. Philadelphia, PA: WB Saunders; 1998:483.
3. Tauber M. Management of acute acromioclavicular joint dislocations: current concepts. *Arch Orthop Trauma Surg*. 2013;133:985–995.
4. Vanarthos WJ, Ekman EF, Bohrer SP. Radiographic diagnosis of acromioclavicular joint separation without weight bearing: importance of internal rotation of the arm. *AJR Am J Roentgenol*. 1994;162:120–122.

RUPTURED AVM
Case 77

1. Al-Shahi R, Bhattacharya JJ, Currie DG, et al. Scottish Intracranial Vascular Malformation Study (SIVMS): evaluation of methods, ICD-10 coding, and potential sources of bias in a prospective, population-based cohort. *Stroke*. 2003;34:1156–1162.
2. Atkinson RP, Awad IA, Batjer HH, et al. Reporting terminology for brain arteriovenous malformation: clinical and radiographic features for use in clinical trials. *Stroke*. 2001;32:1430–1442.

3. Meyer-Heim AD, Bolthauser E. Spontaneous intracranial hemorrhage in children: etiology presentation, and outcome. *Brain Dev.* 2003;25:416–421.

4. Perret G, Nishioka H. Report on the cooperative study of intracranial aneurysms and subarachnoid hemorrhage. Section VI. Arteriovenous malformations: an analysis of 545 Cases of cranio-cerebral arteriovenous malformations and fistulae reported to the cooperative study. *J Neurosurg.* 1966;25:467–490.

5. Pollock BE, Flickinger JC. Modification of the radiosurgery-bases arteriovenous malformation grading system. *Neurosurgery.* 2008;63:239–243.

6. Spetzler RF, Martin NA. A proposed grading system for arteriovenous malformation. *J Neurosurg.* 1986;65:476–483.

7. Starke RM, Yen CP, Ding D, et al. A practical grading scale for predicting outcome after radiosurgery for arteriovenous malformation: analysis of 1012 treated patients. *J Neurosurg.* 2013;119:981–987.

TENSION PNEUMOTHORAX
Case 78

1. Collins J, Stern EJ. *Chest Radiology: The Essentials.* Philadelphia, PA: Lippincott Williams & Wilkins; 2007.

2. Hsu C-W, Sun S-F. Iatrogenic pneumothorax related to mechanical ventilation. *World J Crit Care Med.* 2014;3(1):8–14. doi:10.5492/wjccm.v3.i1.8.

3. Srichai MB. *Computed Tomography and Magnetic Resonance of the Thorax.* Philadelphia, PA: Lippincott Williams & Wilkins; 2007.

ACUTE MESENTERIC ISCHEMIA
Case 79

1. Furukawa A, Kanasaki S, Kono N, et al. CT diagnosis of acute mesenteric ischemia from various causes. *AJR Am J Roentgenol.* 2009;192(2):408–416.

2. Shih MP, Hagspiel KD. CTA and MRA in mesenteric ischemia. Part I: role in diagnosis and differential diagnosis. *AJR Am J Roentgenol.* 2007;188(2):452–461.

RADIO-OCCULT HIP FRACTURE
Case 80

1. Brauer CA, Coca-Perraillon M, Cutler DM, et al. Incidence and mortality of hip fractures in the United States. *JAMA.* 2009;302:1573–1579.

2. Kirby MW, Spritzer C. Radiographic detection of hip and pelvic fractures in the emergency department. *AJR Am J Roentgenol.* 2010;194(4):1054–1060.

3. Sankey RA, Turner J, Lee J, et al. The use of MRI to detect occult fractures of the proximal femur: a study of 102 consecutive cases over a ten-year period. *J Bone Joint Surg Br.* 2009;91(8):1064–1068.

4. Ward RJ, Weissman BN, Kransdorf MJ, et al. ACR appropriateness criteria acute hip pain-suspected fracture. *J Am Coll Radiol.* 2014;11(2):114–120.

PYOGENIC DISCITIS AND EPIDURAL ABSCESS
Case 81

1. Cottle L, Riordan T. Infectious spondylodiscitis. *J Infect.* 2008;56:401–412.

2. Go JL, Rothman S, Prosper A, et al. Spine infections. *Neuroimaging Clin N Am.* 2012;22(4):755–772.

3. Gouliouris T, Aliyu SH, Brown NM. Spondylodiscitis: update on diagnosis and management. *J Antimicrob Chemother.* 2010;65(suppl 3):iii11–iii24.

4. Ledermann HP, Schweitzer ME, Morrison WB, et al. MR imaging findings in spinal infections: rules or myths? *Radiology.* 2003;228:506–514.

KNEE DISLOCATION
Case 82

1. Henrichs A. A review of knee dislocations. *J Athl Train.* 2004;39(4):365–369.

2. Medina O, Arom GA, Yeranosian MG, et al. Vascular and nerve injury after knee dislocation: a systematic review. *Clin Orthop Relat Res.* 2014;472(9):2621–2629.

3. Walker RE, McDougall D, Patel S, et al. Radiologic review of knee dislocation: from diagnosis to repair. *AJR Am J Roentgenol.* 2013;201(3):483–495.

SHOTGUN WOUNDS
Case 83

1. Bartlett CS. Clinical update: gunshot wound ballistics. *Clin Orthop Relat Res.* 2003;408:28–57.

2. Vedelago J, Dick E, Thomas R, et al. Look away: arterial and venous intravascular embolization following shotgun injury. *J Trauma Manag Outcomes.* 2014;8:19.

SCAPHOID FRACTURE
Case 84

1. Fowler JR, Hughes TB. Scaphoid fractures. *Clin Sports Med.* 2015;34(1):37–50.

2. Herbert TJ, Fisher WE. Management of the fractured scaphoid using a new bone screw. *J Bone Joint Surg Br.* 1984;66(1):114–123.

3. Tiel Van-Buul MMC, Van Beek EJR, Borm JJJ, et al. The value of radiographs and bone scintigraphy in suspected scaphoid fracture. A statistical analysis. *J Hand Surg Br.* 1993;18(3):403–406.

4. Yin Z-G, Zhang J-B, Kan S-L, et al. Diagnostic accuracy of imaging modalities for suspected scaphoid fractures. *J Bone Joint Surg Br.* 2012;94:1077–1085.

ACUTE MULTIPLE SCLEROSIS FLARE
Case 85

1. Filippi M, Rocca MA. MR imaging of multiple sclerosis. *Radiology.* 2011;259(3):659–681.

2. Lövblad KO, Anzalone N, Dörfler A, et al. MR imaging in multiple sclerosis: review and recommendations for current practice. *AJNR Am J Neuroradiol.* 2010;31(6):983–989.

3. Wingerchuk DM, Carter JL. Multiple sclerosis: current and emerging disease-modifying therapies and treatment strategies. *Mayo Clin Proc.* 2014;89(2):225–240.

4. Yousem DM, Grossman RI. Multiple sclerosis. In: *Neuroradiology: The Requisites.* St Louis, MO: Mosby; 2010: 227–236.

FOREIGN BODY—ULTRASOUND
Case 86

1. Anderson M, Newmeyer W, Kilgore E. Diagnosis and treatment of retained foreign bodies in the hand. *Am J Surg.* 1982;144:63–67.

2. Boyse T, Fessell D, Jacobson J, et al. US of soft-tissue foreign bodies and associated complications with surgical correlation. *Radiographics.* 2001;21(5):1251–1256.

3. Courter B. Radiographic screening for retained foreign bodies—what does a "negative" foreign body series really mean? *Ann Emerg Med.* 1990;19(9):997–1000.

4. Davis J, Czerniski B, Au A, et al. Diagnostic accuracy of ultrasonography in retained soft tissue foreign bodies: a systematic review and meta-analysis. *Acad Emerg Med.* 2015;22(7):777–787.

5. Halverson M, Servaes S. Foreign bodies: radiopaque compared to what? *Pediatr Radiol.* 2013;43(9):1103–1107.

6. Ingraham C, Mannelli L. Radiology of foreign bodies: how do we image them? *Emerg Radiol.* 2015;22(4): 425–430.

7. Jacobson J, Powell A, Craig J, et al. Wooden foreign bodies in soft tissue: detection at US. *Radiology.* 1998;206(1):45–48.

8. Tandberg D. Glass in the hand and foot. Will an X-ray film show it? *JAMA.* 1982;248(15):1872–1874.

FOREIGN BODY URETHRA
Case 87

1. Bedi N, El-Husseiny T, Buchholz N, et al. 'Putting lead in your pencil': self-insertion of an unusual urethral foreign body for sexual gratification. *JRSM Short Rep.* 2010;1(2):18.

2. Rahman NU, Elliott SP, McAninch JW. Self-inflicted male urethral foreign body insertion: endoscopic management and complications. *BJU Int.* 2004;94(7): 1051–1053.

3. Van Ophoven A, DeKernion JB. Clinical management of foreign bodies of the genitourinary tract. *J Urol.* 2000;164:274–287.

SEPTIC ARTHRITIS (KNEE)
Case 88

1. Karchevsky M, Schweitzer ME, Morrison WB, et al. MRI findings of septic arthritis and associated osteomyelitis in adults. *AJR Am J Roentgenol.* 2004;182(1):119–122.

2. Lin HM, Learch TJ, White EA, et al. Emergency joint aspiration: a guide for radiologists on call. *Radiographics.* 2009;29(4):1139–1158.

CRANIOCERVICAL DISSOCIATION
Case 89

1. Bellabarba C, Mirza SK, West GA, et al. Diagnosis and treatment of craniocervical dislocation in a series of 17 consecutive survivors during an 8-year period. *J Neurosurg Spine.* 2006;4:429–440.

2. Bransford RJ, Alton TB, Patel AR, et al. Upper cervical spine trauma. *J Am Acad Orthop Surg.* 2014;22:718–729.

3. Chaput CD, Torres E, Davis M, et al. Survival of atlanto-occipital dissociation correlates with atlanto-occipital distraction, injury severity score, and neurologic status. *J Trauma.* 2011;71(2):393–395.

4. Chaput CD, Walgama J, Torres, et al. Defining and detecting missed ligamentous injuries of the occipitocervical complex. *Spine (Phila Pa 1976).* 2011;36(9): 709–714.

5. Deliganis AV, Baxter AB, Hanson JA, et al. Radiologic spectrum of craniocervical distraction injuries. *Radiographics.* 2000;20:S237–S250.

6. Labbe JL, Leclair O, Duparc B. Traumatic atlanto-occipital dislocation with survival in children. *J Pediatr Orthop B.* 2001;10(4):319–327.

7. Pang D, Nemzek WR, Zovickian J. Atlanto-occipital dislocation—part 2: the clinical use of (occipital) condyle-C1 interval, comparison with other diagnostic methods, and the manifestation, management, and outcome of atlanto-occipital dislocation in children. *Neurosurgery.* 2007;61(5):995–1015.

8. Rojas CA, Bertozzi JC, Martinez CR, et al. Reassessment of the craniocervical junction: normal values on CT. *AJNR Am J Neuroradiol.* 2007;28(9):1819–1823.

RIB FRACTURE WITH HEMOPNEUMOTHORAX
Case 90

1. Bansishar BJ, Lagares-Garcia JA, Miller SL. Clinical rib fractures: are follow-up chest X-rays a waste of resources? *Am Surg.* 2002;68(5):449–453.

2. Henry TS, Kirsch J, Kanne JP, et al. ACR appropriateness criteria rib fractures. *J Thorac Imaging.* 2014;29(6): 364–366.

3. Sirmali M, Türüt H, Topçu S, et al. A comprehensive analysis of traumatic rib fractures: morbidity, mortality, and management. *Eur J Cardiothorac Surg.* 2003;24(1): 133–138. doi:10.1016/S1010-7940(03)00256-2.

PYLORIC STENOSIS
Case 91

1. Blumhagen JD, Maclin L, Krauter D, et al. Sonographic diagnosis of hypertrophic pyloric stenosis. *AJR Am J Roentgenol.* 1988;150(6):1367–1370.

2. Hernanz-Schulman M. Infantile hypertrophic pyloric stenosis. *Radiology.* 2003;227:319–331.

3. Maheshwari P, Abograra A, Shamam O. Sonographic evaluation of gastrointestinal obstruction in infants: a pictorial essay. *J Pediatr Surg.* 2009;44(10):2037–2042.

POSTERIOR HIP DISLOCATION WITH INTRA-ARTICULAR FRAGMENT
Case 92

1. Foulk DM, Mullis BH. Hip dislocation: evaluation and management. *J Am Acad Orthop Surg.* 2010;18:199–209.

2. Milenvovic S, Mitkovic M, Saveski J, et al. Avascular necrosis of the femoral head in the patients with posterior wall acetabular fractures associated with dislocations of the hip. *Acta Chir Iugosi.* 2013;60(2):65–69.

3. Pascarella R, Maresca A, Reggiani LM, et al. Intra-articular fragments in acetabular fracture-dislocation. *Orthopedics.* 2009;32(6):402–405.

ACUTE TRANSVERSE MYELITIS
Case 93

1. Goh C, Desmond PM, Phal PM. MRI in transverse myelitis. *J Magn Reson Imaging.* 2014;40:1267–1279.

2. Sorte DE, Poretti A, Newsome SD, et al. Longitudinally extensive myelopathy in children. *Pediatr Radiol.* 2015;45:244–257.

3. Tobin WO, Weinshenker BG, Lucchinetti CF. Longitudinally extensive transverse myelitis. *Curr Opin Neurol.* 2014;27:279–289.

4. Wolf VL, Lupo PJ, Lotze TE. Pediatric acute transverse myelitis: overview and differential diagnosis. *J Child Neurol.* 2012;27(11):1426–1436.

MEDIAL HEAD OF GASTROCNEMIUS MUSCLE TEAR
Case 94

1. Bianchi S, Martinoli C, Abdelwahab IF, et al. Sonographic evaluation of tears of the gastrocnemius medial head ("tennis leg"). *J Ultrasound Med.* 1998;17(3):157–162.

2. Cheng Y, Yang H-L, Sun Z-Y, et al. Surgical treatment of gastrocnemius muscle ruptures. *Orthop Surg.* 2012;4(4):253–257.

3. Delgado G, Chung C, Lektrakul N, et al. Tennis leg: clinical US study of 141 patients and anatomic investigation of four cadavers with MR imaging and US. *Radiology.* 2002;224:112–119.

4. Kwak HS, Lee KB, Han YM. Ruptures of the medial head of the gastrocnemius ("tennis leg"): clinical outcome and compression effect. *Clin Imaging.* 2006;30(1):48–53.

5. Noonan TJ, Garrett WE Jr. Muscle strain injury: diagnosis and treatment. *J Am Acad Orthop Surg.* 1999;7:262–269.

GASTRIC VOLVULUS
Case 95

1. Altintoprak F, Yalkin O, Dikicier E, et al. A rare etiology of acute abdominal syndrome in adults: gastric volvulus—cases series. *Int J Surg Case Rep.* 2014;5:731–734.

2. Peterson CM, Anderson JS, Hara AK, et al. Volvulus of the gastrointestinal tract: appearances at multi-modality imaging. *Radiographics.* 2009;29:1281–1293.

3. Rashid F, Thangarajah T, Mulvey D, et al. A review article on gastric volvulus: a challenge to diagnosis and management. *Int J Surg.* 2010;8:18–24.

PATELLAR TENDON RUPTURE
Case 96

1. Dupuis CS, Westra SJ, Makris J, et al. Injuries and conditions of the extensor mechanism of the pediatric knee. *Radiographics.* 2009;29:877–886.

2. Hunt DM, Somashekar N. A review of sleeve fractures of the patella in children. *Knee.* 2005;12(1):3–7.

3. Zernicke RF, Garhammer J, Jobe FW. Human patellar tendon rupture. *J Bone Joint Surg Am.* 1977;59:179–183.

HYPERTENSIVE BASAL GANGLIA HEMORRHAGE
Case 97

1. Castellanos M, Leira R, Tejada J, et al. Predictors of good outcome in medium to large spontaneous supratentorial intracerebral haemorrhages. *J Neurol Neurosurg Psychiatry.* 2005;76:691–695.

2. Mendelow AD, Gregson BA, Fernandes HM, et al. Early surgery versus initial conservative treatment in patients with spontaneous supratentorial intracerebral haematomas in the International Surgical Trial in Intracerebral Haemorrhage (STICH): a randomised trial. *Lancet.* 2005;365:387–397.

3. Sacco RL, Kasner SE, Broderick JP, et al. An updated definition of stroke for the 21st century: a statement for healthcare professionals from the American Heart Association/American Stroke Association. *Stroke.* 2013;44(7):2064–2089.

4. Wang K, Xue Y, Chen X, et al. Transtentorial herniation in patients with hypertensive putaminal haemorrhage is predictive of elevated intracranial pressure following haematoma removal. *J Clin Neurosci.* 2012;19(7):975–979.

VENTRICULOPERITONEAL SHUNT MALFUNCTION
Case 98

1. Wallace AN, McConathy J, Menias CO, et al. Imaging evaluation of CSF shunts. *AJR Am J Roentgenol.* 2014;202:38–53.

ACUTE CHOLECYSTITIS
Case 99

1. Hanbidge AE, Buckler PM, O'Malley ME, et al. Imaging evaluation for acute pain in the right upper quadrant. *Radiographics.* 2004;24:1117–1135.

2. Harvey RT, Miller WT. Acute biliary disease: initial CT and follow-up US versus initial US and follow-up CT. *Radiology.* 1999;213:831–836.

3. Smith EA, Dillman JR, Elsayes KM, et al. Cross-sectional imaging of acute and chronic gallbladder inflammatory disease. *AJR Am J Roentgenol.* 2009;192:188–196.

DIABETIC FOOT WITH GAS-FORMING INFECTION
Case 100

1. Fugitt JB, Puckett ML, Quigley MM, et al. Necrotizing fasciitis. *Radiographics*. 2004;24:1472–1476.
2. Kaafarani HMA, King DR. Necrotizing skin and soft tissue infections. *Surg Clin North Am*. 2014;94:155–163.
3. Lipsky BA, Berendt AR, Deery HG, et al. Diagnosis and treatment of diabetic foot infections. *Clin Infect Dis*. 2004;39:885–910.

Note: Page numbers followed by "*f*" refer to figures.